Applications of Orthodontic Mini-Implants

Applications of
Orthodontic
Mini-Implants

Jong Suk Lee, DDS, MS, PhD

Adjunct Assistant Professor
Department of Orthodontics
University of Pennsylvania
School of Dental Medicine
Philadelphia, Pennsylvania

Jung Kook Kim, DDS, MS, PhD

Adjunct Associate Professor
Department of Orthodontics
University of Pennsylvania
School of Dental Medicine
Philadelphia, Pennsylvania

Young-Chel Park, DDS, MS, PhD

Dean, College of Dentistry
Professor, Department of Orthodontics
Yonsei University, Seoul, Korea

Robert L. Vanarsdall, Jr, DDS

Professor and Chairman
Department of Orthodontics
University of Pennsylvania
School of Dental Medicine
Philadelphia, Pennsylvania

Quintessence Publishing Co, Inc

Chicago, Berlin, Tokyo, London, Paris, Milan, Barcelona, Istanbul, São Paulo, Mumbai, Moscow, Prague, and Warsaw

Library of Congress Cataloging-in-Publication Data

Applications of orthodontic mini implants / Jong Suk Lee ... [et al.].
   p. ; cm.
  ISBN 978-0-86715-465-8 (hardcover)
  1. Dental implants. 2. Orthodontics. I. Lee, Jong Suk.
  [DNLM: 1. Dental Implantation--methods. 2. Orthodontic Anchorage Procedures--methods.
3. Dental Implants. WU 640 A652 2007]
  RK667.I45A67 2007
  617.6'93--dc22

                  2007001922

quintessence
books

Quintessence Publishing Co, Inc
4350 Chandler Drive
Hanover Park, IL 60133
www.quintpub.com

Editor: Lisa C. Bywaters
Design: Dawn Hartman
Production: Sue Robinson

Printed in Canada

TABLE OF CONTENTS

PREFACE

When Dr Edward Angle developed the edgewise bracket for three-dimensional control of teeth, he set the stage for those who followed to design techniques that allowed for more efficient treatment and better outcomes. Their common objective was to minimize unwanted tooth movements and at the same time promote control of practical three-dimensional tooth movements. Development of the simple, stable, and easy-to-use orthodontic mini-implant represents a critical turning point in the search for effortless control of orthodontic anchorage.

The effectiveness of orthodontic mini-implants does not diminish concerns about loss of anchorage, nor does it solve the problem of loss of anchorage. The orthodontic mini-implant does, however, provide rigid anchorage that makes treatment more efficient, and it also makes biologically permissible movements possible as well. In particular, intrusion of the molars is now practical, in turn allowing vertical disharmony to be corrected with predictability and control.

Of course, many problems remain unresolved. Given the relatively short (10-year) history of the use of mini-implants in orthodontic treatment, long-term data is necessarily limited. More research is needed, particularly

with regard to orthopedic applications. Today we find ourselves at the clinical stage of development, which calls for further systematic and prospective research.

This textbook is based on the clinical data we have collected thus far. It describes precise conditions and techniques for clinical application of orthodontic mini-implants and serves as a foundation upon which future treatment using mini-implants can be supported. Despite the need for additional basic and clinical research, we offer this book as an introduction to the new treatment concept of mini-implant orthodontics for those orthodontists and students who have been searching for better treatment results.

This textbook provides an alternative to surgical orthodontics in selected cases. Because the success of this treatment modality depends on new treatment principles and a more precise diagnosis, treatment on the basis of biologic principles is imperative. Can this tiny implant complete the evolutionary advances in mechanotherapy of the past 100 years, transform the treatment paradigm, extend the scope of nonsurgical therapy, and usher in a new era in orthodontic treatment? We believe so, and we think you will too after reading this book.

ACKNOWLEDGMENTS

We would like to express our appreciation to Dr Kee Joon Lee of the Department of Orthodontics and Dr Hee Jin Kim of the Department of Anatomy at the College of Dentistry, Yonsei University, for their contributions in scientific background and basic data.

Also, we owe many thanks to Dr Doo Hyung Kim, Dr Hee Sun Yoon, and Dr Jae Hyung Cho for their wonderful research efforts, as well as to Dr Joong Ki Lim and Dr Byung Soo Yoon for permitting us to use their fantastic clinical cases. This book would not have been possible without the support of Dr Yoon Jung Choi, Dr Uk Joo, Dr Ju Young Park, Dr Nak Chun Choi, and other members of the Department of Orthodontics at the College of Dentistry, Yonsei University; and Dr Chun-Hsi Chung, Dr Antonino Secchi, and the Department of Orthodontics at the University of Pennsylvania School of Dental Medicine.

Finally, we would like to thank Ms Ji Young Kim for her translation work and Dr Jeong Moon Kim of Ortholution Co, Ltd, for his endless support in the research and development of the Orlus mini-implant.

This book was made possible by the help of the incredible staff at Quintessence Publishing Company.

EVOLUTION OF THE ORTHODONTIC MINI-IMPLANT

1

A goal of any orthodontic treatment is to achieve desired tooth movement with a minimum number of undesirable side effects.[1] Strategies for anchorage control have been a major factor in achieving successful orthodontic treatment since the specialty began. Edward Angle,[2] writing in 1900, was one of the earliest to advocate the use of equal and opposite appliance forces to control anchorage. Traditionally, anchorage is reinforced by increasing the number of teeth bilaterally or using the musculature, extraoral devices, and the alveolar processes.

Prevention of undesirable tooth movement in both arches is now possible. The use of small titanium bone screws has increased the envelope of orthodontic treatment, providing an alternative to orthognathic surgery (particularly in the vertical dimension) and allowing asymmetric tooth movement in three planes of space. Miniscrews provide the biomechanical advantage that allows more effective and efficient treatment with fewer auxiliaries and other appliances. Predicting resistance to tooth movement can minimize adverse responses, lead to more successful treatment of complicated problems, and provide efficient care in less time. Teeth can be moved directly (en masse without anchorage loss) to their final positions.

Improved techniques and information over the last two decades have enabled clinicians to obtain more ideal tooth positioning. Much of this has come from case reports published outside the United States. Miniscrews can be used in conjunction with all types of orthodontic systems (edgewise, self-ligation, expansion devices, etc).

While biomechanical techniques have been simplified over the last century, they nonetheless remain complicated. The second half of this text presents chapters that address mechanotherapy in specific detail with regard to various types of predictable tooth movement.

HISTORICAL BACKGROUND

The concept of skeletal anchorage is not new. Basal bone anchorage was suggested more than 60 years ago as an alternative to increasing the number of teeth to achieve conventional anchorage. Because of the limitations of headgear, clinicians sought other means of anchorage. For example, orthopedists have used stainless steel bone screws for leg lengthening since before 1905.[3] In 1945, research into the concept of using a pin or screw attachment to the ramus was initiated not only for moving teeth, but also for "exerting a pull on the mandible."[4] One study involved placing Vitallium screws (Dentsply) in dogs. Using basal bone for anchorage, tooth movement was successful; however, it was found that an effective force could be maintained for no longer than 31 days. The loss of all screws was attributed to infection from communication between the Vitallium screw and the oral cavity. Nonetheless, the authors concluded that "anchorage may be obtained for orthodontic movement in the future."[4]

It has taken 60 years to progress from stainless steel to Vitallium to the current standard, titanium. Although it ranks ninth among the earth's most abundant elements, titanium was not discovered until 1791 and was not mass produced until 1948, when the technology to separate it from compounded materials was developed. Titanium has many valuable properties: it is three times stronger than stainless steel; exhibits little response to electricity, heat, or magnetic force; is highly biocompatible; and is inert. Type V titanium has the smallest amount of alloy (6% aluminium and 4% vanadium) of all titanium grades and hence the highest tensile strength, making it the material of choice for bone screws.

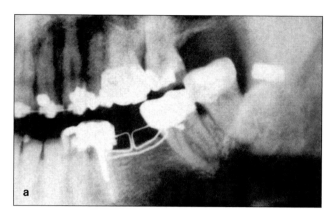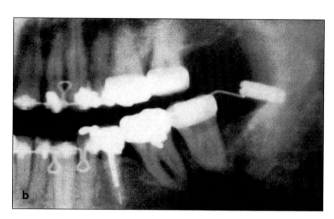

Figs 1-1a and 1-1b (a) Placement of a rigid endosseous implant in the retromolar area for space closure between the mandibular left first and second molars. **(b)** Through mesial translation of the second and third molars, 10 to 12 mm of space closure was accomplished. The retromolar implant was later removed with a trephine. (From Roberts et al.[7] Reprinted with permission.)

Screw head and bracket designs have changed dramatically during the past several decades. When Brainerd Swain designed the edgewise twin bracket that remains in use today, he used the head of a wood screw; by 1986, 90% of the orthodontists in the United States were using the pre-adjusted system with twin brackets favored for all teeth.

OSSEOINTEGRATION AND DENTAL IMPLANTS

Since 1969, when Brånemark et al[5] introduced dental implants for tooth replacement and prosthetic rehabilitation, osseointegration has remained the singular goal. In the last 25 years, dental implants have been used successfully in combined management of orthodontic-restorative patients, particularly in partially edentulous adults. Osseointegrated dental implants are used for orthodontic anchorage and then later serve as abutments for tooth replacement. This type of anchorage is very effective in treating patients with hypodontia, congenitally missing teeth, or periodontal disease, who lack sufficient teeth for conventional anchorage. Additionally, implants have been used for presurgical tooth movement, space opening/closing, and generally as a means to achieve better functional, biologic, and esthetic results in multidisciplinary treatment.

For orthodontic purposes, however, standard implants of 3.25 to 7.0 mm in diameter were less than ideal. They required multiple-stage surgical procedures and a wait-ing period of 4 to 6 months for osseointegration before orthodontic loading could be activated. Lack of adequate bone to place the large-diameter dental implants restricted their use in some patients. In others, anatomic limitations (soft tissue, sinus, nerves, unerupted teeth in children, etc) were problems. Another disadvantage of osseointegrated implants involved the need to place them in edentulous areas, retromolar regions (Fig 1-1), along the palatine suture, or pterygoid areas.[6–8] Finally, dental implant surgical protocols were invasive, expensive, uncomfortable for patients, and lengthy, and they excluded children under the age of 16 years.

Anchorage without osseointegration

Over the last decade, a dynamic effort has been underway in Europe and Asia to achieve skeletal or absolute anchorage with the use of a variety of small titanium screws (miniscrews and microscrews), palatal implants, and plates or miniplates with screws. Many animal studies (rabbit, dog, and monkey) and human case reports were published,[9–11] but lack of Food and Drug Administration (FDA) clearance discouraged pursuit of this research topic in the United States. The published reports found that screws and smaller devices used for skeletal anchorage are less invasive (flapless surgery); have few anatomic limitations; are easy to place and remove; allow for immediate loading since osseointegration is not a prerequisite; cost less than conventional implants; may be used in children; and generally improve the orthodontic result while increasing patient compliance.

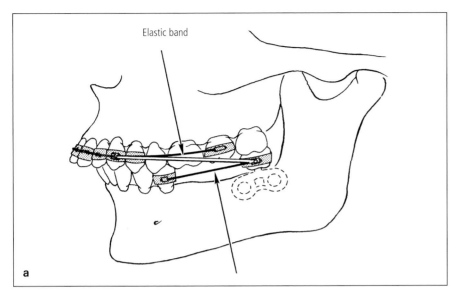
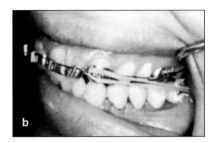
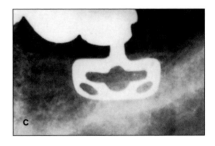

Figs 1-2a to 1-2c **(a)** Skeletal anchorage to correct Class II malocclusion using class II elastics from the maxillary canine to the blade implant placed in the mandibular molar area. **(b)** Left lateral view of Class II malocclusion. **(c)** Radiographic view of a blade implant supporting the posterior portion of the prosthesis. (From Linkow.[12] Reprinted with permission.)

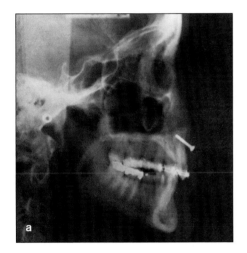
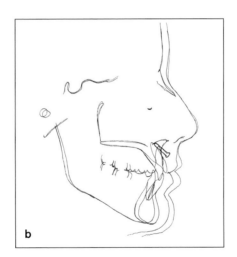
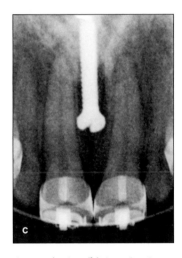

Figs 1-3a to 1-3c **(a)** The cephalometric radiograph reveals the Vitallium bone screw placed below the anterior nasal spine. **(b)** A tracing 1 year later *(red)* shows 6 mm of intrusion and 25 degrees of torque following continuous elastic thread tied to the screw, allowing for intrusion. **(c)** Periapical view of Vitallium screw at time of placement. (From Creekmore and Eklund.[13] Reprinted with permission.)

Improvements in design and application

Several innovations in anchorage design slowly led to improved outcomes and the treatment protocol widely used today. Linkow,[12] in 1970, was among the first to propose use of the blade implant as anchorage for class II elastics (Fig 1-2). Creekmore and Eklund[13] used a bone screw to intrude maxillary incisors as early as 1983 (Fig 1-3). Block[14] promoted the use of an "onplant" palatal anchorage device (Fig 1-4), and Wehrbein et al[15] introduced the so-called Orthosystem (Straumann) (Fig 1-5), both of which require an osseointegrated interface. Palatal

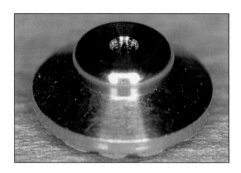

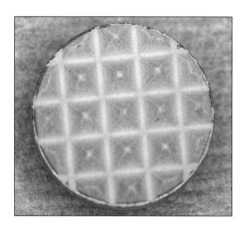

Fig 1-4a Superficial surface of a titanium onplant.

Fig 1-4b Textured/hydroxyapatite-coated under-surface of the onplant, which is placed directly on bone (under periosteum).

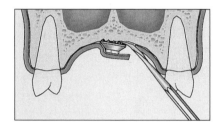

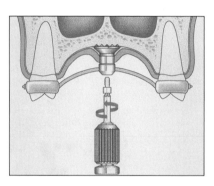

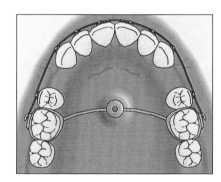

Fig 1-4c Subperiosteal placement of the onplant in the central portion of the palate.

Fig 1-4d A transpalatal wire is secured to the onplant with a screw. The wire is shaped and soldered to bands on the anchor teeth.

Fig 1-4e The transpalatal arch connected to molars serves as anchorage to move anterior teeth posteriorly without loss of molar anchorage. (Figs 1-4a to 1-4e from Block.[14] Reprinted with permission.)

implants require a three-stage procedure—surgery, abutment placement, and removal—that subjects patients to the risk of developing an osseous defect (Fig 1-6). In addition, a healing period of 4 months and the placement of transfer molar bands or transpalatal bars may be required as part of the protocol for these palatal devices.

Like the palatal device, bone screws can be placed on the palate, but they are much easier to use (Fig 1-7) and can be placed in the paramedian areas of the palate in growing children[16] (Fig 1-8). Studies using bone screws with immediate loading have reported effective molar distalization (88%) without major anchorage loss (12%) when the first and second molars are present.[17] Osseointegration, as noted earlier, requires delayed loading and thus greatly increases treatment time.

As recently as 1998, zygoma ligatures were proposed as an option for maxillary anchorage (Fig 1-9).[18] In 1997, Kanomi[19] reported using the miniscrew for anchorage in an intrusion case (Fig 1-10). In 1999, Umemori et al[20] discussed skeletal anchorage systems and titanium miniplates for correction of open bite (Figs 1-11 to 1-13). The FDA finally cleared the use of titanium screws for anchorage, and, by 2005, 10 to 15 miniscrew systems were available on the United States market.

The screw-type mini-implant is the most commonly used system. Miniplates can be useful for intrusion but require the cooperation of an oral surgeon, and separate procedures are performed for insertion and removal. Some screws are designed with a wide-diameter tapered core and a dual thread for the cortical bone area. A 2005

Figs 1-5a and 1-5b Endosseous (osseo-integrated) palatal implant of reduced length (Orthosystem).

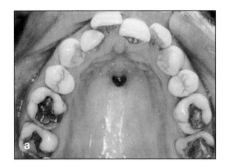
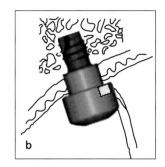

Fig 1-5c A transpalatal arch is bonded to the premolars to distalize the maxillary molars with nickel-titanium coil springs on sectional archwires.

Fig 1-5d Stabilization of the distalized second molars with a transpalatal arch. Retraction of the first molar to complete anterior alignment. (Figs 1-5a to 1-5d from Kinzinger et al.[16] Reprinted with permission.)

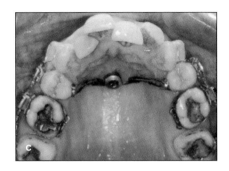
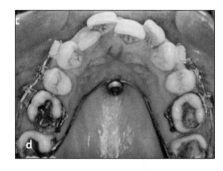

Fig 1-6 An onplant is removed from the palate with a periosteal elevator or osteotome under local anesthetic. A defect (texture) of palatal bone is evident. (From Block.[14] Reprinted with permission.)

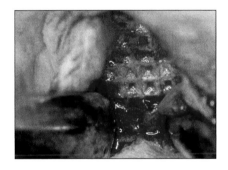

Fig 1-7a Occlusal view of two mini-implants placed in the midline of the palate for indirect anchorage.

Fig 1-7b Cephalometric radiographs are an excellent means of ensuring placement of the implants in sufficient cortical bone.

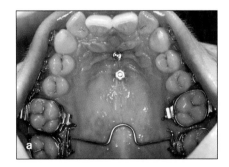
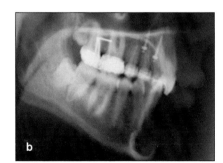

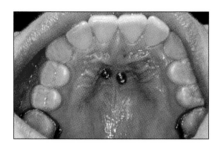

Fig 1-8a Aachen bone implants are placed in the paramedian area of the palate in a growing patient to avoid the midline suture.

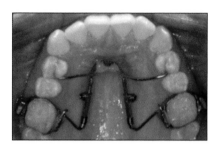

Fig 1-8b Mini-implants support the distal jet after placement.

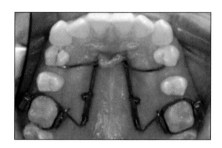

Fig 1-8c Bilateral distalization of the molars without loss of anterior anchorage. (Figs 1-8a to 1-8c from Kinzinger et al.[16] Reprinted with permission.)

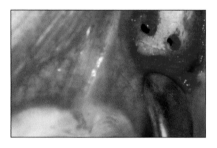

Fig 1-9a A horizontal canal is prepared in the superior part of the infrazygomatic crest. Twisted 0.012-inch stainless steel wire is inserted through canal holes.

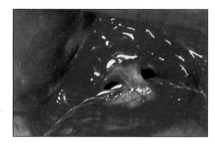

Fig 1-9b Twisted wire is temporarily fixed to the orthodontic appliance in the canine region.

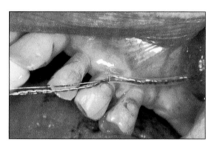

Fig 1-9c The incisors are tied together to be used as a unit for retraction and intrusion by skeletal anchorage. (Figs 1-9a to 1-9c from Melsen et al.[18] Reprinted with permission.)

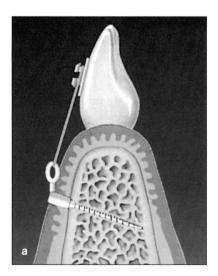

Fig 1-10a Ligature wire or elastic chain is tied to the mini-implant (1.2 mm in diameter) to intrude mandibular incisors.

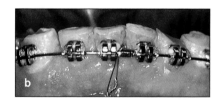

Fig 1-10b Wire is tied to the mandible at the beginning of incisor intrusion.

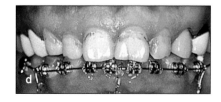

Fig 1-10c Pretreatment anterior view of intrusion of the mandibular incisors in a 44-year-old man.

Fig 1-10d Posttreatment view, 4 months after mandibular anterior intrusion. (Figs 1-10a to 1-10d from Kanomi.[19] Reprinted with permission.)

Fig 1-11 Mechanical setup for correction of open bite by a skeletal anchorage system. The archwire is tied to the first hook of the titanium miniplate by an elastic module. (From Sugawara et al.[21] Reprinted with permission.)

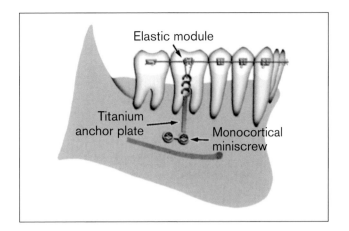

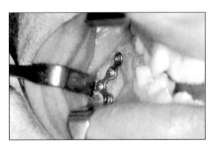

Fig 1-12a Surgical placement of an L-shaped titanium miniplate with bone screws.

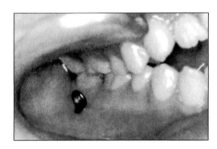

Fig 1-12b Posttreatment view of healing alveolar mucosa.[20]

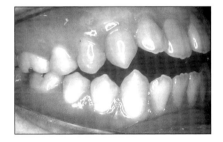

Fig 1-13a Right lateral view prior to treatment.

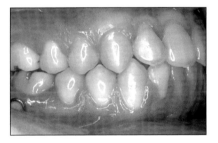

Fig 1-13b Right lateral view at debonding.

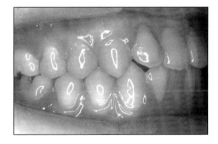

Fig 1-13c Posttreatment view 1 year after debonding. (Figs 1-13a to 1-13c from Sugawara et al.[21] Reprinted with permission.)

study comparing drill-free and self-drilling screws (evaluated in beagle dogs) found better primary stability for early loading with the drill-free screws.[22] In addition, screws in the drill-free group showed less mobility and more bone-metal contact than those in the self-drilling group (Fig 1-14).

Mini-implant anchorage is excellent for adjunctive tooth movement (Fig 1-15); en masse retraction (Fig 1-16); molar distalization or mesialization; molar intrusion or extrusion; correction of canted or tilted occlusal planes; moderate crowding; and vertical control. A thorough review of the biologic aspects, stability, and factors affecting stability of the miniscrew is presented in chapter 3.

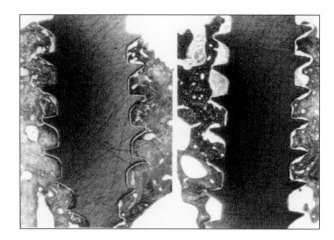

Fig 1-14 Micrographs of a drill-free implant *(left)* and a drilling implant *(right)*. The drill-free implant shows more bone-metal contact and larger bone area than the drilling implant. Drill-free implants provide high stability and result in less bony damage than drilling implants. (From Kim et al.[22] Reprinted with permission.)

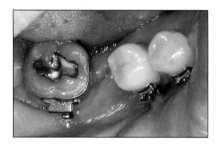

Fig 1-15a Preoperative occlusal view of a mesially inclined mandibular second molar before adjunctive tooth movement using indirect anchorage.

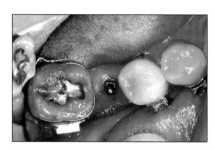

Fig 1-15b A mini-implant is placed in the edentulous area.

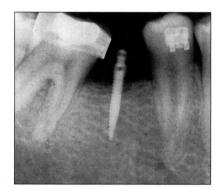

Fig 1-15c Periapical radiograph after placement of the mini-implant.

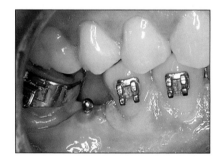

Fig 1-15d Buccal view of the implant before wire and acrylic resin stabilization are attached to the distal surface of the second premolar.

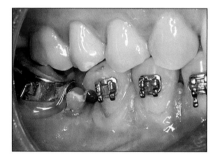

Fig 1-15e Acrylic resin is placed over the implant, and wire is bonded to the distal surface of the second premolar to provide indirect anchorage to upright the second molar.

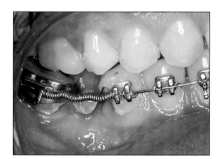

Fig 1-15f A coil spring is placed to move the second molar distally with indirect anchorage without moving the premolar segment forward.

Fig 1-16a Right lateral view with initial activation to retract the mandibular anterior segment.

Fig 1-16b Left lateral view of initial activation of the mandibular anterior segment.

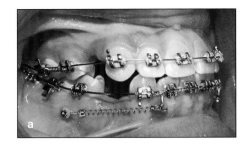
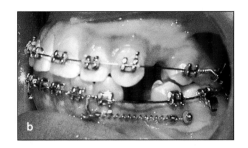

Fig 1-16c Right lateral view after activation to retract the maxillary anterior segment.

Fig 1-16d Left lateral view during maxillary and mandibular retraction.

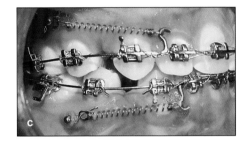
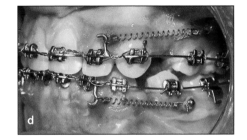

Fig 1-16e Preoperative cephalometric radiograph.

Fig 1-16f Eight-month post-retraction cephalometric radiograph.

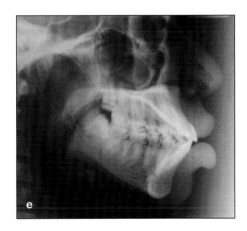
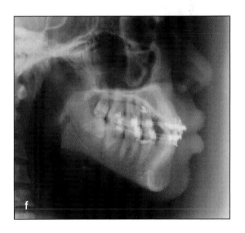

Fig 1-16g Preoperative lateral facial appearance.

Fig 1-16h Eight-month postoperative facial change.

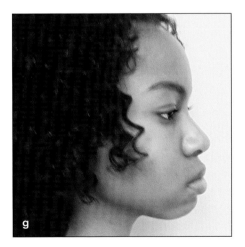
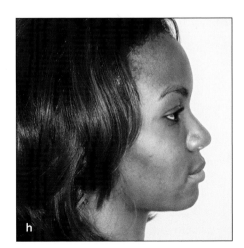

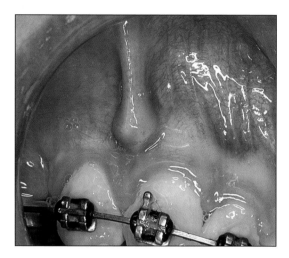

Fig 1-17a The implant is covered by alveolar mucosa when placed below the mucogingival junction; there is also a frenum pull.

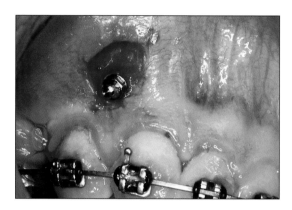

Fig 1-17b The alveolar mucosa is removed to expose the implant.

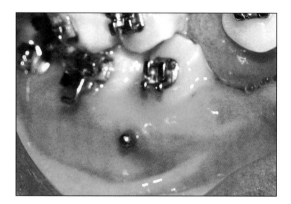

Fig 1-18a On the right side, the implant is placed at the mucogingival junction.

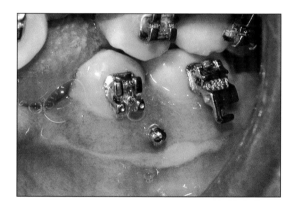

Fig 1-18b A free gingival graft has been placed on the left side of same patient so that the implant can be placed in attached gingiva. Gingival health is easier to maintain.

Implant placement

In preparation for implant placement, good orthodontic records (panoramic, periapical, and cephalometric films, casts, etc) are required along with clinical findings and a definitive orthodontic treatment plan to determine the optimal position for implant placement. Site selection is critical and requires careful consideration of the hard and soft tissues, accessibility, patient comfort, and biomechanical needs. The actual implant placement is atraumatic, nonpainful, and requires minimal anesthesia.

COMPLICATIONS

Potential complications associated with the use of mini-implants include root injury from inadequate interradicular space, vessel injury, and sinus injury. The patient should be carefully instructed in the practice of acceptable oral hygiene to avoid soft tissue inflammation around the implant. Failure is more likely when the device is placed in alveolar mucosa[23] (Figs 1-17 and 1-18). The screw may break during insertion or removal or, if placed on the lingual aspect of the mandible, may be very uncomfortable for the patient. In addition, screws can sometimes loosen and become lost. Sometimes it is difficult to attach elastics and wires to different types of screw heads. Thorough patient evaluation before the selection of candidates is important.

Medical problems have not been correlated with failure of implants. Failure seems to be correlated more with bone quality, bone mass, and surgical technique.[24] However, because complications are minimal, advantages and clinical applications favor the use of the miniscrew for successful treatment. In addition, screws are temporary, easy to remove, and economical (Table 1-1).

The potential for application of the miniscrew is limited only by the imagination and the clinical proficiency of the individual clinician. These devices have provided superior alternatives that previously were not possible in orthodontic treatment.

Table 1-1	Comparison of the properties of implants designed for prosthetic restoration and for orthodontic anchorage	
Property	Prosthodontic implants	Orthodontic implants
Composition	Titanium	Titanium
Duration of use	Permanent	Temporary
Type of load	Axial	Nonaxial
Diameter	Large	Small

REFERENCES

1. Proffit WR. Contemporary Orthodontics, ed 2. St Louis: Mosby-Yearbook, 1993:307.
2. Angle EH. Malocclusion of the Teeth and Fractures of the Maxillae, ed 6. Philadelphia: S.S. White Dental, 1900:110.
3. Codivilla A. On the means of lengthening in the lower limbs, the muscles and tissues which are shortened through deformity. Am J Orthop Surg 1905;2:353–369.
4. Gainsforth BL, Higley LB. A study of orthodontic anchorage possibilities in basal bone. Am J Orthod Oral Surg 1945;31:406–417.
5. Brånemark PI, Adell R, Breine U, Hansson BO, Lindstrom J, Ohlsson A. Intra-osseous anchorage of dental prosthesis. 1. Experimental studies. Scand J Plast Reconstr Surg 1969;3:81–100.
6. Roberts WE, Smith RK, Zilberman Y, Mozsary PG, Smith RS. Osseous adaptation to continuous loading of rigid endosseous implants Am J Orthod Dentofacial Orthop 1984;86:95–111.
7. Roberts WE, Marshall KJ, Mozsary PG. Rigid endosseus implant utilized as anchorage to protract molars and close an atrophic extraction site. Angle Orthod 1990;60:135–152.
8. Higuchi KW, Slack JM. The use of titanium fixtures for intraoral anchorage to facilitate orthodontic tooth movement. Int J Oral Maxillofac Implants 1991;6:338–344.
9. Deguchi T, Takano-Yamamoto T, Kanomi R, Hartsfield JK Jr, Roberts WE, Garetto LP. The use of small titanium screws for orthodontic anchorage. J Dent Res 2003;82:377–381.
10. Kyung HM, Park HS, Bae SM, Sung JH, Kim IB. Development of orthodontic micro-impants for intraoral anchorage. J Clin Orthod 2003;37:321–328.
11. Maino BH, Bednar J, Pagin P, Mura P. The spider screw for skeletal anchorage. J Clin Orthod 2003;37:90–97.
12. Linkow LI. Implant-orthodontics. J Clin Orthod 1970;4:685–690.
13. Creekmore TD, Eklund MK. The possibility of skeletal anchorage. J Clin Orthod 1983;17:266–269.
14. Block M. Orthodontic and orthopedic anchorage using subperiosteal bone anchors. In: Higuchi KW (ed). Orthodontic Applications of Osseointegrated Implants. Chicago: Quintessence, 2000:110–116.
15. Wehrbein H, Metz B, Diedrich P, Glatzmaier J. The use of palatal implants for orthodontic anchorage. Design and clinical applications of the Orthosystem. Clin Oral Implants Res 1996;7:410–416.
16. Kinzinger G, Wehrbein H, Byloff FK, Yildizhan F, Diedrich P. Innovative anchorage alternatives for molar distalization—An overview. J Orofac Orthop 2005;66:397–413.
17. Gelgor IE, Buyukyilmaz T, Karaman AI, Dolanmaz D, Kalayci A. Intraosseous screw-supported upper molar distalization. Angle Orthod 2004;74:838–850.
18. Melsen B, Peterson JK, Costa A. Zygoma ligatures: An alternative form of maxillary anchorage. J Clin Orthod 1998;32:154–158.
19. Kanomi R. Mini-implant for orthodontic anchorage. J Clin Orthod 1997;31:763–767.
20. Umemori M, Sugawara J, Mitani H, Nagasaka H, Kawamura H. Skeletal anchorage system for open-bite correction. Am J Orthod Dentofacial Orthop 1999;115:166–174.
21. Sugawara J, Baik UB, Umemori M, et al. Treatment and posttreatment dentoalveolar changes following intrusion of mandibular molars with application of a skeletal anchorage system (SAS) for open bite correction. Int J Adult Orthodon Orthograth Surg 2002;17:243–253.
22. Kim JW, Ahn SJ, Chang YL. Histomorphometric and mechanical analysis of the drill-free screw as orthodontic anchorage. Am J Orthod Dentofacial Orthop 2005;128:190–194.
23. Cheng SJ, Tseng Y, Lee JJ, Kok SH. A prospective study of the risk factors associated with failure of mini-implants used for orthodontic anchorage. Int J Oral Maxillofac Implants 2004;19:100–106.
24. Moy PK, Medina D, Shetty V, Aghaloo TL. Dental implant failure rates and associated risk factors. Int J Oral Maxillofac Implants 2005;20:569–577.

FUNDAMENTALS OF SKELETAL ANCHORAGE

2

TERMINOLOGY AND BASIC CONCEPTS

An understanding of the biologic background of bone-supported anchorage requires definition of the following terms and concepts.

Bone tissue

Bone is an extremely well-organized tissue, from the modulation of the hydroxyapatite crystal arrangement at the molecular level to the strain pattern of the trabecular cascades at the organ level. The synergy of the molecular, cellular, and tissue arrangements provides a tensile strength nearly equal to that of cast iron, with such an efficient use of material that the skeleton is of surprisingly low weight for such a supportive structure.[1–3]

Under a high-magnification lens, bone can be classified as coarse-fibered *woven bone* or fine-fibered *lamellar bone* (Fig 2-1).[1,2] Coarse-fibered woven, or primary, bone is considered immature or primitive; the collagen fibers in this type of bone do not have a uniform orientation. Lamellar bone is a more mature type of bone that results from the remodeling of woven bone or previously existing bone.

Bone can be classified as *cortical* (*compact* or *dense*) *bone* and *trabecular* (*cancellous* or *spongy*) *bone* (Fig 2-2).[1,2] The presence of a dense outer sheet of cortical bone and a central medullary cavity is characteristic of all bone; the medullary cavity is filled with red or yellow bone marrow in life. This marrow cavity is interrupted, through-

out its length, by a reticular network of trabecular bone, particularly at the ends of long bone. These internal trabeculae act as well-banded reinforcement rods to support the outer (thicker) cortical crust of compact bone. Whether cortical or trabecular, mature bones are histologically identical in that they consist of microscopic layers, or lamellae, which are closely packed in compact bone. Cortical bone is much stronger than trabecular bone[2] (Fig 2-3).

Surrounding all compact bone is the *periosteum*, a two-layered osteogenic (bone cell–forming) connective tissue membrane.[1,2] The inner layer, next to the surface of the bone, consists of bone cells, their precursors, and a rich microvascular supply. Both the internal surface of compact bone and the entire surface of cancellous bone are covered by a single layer, called the *endosteum*, which separates these surfaces physically from the bone marrow within. The endosteum also consists of bone cells and their precursors and a rich microvascular supply.[1,2]

Bone-supported anchorage

Many terms are used to describe bone-supported anchorage systems, including *extradental intraoral osseous anchorage system*,[4] *temporary anchorage device*,[5,6] *osseous anchorage*,[7] *skeletal anchorage*,[8,9] *orthodontic implant*,[10,11] *mini-implant*,[12] *micro-implant*,[13] and *miniscrew*.[14]

The term *screw* can have different meanings, and the term *provisional* may be more appropriate than *temporary*; therefore, terms such as *provisional anchorage devices*, *provisional orthodontic implant*, *orthodontic mini-implant*, or *orthodontic micro-implant* should be used.[15]

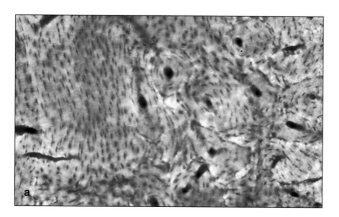

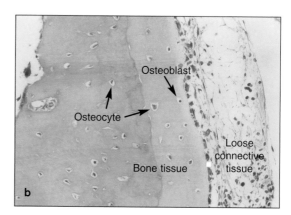

Figs 2-1a and 2-1b **(a)** Low-magnification light micrograph of ground section of mature bone. Lamellar bone has a well-organized structure and load-bearing capacity. **(b)** High-magnification light micrograph of decalcified section of immature bone. Woven bone is less organized and has reduced load-bearing capacity compared with lamellar bone (hematoxylin-eosin stain). (Courtesy of Prof HJ Kim, Seoul, Korea.)

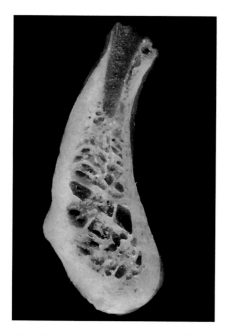

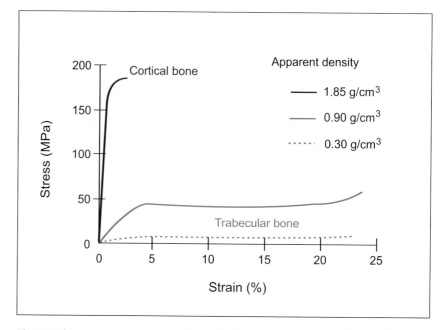

Fig 2-2 A cross section of the mandible at the symphysis clearly indicates that the mechanical support provided by the cortical bone is better than that provided by the cancellous bone.

Fig 2-3 The stress-strain curve reveals the physical properties of cortical bone and trabecular bone. Support of cortical bone is the most important factor in achieving mechanical stabilization. (Modified from Simon[2p157] with permission.)

Implant

Implantation is the transfer of nonliving tissue into a biologic system[16]; this concept differs from *transplantation*, which is the transfer of living tissue.[16]

Implants are classified as *endosteal, subperiosteal,* or *transosseous,* depending on the area of implantation[17] (Fig 2-4). They are also classified as *screw-type, blade-type,* or *cylinder-type implants,* depending on their shapes.[11,16,17] Furthermore, they may be classified as

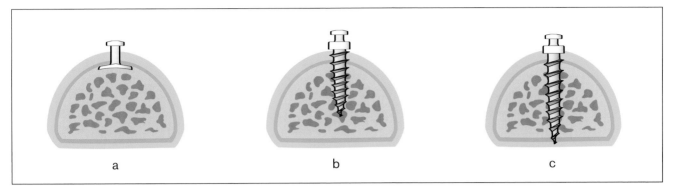

Fig 2-4 There are three types of dental implant: *(a)* The subperiosteal implant is placed under the periosteum and rests on the bone surface without penetrating it; *(b)* the endosteal implant is partially submerged and anchored within the bone; and *(c)* the transosseous implant penetrates the bone completely.

closed implants or *open implants*, based on the condition of exposure.[16] Open implants have contact with the oral cavity, while closed implants are usually used for skeletal fixation.

Screw

A *screw* is a simple machine that converts rotational motion into translational motion while providing a mechanical advantage.[18,19] Generally, a screw has three basic components: a *core*, a *helix* (called the *thread*), and a *head* (Fig 2-5).[18,19] Each component plays an important role in the function of the screw.[16,17]

The head of an orthodontic screw basically serves two purposes: to provide a means for applying twisting torque to the core and thread and to act as an application point for force.

Various means of engaging a screwdriver, including a slot, cross-slot, and recessed hex, are available for bone screws.[20] Bone screws are generally used for closed implants, so they require a less prominent head shape. Therefore, a female-type means of engaging a screwdriver is preferable, and the recessed hex has proved to be the most useful for bone screws.[19,20] On the other hand, orthodontic screws are generally used for open implants, so a male-type means of engaging a screwdriver may be favorable, because it provides the best articulation of a screwdriver and may offer better control during insertion.

The core, which forms the support of the screw, is attached to the head and is wrapped in the helical thread.[18,19] The cross-sectional area of the core (called the *root area* of the screw) determines the torsional

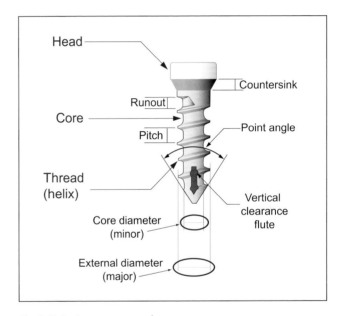

Fig 2-5 Basic components of a screw.

strength of the screw.[18,19,21] Because the torsional strength is proportional to the cube of the core diameter,[21] a very small enhancement of core diameter can greatly increase the strength of a screw. The greater the core diameter, the lower the incidence of screw failure arising from fracture during insertion of the screw. The *shank* is the part of the screw that extends from the head to the beginning of the threads. The spacing between adjacent threads is called the *pitch*. The *lead* of a screw refers to the distance that the screw will advance with each turn.[18,19] In a screw with a single thread, the pitch will equal the lead.[18,19] The cross-sectional shape of the thread is important as well because it is related to insertion methods and stress distribution.[18,19,22–25]

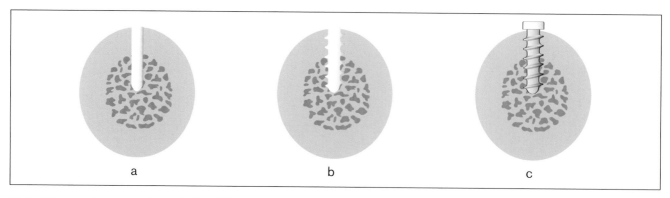

Fig 2-6 Pretapped screws are inserted after *(a)* drilling and *(b)* tapping procedures. The drilling procedure is omitted when self-tapping screws are used, while all drilling and tapping procedures are omitted with the use of self-drilling screws, which involve only *(c)* an insertion procedure.

Screws are classified as *pretapped screws*, *self-tapping screws*, or *self-drilling screws*, according to the method of insertion (Fig 2-6).[19,22–25] The insertion method is also related to the physical properties of materials. Pretapped screws are used in harder, less compressible materials, such as in metal or in cortical bone.[18,19,22] Because the screw threads cannot readily compress these firm materials, pretapped screws require the use of a tap to precut the thread. Pretapped screws are not suitable for thin bone, such as the maxilla.[22,24]

Self-tapping screws are used in softer, less compressible materials and form threads by compressing and cutting the surrounding materials. They have a fluted leading edge and require only a predrilling procedure, meaning that the tapping procedure is omitted.[22,23,25]

Self-drilling screws, also referred to as *drill-free screws*, have a corkscrew-like tip; therefore, neither predrilling nor tapping procedures are needed.[24,25]

Skeletal anchorage

Skeletal anchorage, or support obtained from bone tissues, has been used extensively in many areas, including orthodontics. As described in chapter 1, Creekmore and Eklund[8] used *skeletal anchorage* as a general term for obtaining bone anchorage when they reported treatment of maxillary anterior intrusion with Vitallium (Dentsply) bone screws placed under the anterior nasal spine as orthodontic anchorage. In 1999, Umemori et al[9] reported a case of molar intrusion for which titanium plates and screws were used as orthodontic anchorage and coined the term *skeletal anchorage system* for the titanium plate and screws. In a broad sense, use of the term *skeletal*

anchorage system in orthodontics refers to a bone-supported orthodontic implant system. In a narrower sense, the specific use of the abbreviation *SAS* indicates a bone-supported implant system that consists of plates and screws. *Bone anchorage* is another term for *skeletal anchorage*.

Osteoinduction

Osteoinduction refers to the process by which primitive, undifferentiated, and pluripotent cells are stimulated to develop into bone-forming cell lineages.[26–28] Bone morphogenetic proteins, which belong to the transforming growth factor β family of growth factors, are the only known inductive agents.[26,29] Bone morphogenetic proteins are naturally released in response to trauma or during bone remodeling. The alloplastic implant itself is not osteoinductive.

Osteoconduction

Osteoconduction indicates the growth of bone on a surface, and an osteoconductive surface is one that permits bone growth on its surface or down into pores, channels, or tubules.[26–28] In the case of implants, bone conduction is dependent on the characteristics of the biomaterials used.[26,27,30] Bone conduction is not possible with materials with poor biocompatibility, such as copper and silver, but may occur with biomaterials that are not regarded as ideally biocompatible, such as stainless steel.[26–28]

Osseointegration

Osseointegration is histologically defined as the direct anchorage of an implant by the formation of bony tissue around the implant without the growth of fibrous tissue at the bone-implant interface.[26–28,31–37] Even if direct contact between the bone and the implant occurs on the light microscopic level, it does not actually occur on the electron microscopic level.[36,37] The electron microscope reveals direct contact only when there is chemical bonding between the bone and implants.[36,37] That is, osseointegration encompasses a wide spectrum, including various ultrastructural interfaces, and demonstrates various biomechanical characteristics accordingly.[26–28,31–38] Moreover, it is difficult to define not only qualitatively but quantitatively as well.[37,39]

Rather than being an isolated phenomenon, osseointegration is a series of healing processes that form new bone tissue with the implant surface; it is the process of long-term interface maintenance through continued courses of modeling and remodeling.[27,36,37,40] In this regard, there are several considerations when the concept of osseointegration is applied in the field of orthodontics. The turnover rate (Σ) of cortical bone, 1 Σ, is equal to approximately 4 months in humans,[41] and implants are usually used only during 2 to 3 Σ in orthodontic treatment. Thus, it would be prudent to use the term *osseointegration concept*, including the meaning of long-term stability of the implant.

BIOLOGIC ASPECTS OF ORTHODONTIC IMPLANTATION

Healing process and results: Formation of the tissue-implant interface

In any kind of insertion procedure, surgical trauma and consequent damage to the adjacent bone are inevitable. The damage to the cell and matrix that results from surgical trauma triggers the healing process of the bone tissue, and typical bone wound-healing processes are initiated (Figs 2-7 and 2-8).[42,43] The healing process progresses in three phases: the inflammation phase, the reparative phase, and the remodeling phase. Many factors may influence the healing process (see Fig 2-7).[44–46]

Depending on healing conditions, the healing process results in a broad spectrum of interfaces between the implant and the tissue (Fig 2-9).[32,34] The biomechanical characteristics of this interface also affect the stability of implants.[32,37] Most important, for the composite structure of bone tissue and implants to function properly, the mechanical integrity of this interface should be maintained stably.[33] Both the formation of the interface after the healing process and the maintenance of the interface occur in a predictable manner. From the viewpoint of stability, an osseous interface is more desirable than a fibrous interface (Fig 2-10).[47,48]

Healing with new bone requires adequate numbers of cells, delivery of sufficient nutrition to these cells, an appropriate stimulus for bone repair, and optimized healing conditions.[32] Local circulation is essential for the recruitment of adequate cells, the supply of sufficient nutrition, and the removal of necrotic bone[32] (Fig 2-11). Bone repair will not begin before local circulation has been reestablished.[1,49–51]

Factors affecting formation of the interface

Structural and tissue repair necessitate a complex process under favorable conditions, because bone is an extremely well-organized, highly differentiated tissue (Fig 2-12).[44,47,52,53] This healing process is affected by many factors, including the degree of surgical trauma, implant biocompatibility, healing conditions, and initial stabilization.

General conditions

Calcium metabolism; metabolic diseases such as osteoporosis, osteopenia, or hyperparathyroidism; and irradiation therapy may affect the healing process of bone tissue.[54–58] Clinically, however, local bone density seems more important than systemic bone density,[54,55] and orthodontic mini-implants can be used as long as sufficient primary stability can be obtained from the existing cortical bone.

Local conditions

The quantity and quality of the host bone bed of the implantation site also greatly influence primary stability[59,60] (ie, the mechanical stabilization immediately after implantation). Primary stability is closely related to healing

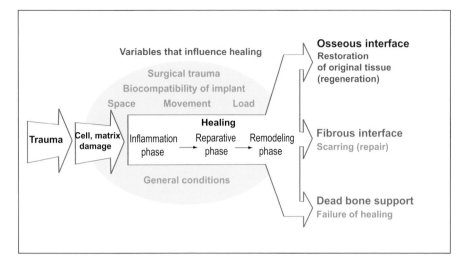

Fig 2-7 Surgical trauma, such as frictional heat and pressure, initiate the healing process. The healing process progresses in three phases: an inflammation phase, a reparative (modeling) phase, and a remodeling phase. The results of healing can be grouped into three overlapping categories: restoration of the original tissue, scarring (poorly differentiated tissue), and repair failure.

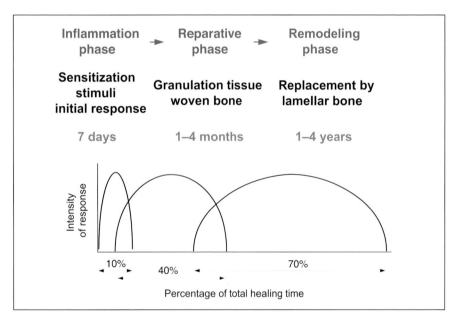

Fig 2-8 Phases of healing. In the reparative (modeling) phase, woven bone is formed. In the remodeling phase, woven bone, which cannot bear a functional load, is converted to lamellar bone. Approximate time periods for each phase in the human healing process are provided.

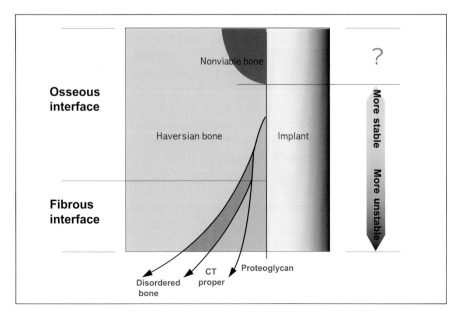

Fig 2-9 Tissue-implant interface after the healing process. During the healing process, a broad spectrum of interface types is formed between the implant and tissue. The biomechanical characteristics differ, depending on the interface. A direct biochemical attachment to the bone surface has the strongest bond strength at the interface. Cell viability is not essential for the composite structure of a bone-implant interface to function. Dead bone can support the implant, but it also has the potential to become unstable as microdamage becomes more concentrated. (CT) connective tissue.

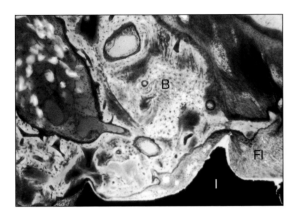

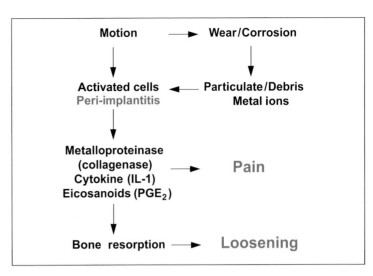

Fig 2-10a The fibrous interface is different from the periodontal ligament in that the latter is well organized while the former is not. (B) bone; (FI) fibrous interface; (I) implant.

Fig 2-10b With a fibrous interface, there is a risk of instability with increasing mobility.[2] Motion may induce peri-implant inflammation of fibrous tissue, which causes pain and bone resorption. (IL-1) interleukin 1; (PGE$_2$) prostaglandin E$_2$.

Fig 2-11a Remodeling process of trabecular bone. Revascularization of the necrotic zone and the healing process are similar to the normal remodeling process. If revascularization of the necrotic zone is prevented, healing will not occur. *(left)* In trabecular bone, blood supply is abundant compared with that of cortical bone. *(center)* Osteoclasts are recruited to resorb old or necrotic bone. *(right)* Osteoblasts synthesize and mineralize new osteoid. (OC) osteocyte; (OB) osteoblast; (EC) epithelial cell; (RBC) red blood cell; (OCL) osteoclast.

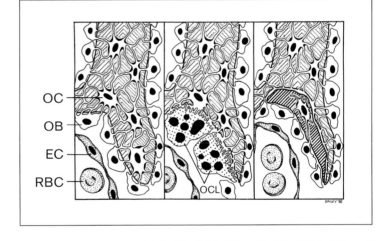

Fig 2-11b Remodeling process of cortical bone. *(top)* Old or necrotic bone is being removed in segment α by osteoclasts forming a cutting cone. In segment β, osteoblasts begin to synthesize osteoid (ie, form a filling cone). Osteoid then mineralizes, becoming new bone. *(bottom)* Turnover of old bone progresses from left to right as osteoclasts continue to resorb old bone, osteoblasts continue to synthesize osteoid, and new osteoid is mineralized. (Figs 2-11a and 2-11b from Ten Cate.[1] Reprinted with permission.)

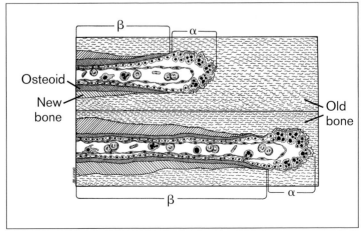

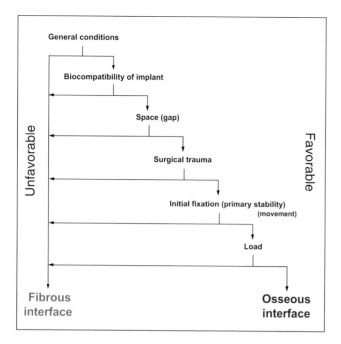

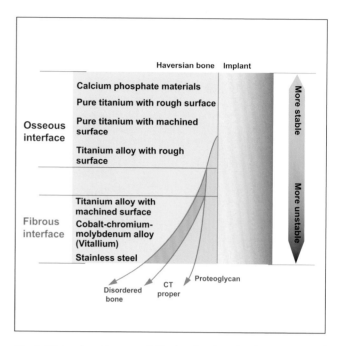

Fig 2-12 The formation of the osseous interface is a complex process. Each condition that affects the formation of the interface must be favorable for healing with highly differentiated bone tissue in order for an osseous interface to form. Under any unfavorable condition, the healing process results in fibrous tissue formation instead of bone tissue formation. The dead bone will remain and, like the dead branch of a tree, will be capable of some load-bearing. Healing will occur with new bone only if certain local conditions are optimized.

Fig 2-13 Implant biocompatibility is related to the characteristics of the implant surface. The materials with the greatest biocompatibility are calcium phosphate ceramics and titanium with a rough surface, followed by titanium alloy with a machined surface; titanium alloy with a rough surface and pure titanium with a machined surface; cobalt-chromium-molybdenum alloy (Vitallium); and stainless steel.[27,30,61–67] Fibrous tissue formation is thought to be inevitable when Vitallium and stainless steel implants are used. For long-term stability, implants should be made of materials that are more biocompatible than titanium alloy. (CT) connective tissue.

conditions and loading conditions; the blood supply also influences the healing process.

Biocompatibility

Implants for orthodontic anchorage are made of alloplastic materials. Each material has its own advantages and disadvantages with regard to physical properties, such as biocompatibility, mechanical strength, machinability, and elasticity.[27,30,61–70] The biocompatibility of the material is the most important of these characteristics (Fig 2-13). Biocompatibility is strongly influenced by the surface characteristics of the materials, because the primary chemical interaction between an implant and its host tissue takes place over a few atomic radii.[62,71] In other words, the biocompatibility of the surface texture greatly influences which type of interface is formed or how fast the adjacent tissue reacts. Moreover, it is also strongly related to the long-term maintenance of the interface.[27,30,65–68]

Implant materials can be classified by their biocompatibility into *bioactive*, *bioinert*, and *biotolerant* materials.

Bioactive materials, such as hydroxyapatite or aluminum oxide, can create chemical bonds with bone.[16,69] Meanwhile, fibrous tissue formation is thought to be an inevitable phenomenon with Vitallium and stainless steel implants.[16,48,61–63]

Additionally, implants have sufficient strength, and mechanical failure or fatigue failure should not occur during the functioning of implants. There should be no ional leakage or corrosion products in vivo. Generally, stainless steel and chrome-cobalt alloy are considered stabilized materials, but these materials do not show long-term inertness in vivo.[61–63] Chronic inflammation and fibrous encapsulation can result from corrosion products.

Size of the implant-bone space

Shortly after implantation, the implant-bone space fills with a blood clot and host bone chips that arise from the surgical procedure.[51,72,73] The dimension of the implant-bone space influences the results of the healing process and the mode of ossification.[40,51,73–77] As the space is

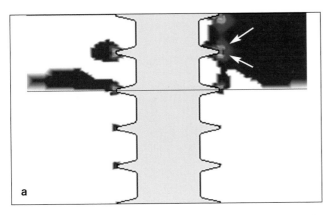

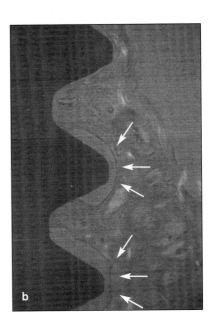

Figs 2-14a and 2-14b **(a)** Stress is primarily concentrated in the vicinity of the screws *(arrows)*. **(b)** Appropriate loading can accelerate bone formation, and new bone is formed at the tip of the thread *(arrows)*. (Fig 2-14b from Wehrbein and Diedrich.[88] Reprinted with permission.)

widened over the critical threshold, the amount of bone-implant contact decreases.[74] For areas where new bone formation occurs, the appropriate implant-bone space may enhance establishment of circulation for bone formation.[40,73] In addition, the effect of the space on bone healing may differ depending on whether bone growth occurs *toward* or *from* implant surfaces,[69] which is influenced by the biocompatibility of the implant. On the other hand, for areas where existing bone provides initial mechanical stabilization, the dimension of the implant-bone space should be minimal.[40]

Surgical trauma

Bone will permanently heal with fibrous tissue as a response to severe trauma, whether it is of a physical, a chemical, or another nature. The characteristics of bone cause the healing process to progress very slowly.[1,35] The larger the area of injury, the greater the chance that healing will result in poorly differentiated fibrous tissue instead of highly differentiated bone tissue.[32,78] Even a 0.5-mm necrotic zone requires several months to be replaced with newly formed hard tissue.[32]

Mature bone is temperature sensitive.[79,80] If the temperature rises, an element of bone, alkaline phosphatase, is destroyed; as a result, alkaline calcium synthesis and bone formation do not occur. It has been found that bone tissue damage occurs when the bone temperature reaches 47°C for 1 to 5 minutes.[79,80] Excessive pressure during surgical procedures may also cause injury of bone tissue.[23,56] Surgical trauma can be reduced with the use

of well-sharpened drills under flowing saline cooling at a high speed during the drilling procedures and at a low speed during the insertion procedures.[81-84]

Healing conditions

Excessive movement or excessive micromotion adversely affects the healing sequence that leads to direct bone anchorage of implants.[67,85-87] Low levels of micromotion may be tolerated or may even stimulate bone formation, but micromotion over the critical threshold may prevent bone ingrowth and depress bone formation.[86] This threshold can be determined according to the implant surface and design.[66,87]

Loading conditions

Bone healing around endosseous dental implants is affected by peri-implant loading conditions[33,34,88-99]; orthodontic loading may affect the modeling and remodeling activity of the peri-implant bone tissue[70,88-112] (ie, bone-to-implant contact, marginal bone level, marginal bone apposition, bone density, and turnover rate of the bone). Whereas appropriate loading may stimulate increased bone formation (Fig 2-14),[88-99] early loading or excessive loading could have detrimental effects on bone formation (Fig 2-15).[31,32,100] However, it is not the loading itself or its timing but rather the strain applied to bone that affects the healing process (Fig 2-16).[113] If loading is well controlled clinically, immediate loading will not compromise stability in cases where mechanical stabilization

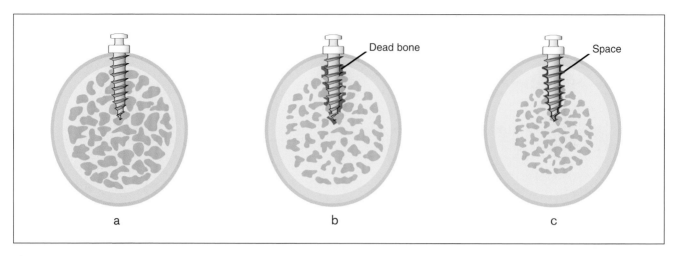

Fig 2-15 The same orthodontic load may lead to different bone reactions, depending on the primary stability (mechanical stabilization after implant placement). Even a light force can cause excessive strain, so that the mechanical integrity of bone tissue cannot be maintained, in the presence of *(a)* poor bone quality and quantity, *(b)* excessive surgical trauma, and *(c)* "eccentric" insertion.

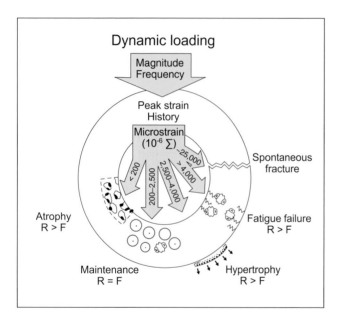

Fig 2-16 Frost[44] modeled four zones for bone adaptation to mechanical strain. The acute disuse window (atrophy) indicates the lowest amount of microstrain. The adapted window (maintenance) is an ideal physiologic loading zone. The mild overload zone (hypertrophy) causes microfracture and triggers an increase in bone remodeling, which produces more woven bone. The pathologic overload zone (fatigue failure) causes an increase in fatigue fracture, remodeling, and bone resorption. In brief, if too little or too much strain occurs, bone is resorbed, and if appropriate strain is delivered, bone formation may be accelerated. (R) resorption; (F) formation.

of implants from the existing cortical bone ensures sufficient primary stability.[95,96,98,114] Even the same loading conditions may induce different bone responses depending on the biocompatibility of the implants.

Factors affecting maintenance of the interface

The maintenance of the interface is strongly related to the biomechanical characteristics of the interface and the

stress applied to the implant. The bone-implant interface has low tolerance for shear stress and impact stress.

Bone is dynamic tissue, and the adaptation of bone to environmental changes continues through two distinct physiologic processes: modeling (change in shape and form) and remodeling (turnover).[1,28,32,40,43,44,113] Even when healing has resulted in the formation of an osseous interface, the balance between bone formation and bone resorption may be interrupted, and the osseous interface cannot be maintained[32] (Figs 2-17 and 2-18).

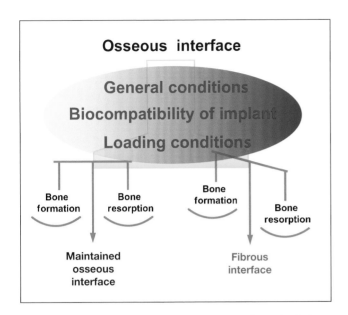

Fig 2-17 For maintenance of the osseous interface, the balance between formation and resorption should be maintained.

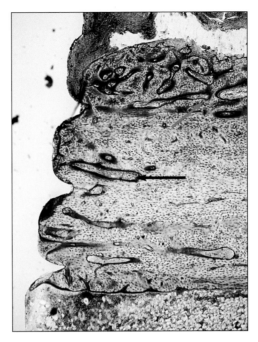

Fig 2-18 Histologic examination of a loaded implant in the femur of a rabbit. New bone formation occurred under the periosteum *(red arrow)*. The process of remodeling also occurred in the existing cortical bone *(black arrow)*.

Biomechanical characteristics of the interface

The bond strength at the interface varies widely.[38,64,66,114-119] There may be Van der Waals bonding or physisorption bonding, hydrobonding, and chemical bonding at the interface, depending on the characteristics of surface composition on an atomic scale.[62,66,71] Strong bonds at the interface can certainly facilitate load distribution.

Biocompatibility

The biocompatibility of materials is most important not only for formation of the interface but also for maintenance of the interface.[27,30,61-68] Leakage of ions or corrosion products from implants leads to bone resorption and fibrous encapsulation.[61-63]

Loading conditions

The type and the amount of stress put on the bone tissue also influence maintenance. Bone tissue is weaker against tensile stress than compressive stress and weakest against shear stress.[2,25,66,95] In cases in which stress is concentrated at one site and where stress is over the physiologic threshold of bone, the structural integrity of the surrounding bone tissue cannot be maintained. The type and the distribution of this stress are related to the screw-thread design and the implant-bone interface.[120]

Implant design

Implant design parameters, including length, diameter, and thread shape, directly influence the distribution of orthodontic load.[25,95,121-124] This will be described in more detail in chapter 3.

Mechanisms of orthodontic implantation

The arena of dental implants includes osseointegrated prosthodontic implants, surgical bone screws, and orthodontic mini-implants. Because their roles in treatment differ, their requirements for success also vary. For example, osseointegrated prosthodontic implants must be stable for a long period of time under strong masticatory loads; conversely, surgical bone screws need only be stable for 4 to 6 weeks, until callus formation. In other words, osseointegrated prosthodontic implants require stricter criteria for success to attain proper functioning. However, all implants are based on the same biologic princi-

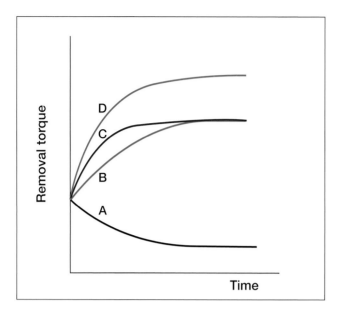

Fig 2-19 Chronologic changes in the bond strength at the bone-implant interface according to the biocompatibilities of implant materials. Biocompatibility influences how fast the healing process progresses and the eventual bond strength. (A) As time passes, the bond strength decreases. The torque required for removal of stainless steel implants is much less than that needed for insertion because of the fibrous tissue formed at the interface. (B) The bond strength increases because of the formation of new bone at the interface. (C) With increased biocompatibility and optimized healing conditions, the healing period can be shortened. (D) More biocompatible implants are used so that bonding at the interface can be strengthened. For example, implants coated with hydroxyapatite can create chemical bonds at the interface.[117–119]

ples and differ only in that they use different tissue-implant interfaces as criteria for success.

For any type of implant to function, it is essential that adequate support be obtained from the surrounding tissues, although an orthodontic implant is loaded by light forces for a short period of time compared to a prosthodontic implant.

Support from fibrous connective tissue is advantageous in procedures for removal of implants. An implant supported by fibrous connective tissue can remain stable for a certain period of time. However, there is a risk of instability because of increased mobility, and fibrous connective tissue is not appropriate for supporting a load.[2,48] Fibrous tissue formation at the bone-implant interface is regarded as the most important risk factor in implant loosening; thus, for an implant to be used for stable and reliable anchorage, it is important that sufficient support be obtained from bone tissue rather than the other tissues. Lamellar bone is more appropriate than woven bone on the microscopic level; with regard to physical strength and characteristics, support from cortical bone is more important than that from cancellous bone on the macroscopic level.

An implant can be supported by newly formed bone and older existing bone (Fig 2-19).[35,47,114,125–127] The maintenance of bone support is also important. The support from existing cortical bone is key to early stability, while support from newly formed bone and maintenance of the interface are important for later stability.

Support from existing bone

Healthy bone, especially cortical bone, can bear considerable loads. Intact, healthy bone resists appreciable amounts of loading without failure. For example, a standard 4.5-mm cortical screw anchored in only one cortex of the femur can withstand 250 kg in terms of the holding strength of a screw.[2,3] However, surgical trauma is inevitable during implantation procedures, and it may compromise the support from existing bone.

Support from newly formed bone

Under optimum conditions, at least 2 to 4 weeks are needed for bone formation to occur around implants in humans.[40,66,72–74] The bone tissue formed at this time is woven bone, which cannot withstand any load.[43–46,56,66,125] Therefore, 3 to 6 months are needed for the formation of lamellar bone that is capable of withstanding orthodontic forces.

SUMMARY

Skeletal anchorage in orthodontics involves the use of implanted devices to control tooth movement and provide support. Surgical trauma and consequent damage to the adjacent bone during implantation procedures trigger the healing process of the bone tissue. The healing conditions determine the nature of the interface between the implant and the tissue, and the biomechanical characteristics of this interface affect the stability of the implant.

Mechanical stabilization from the existing cortical bone is important for primary stability and optimal healing conditions within the 3 months following implantation. Support from the newly formed bone is not available for at least 3 months postimplantation. Fibrous connective tissue is not appropriate for supporting a load. For an implant to provide stable and reliable anchorage, it is important that sufficient support be obtained from bone tissue rather than other tissues. Microscopically, lamellar bone is more appropriate than woven bone; macroscopically, support from cortical bone is more important than that from cancellous bone.

REFERENCES

1. Ten Cate AR. Oral Histology: Development, Structure, and Function, ed 4. St Louis: Mosby, 1994.
2. Kaplan FS, Hayes WC, Keaveny TM, Boskey A, Einhorn TA, Iannotti JP. Form and function of bone. In: Simon SR (ed). Orthopaedic Basic Science, ed 1. Rosemont, IL: American Academy of Orthopaedic Surgeons, 1994:127–174.
3. Muller ME, Perren SM. Manual of Internal Fixation: Techniques Recommended by the AO-ASIF Group, ed 3. Berlin: Springer-Verlag, 1991.
4. Costa A, Raffainl M, Melsen B. Miniscrews as orthodontic anchorage: A preliminary report. Int J Adult Orthodon Orthognath Surg 1998;13:201–209.
5. Cope JB. Temporary anchorage devices in orthodontics: A paradigm shift. Semin Orthod 2005;11:3–9.
6. Mah J, Bergstrand F. Temporary anchorage devices: A status report. J Clin Orthod 2005;39:132–136.
7. Roberts WE, Smith RK, Zilberman Y, Mozsary PG, Smith RS. Osseous adaptation to continuous loading of rigid endosseous implants. Am J Orthod 1984;86:95–111.
8. Creekmore TD, Eklund MK. The possibility of skeletal anchorage. J Clin Orthod 1983;17:266–269.
9. Umemori M, Sugawara J, Mitani H, Nagasaka H, Kawamura H. Skeletal anchorage system for open-bite correction. Am J Orthod Dentofacial Orthop 1999;115:166–174.
10. Favero L, Brollo P, Bressan E. Orthodontic anchorage with specific fixtures: Related study analysis. Am J Orthod Dentofacial Orthop 2002;122:84–94.
11. Huang LH, Shotwell JL, Wang HL. Dental implants for orthodontic anchorage. Am J Orthod Dentofacial Orthop 2005;127:713–722.
12. Park YC, Lee SY, Kim DH, Jee SH. Intrusion of posterior teeth using mini-screw implants. Am J Orthod Dentofacial Orthop 2003;123:690–694.
13. Melsen B. Mini-implants: Where are we? J Clin Orthod 2005;39:539–547.
14. Kyung HM, Park HS, Bae SM, Sung JH, Kim IB. Development of orthodontic micro-implants for intraoral anchorage. J Clin Orthod 2003;37:321–328.
15. Carano A, Melsen B. Implants in orthodontics. Interview. Prog Orthod 2005;6:62–69.
16. Spiekermann H. Implantology, ed 1. Stuttgart: Thieme, 1995:38.
17. Phillips RW. Phillips' Science of Dental Materials, ed 10. Philadelphia: Saunders, 1996:655–657.
18. Uhl RL. The biomechanics of screws. Orthop Rev 1989;18:1302–1307.
19. Perry CR, Gilula LA. Basic principles and clinical uses of screws and bolts. Orthop Rev 1992;21:709–713.
20. Saka B. Mechanical and biomechanical measurements of five currently available osteosynthesis systems of self-tapping screws. Br J Oral Maxillofac Surg 2000;38:70–75.
21. Perren SM. Force measurements in screw fixation. J Biomech 1976;9:669–675.
22. Bahr W. Pretapped and self-tapping screws in the human midface. Torque measurements and bone screw interface. Int J Oral Maxillofac Surg 1990;19:51–53.
23. Sowden D, Schmitz JP. AO self-drilling and self-tapping screws in rat calvarial bone: An ultrastructural study of the implant interface. J Oral Maxillofac Surg 2002;60:294–299.
24. Heidemann W, Gerlach KL, Grobel KH, Kollner HG. Drill free screws: A new form of osteosynthesis screw. J Craniomaxillofac Surg 1998;26:163–168.
25. Hitchon PW, Brenton MD, Coppes JK, From AM, Torner JC. Factors affecting the pullout strength of self-drilling and self-tapping anterior cervical screws. Spine 2003;28:9–13.
26. Albrektsson T, Johansson C. Osteoinduction, osteoconduction and osseointegration. Eur Spine J 2001;10(suppl 2):S96–S101.
27. Cooper LF. Biologic determinants of bone formation for osseointegration: Clues for future clinical improvements. J Prosthet Dent 1998;80:439–449.
28. Ostrum RF, Chao EYS, Bassett CAL, et al. Bone injury: Regeneration and repair. In: Simon SR (ed). Orthopaedic Basic Science, ed 1. Rosemont, IL: American Academy of Orthopaedic Surgeons, 1994:284–286.
29. Lind M. Growth factors: Possible new clinical tools. A review. Acta Orthop Scand 1996;67:407–417.
30. Puleo DA, Nanci A. Understanding and controlling the bone-implant interface. Biomaterials 1999;20:2311–2321.
31. Brånemark PI. Osseointegration and its experimental background. J Prosthet Dent 1983;50:399–410.
32. Brånemark PI, Zarb GA, Albrektsson T. Tissue-integrated Prostheses: Osseointegration in Clinical Dentistry. Chicago: Quintessence, 1985.
33. Albrektsson T, Jacobsson M. Bone-metal interface in osseointegration. J Prosthet Dent 1987;57:597–607.
34. Albrektsson TO, Johansson CB, Sennerby L. Biological aspects of implant dentistry: Osseointegration. Periodontol 2000 1994;4:58–73.
35. Schenk RK, Buser D. Osseointegration: A reality. Periodontol 2000 1998;17:22–35.
36. Newman MG, Takei HH, Carranza FA. Carranza's Clinical Periodontology. Philadelphia: Saunders, 2002.
37. Lindhe J, Karring T, Lang NP. Clinical Periodontology and Implant, ed 4. Oxford: Blackwell, 2003.
38. Wong M, Eulenberger J, Schenk R, Hunziker E. Effect of surface topology on the osseointegration of implant materials in trabecular bone. J Biomed Mater Res 1995;29:1567–1575.
39. Roberts WE, Helm FR, Marshall KJ, Gongloff RK. Rigid endosseous implants for orthodontic and orthopedic anchorage. Angle Orthod 1989;59:247–256.

40. Berglundh T, Abrahamsson I, Lang NP, Lindhe J. De novo alveolar bone formation adjacent to endosseous implants. Clin Oral Implants Res 2003;14:251–262.

41. Roberts WE, Turley PK, Brezniak N, Fielder PJ. Implants: Bone physiology and metabolism. CDA J 1987;15:54–61.

42. Rockwood CA, Green DP. Rockwood and Green's Fractures in Adults. Philadelphia: Lippincott-Raven, 1996.

43. Higuchi KW. Orthodontic Applications of Osseointegrated Implants. Chicago: Quintessence, 2000.

44. Frost HM. The biology of fracture healing. An overview for clinicians. Part I. Clin Orthop 1989;248:283–293.

45. Einhorn TA. The cell and molecular biology of fracture healing. Clin Orthop Relat Res 1998;(355 suppl):S7–21.

46. Browner BD. Skeletal Trauma: Fractures, Dislocations, Ligamentous Injuries, ed 2. Philadelphia: Saunders, 1998.

47. Albrektsson T, Albrektsson B. Osseointegration of bone implants. A review of an alternative mode of fixation. Acta Orthop Scand 1987;58:567–577.

48. Moroni A, Vannini F, Mosca M, Giannini S. State of the art review: Techniques to avoid pin loosening and infection in external fixation. J Orthop Trauma 2002;16:189–195.

49. Albrektsson T. The healing of autologous bone grafts after varying degrees of surgical trauma. A microscopic and histochemical study in the rabbit. J Bone Joint Surg Br 1980;62:403–410.

50. Matsuo M, Nakamura T, Kishi Y, Takahashi K. Microvascular changes after placement of titanium implants: Scanning electron microscopy observations of machined and titanium plasma-sprayed implants in dogs. J Periodontol 1999;70:1330–1338.

51. Franchi M, Fini M, Martini D, et al. Biological fixation of endosseous implants. Micron 2005;36:665–671.

52. Cooper LF, Masuda T, Yliheikkila PK, Felton DA. Generalizations regarding the process and phenomenon of osseointegration. Part II. In vitro studies. Int J Oral Maxillofac Implants 1998;13:163–174.

53. Albrektsson T. Direct bone anchorage of dental implants. J Prosthet Dent 1983;50:255–261.

54. Roberts WE, Simmons KE, Garetto LP, DeCastro RA. Bone physiology and metabolism in dental implantology: Risk factors for osteoporosis and other metabolic bone diseases. Implant Dent 1992;1:11–21.

55. Tonetti MS. Risk factors for osseodisintegration. Periodontol 2000; 17:55–62.

56. Esposito M, Hirsch JM, Lekholm U, Thomsen P. Biological factors contributing to failures of osseointegrated oral implants (II). Etiopathogenesis. Eur J Oral Sci 1998;106:721–764.

57. Cooper LF. Systemic effectors of alveolar bone mass and implications in dental therapy. Periodontol 2000 2000;23:103–109.

58. Bryant SR. The effects of age, jaw site, and bone condition on oral implant outcomes. Int J Prosthodont 1998;11:470–490.

59. Bischof M, Nedir R, Szmukler-Moncler S, Bernard JP, Samson J. Implant stability measurement of delayed and immediately loaded implants during healing. Clin Oral Implants Res 2004;15:529–539.

60. Gedrange T, Hietschold V, Mai R, Wolf P, Nicklisch M, Harzer W. An evaluation of resonance frequency analysis for the determination of the primary stability of orthodontic palatal implants. A study in human cadavers. Clin Oral Implants Res 2005;16:425–431.

61. Litsky AS, Spector M. Biomaterials. In: Simon SR (ed). Orthopaedic Basic Science, ed 1. Rosemont, IL: American Academy of Orthopaedic Surgeons, 1994:447–486.

62. Brånemark PI, Zarb GA, Albrektsson T (eds). Tissue-Integrated Prostheses: Osseointegration in Clinical Dentistry. Chicago: Quintessence, 1985.

63. Misch CE. Dental Implant Prosthetics. St Louis: Elsevier Mosby, 2005.

64. Steinemann SG. Titanium—The material of choice? Periodontol 2000 1998;17:7–21.

65. Glantz PO. The choice of alloplastic materials for oral implants: Does it really matter? Int J Prosthodont 1998;11:402–407.

66. Moroni A, Faldini C, Chilo V, Rocca M, Stea S, Giannini S. The effect of surface material and roughness on bone screw stability. J Orthop Trauma 1999;13:477–482.

67. Brunski JB, Puleo DA, Nanci A. Biomaterials and biomechanics of oral and maxillofacial implants: Current status and future developments. Int J Oral Maxillofac Implants 2000;15:15–46.

68. Albrektsson T, Wennerberg A. Oral implant surfaces: Part 2—Review focusing on clinical knowledge of different surfaces. Int J Prosthodont 2004;17:544–564.

69. Davies JE. Mechanisms of endosseous integration. Int J Prosthodont. 1998;11:391–401.

70. Aldikacti M, Acikgoz G, Turk T, Trisi P. Long-term evaluation of sandblasted and acid-etched implants used as orthodontic anchors in dogs. Am J Orthod Dentofacial Orthop 2004;125:139–147.

71. Kasemo B, Lausmaa J. Biomaterial and implant surfaces: On the role of cleanliness, contamination, and preparation procedures. J Biomed Mater Res 1988;22(A2 suppl):145–158.

72. Dhert WJ, Thomsen P, Blomgren AK, Esposito M, Ericson LE, Verbout AJ. Integration of press-fit implants in cortical bone: A study on interface kinetics. J Biomed Mater Res 1998;41:574–583.

73. Futami T, Fujii N, Ohnishi H, et al. Tissue response to titanium implants in the rat maxilla: Ultrastructural and histochemical observations of the bone-titanium interface. Periodontol 2000;71: 287–298.

74. Carlsson L, Rostlund T, Albrektsson B, Albrektsson T. Implant fixation improved by close fit. Cylindrical implant-bone interface studied in rabbits. Acta Orthop Scand 1988;59:272–275.

75. Dalton JE, Cook SD, Thomas KA, Kay JF. The effect of operative fit and hydroxyapatite coating on the mechanical and biological response to porous implants. J Bone Joint Surg Am 1995;77: 97–110.

76. Ivanoff CJ, Sennerby L, Lekholm U. Influence of initial implant mobility on the integration of titanium implants. An experimental study in rabbits. Clin Oral Implants Res 1996;7:120–127.

77. Akimoto K, Becker W, Persson R, Baker DA, Rohrer MD, O'Neal RB. Evaluation of titanium implants placed into simulated extraction sockets: A study in dogs. Int J Oral Maxillofac Implants 1999; 14:351–360.

78. Hoshaw SJ, Fyhrie DP, Schaffler MB. The effect of implant insertion and design on bone microdamage. In: Davidovitch Z (ed). The Biological Mechanism of Tooth Eruption, Resorption and Replacement by Implants. Boston: Harvard Society for the Advancement of Orthodontics, 1994:735–741.

79. Eriksson AR, Albrektsson T. Temperature threshold levels for heat-induced bone tissue injury: A vital-microscopic study in the rabbit. J Prosthet Dent 1983;50:101–107.

80. Eriksson RA, Albrektsson T. The effect of heat on bone regeneration: An experimental study in the rabbit using the bone growth chamber. J Oral Maxillofac Surg 1984;42:705–711.

81. Sharawy M, Misch CE, Weller N, Tehemar S. Heat generation during implant drilling: The significance of motor speed. J Oral Maxillofac Surg 2002;60:1160–1169.

82. Iyer S, Weiss C, Mehta A. Effects of drill speed on heat production and the rate and quality of bone formation in dental implant osteotomies. Part I: Relationship between drill speed and heat production. Int J Prosthodont 1997;10:411–414.

83. Iyer S, Weiss C, Mehta A. Effects of drill speed on heat production and the rate and quality of bone formation in dental implant osteotomies. Part II: Relationship between drill speed and healing. Int J Prosthodont 1997;10:536–540.

84. Tehemar SH. Factors affecting heat generation during implant site preparation: A review of biologic observations and future considerations. Int J Oral Maxillofac Implants 1999;14:127–136.

85. Goodman SB. The effects of micromotion and particulate materials on tissue differentiation. Bone chamber studies in rabbits. Acta Orthop Scand Suppl 1994;258:1–43.

86. Soballe K, Hansen ES, B-Rasmussen H, Jorgensen PH, Bunger C. Tissue ingrowth into titanium and hydroxyapatite-coated implants during stable and unstable mechanical conditions. J Orthop Res 1992;10:285–299.

87. Szmukler-Moncler S, Salama H, Reingewirtz Y, Dubruille JH. Timing of loading and effect of micromotion on bone-dental implant interface: Review of experimental literature. J Biomed Mater Res 1998;43:192–203.

88. Wehrbein H, Diedrich P. Endosseous titanium implants during and after orthodontic load–An experimental study in the dog. Clin Oral Implants Res 1993;4(2):76–82.

89. Majzoub Z, Finotti M, Miotti F, Giardino R, Aldini NN, Cordioli G. Bone response to orthodontic loading of endosseous implants in the rabbit calvaria: Early continuous distalizing forces. Eur J Orthod 1999;21:223–230.

90. Brunski JB. In vivo bone response to biomechanical loading at the bone/dental-implant interface. Adv Dent Res 1999;13:99–119.

91. Melsen B, Lang NP. Biological reactions of alveolar bone to orthodontic loading of oral implants. Clin Oral Implants Res 2001;12:144–152.

92. Duyck J, Ronold HJ, Van Oosterwyck H, Naert I, Vander Sloten J, Ellingsen JE. The influence of static and dynamic loading on marginal bone reactions around osseointegrated implants: An animal experimental study. Clin Oral Implants Res 2001;12:207–218.

93. Romanos GE, Toh CG, Siar CH, Swaminathan D. Histologic and histomorphometric evaluation of peri-implant bone subjected to immediate loading: An experimental study with Macaca fascicularis. Int J Oral Maxillofac Implants 2002;17:44–51.

94. Romanos GE, Toh CG, Siar CH, Wicht H, Yacoob H, Nentwig GH. Bone-implant interface around titanium implants under different loading conditions: A histomorphometrical analysis in the Macaca fascicularis monkey. J Periodontol 2003;74:1483–1490.

95. Gapski R, Wang HL, Mascarenhas P, Lang NP. Critical review of immediate implant loading. Clin Oral Implants Res 2003;14:515–527.

96. Romanos GE. Present status of immediate loading of oral implants. J Oral Implantol 2004;30:189–197.

97. De Smet E, Jaecques S, Vandamme K, Vander Sloten J, Naert I. Positive effect of early loading on implant stability in the bicortical guinea-pig model. Clin Oral Implants Res 2005;16:402–407.

98. Trisi P, Rebaudi A. Peri-implant bone reaction to immediate, early, and delayed orthodontic loading in humans. Int J Periodontics Restorative Dent 2005;25:317–329.

99. Buchter A, Wiechmann D, Koerdt S, Wiesmann HP, Piffko J, Meyer U. Load-related implant reaction of mini-implants used for orthodontic anchorage. Clin Oral Implants Res 2005;16:473–479.

100. Hoshaw SJ, Brunski JB, Cochran GVB. Mechanical loading of Brånemark implants affects interfacial bone remodeling and remodeling. Int J Oral Maxillofac Implants. 1994;9:345–360.

101. Wehrbein H, Glatzmaier J, Yildirim M. Orthodontic anchorage capacity of short titanium screw implants in the maxilla. An experimental study in the dog. Clin Oral Implants Res 1997;8:131–141.

102. Akin-Nergiz N, Nergiz I, Schulz A, Arpak N, Niedermeier W. Reactions of peri-implant tissues to continuous loading of osseointegrated implants. Am J Orthod Dentofacial Orthop 1998;114:292–298.

103. Wehrbein H, Merz BR, Hammerle CH, Lang NP. Bone-to-implant contact of orthodontic implants in humans subjected to horizontal loading. Clin Oral Implants Res 1998;9:348–353.

104. De Pauw GA, Dermaut L, De Bruyn H, Johansson C. Stability of implants as anchorage for orthopedic traction. Angle Orthod 1999;69:401–407.

105. Wehrbein H, Yildirim M, Diedrich P. Osteodynamics around orthodontically loaded short maxillary implants. An experimental pilot study. J Orofac Orthop 1999;60:409–415.

106. Gotfredsen K, Berglundh T, Lindhe J. Bone reactions adjacent to titanium implants subjected to static load. A study in the dog (I). Clin Oral Implants Res 2001;12:1–8.

107. Gotfredsen K, Berglundh T, Lindhe J. Bone reactions adjacent to titanium implants with different surface characteristics subjected to static load. A study in the dog (II). Clin Oral Implants Res 2001;12:196–201.

108. Gotfredsen K, Berglundh T, Lindhe J. Bone reactions adjacent to titanium implants subjected to static load of different duration. A study in the dog (III). Clin Oral Implants Res 2001;12:552–558.

109. Gedrange T, Bourauel C, Kobel C, Harzer W. Three-dimensional analysis of endosseous palatal implants and bones after vertical, horizontal, and diagonal force application. Eur J Orthod 2003;25:109–115.

110. Fritz U, Diedrich P, Kinzinger G, Al-Said M. The anchorage quality of mini-implants towards translatory and extrusive forces. J Orofac Orthop 2003;64:293–304.

111. Oyonarte R, Pilliar RM, Deporter D, Woodside DG. Peri-implant bone response to orthodontic loading: Part 1. A histomorphometric study of the effects of implant surface design. Am J Orthod Dentofacial Orthop 2005;128:173–181.

112. Oyonarte R, Pilliar RM, Deporter D, Woodside DG. Peri-implant bone response to orthodontic loading: Part 2. Implant surface geometry and its effect on regional bone remodeling. Am J Orthod Dentofacial Orthop 2005;128:182–189.

113. Frost HM. Bone's mechanostat: A 2003 update. Anat Rec A Discov Mol Cell Evol Biol 2003;275:1081–1101.

114. Crismani AG, Bernhart T, Schwarz K, Celar AG, Bantleon HP, Watzek G. Ninety percent success in palatal implants loaded 1 week after placement: A clinical evaluation by resonance frequency analysis. Clin Oral Implants Res 2006;17:445–550.

115. Brånemark R, Ohrnell LO, Skalak R, Carlsson L, Brånemark PI. Biomechanical characterization of osseointegration: An experimental in vivo investigation in the beagle dog. J Orthop Res 1998;16:61–69.

116. Skripitz R, Aspenberg P. Tensile bond between bone and titanium: A reappraisal of osseointegration. Acta Orthop Scand 1998;69:315–319.

117. Magyar G, Toksvig-Larsen S, Moroni A. Hydroxyapatite coating of threaded pins enhances fixation. J Bone Joint Surg Br 1997;79:487–489.

118. Moroni A, Aspenberg P, Toksvig-Larsen S, et al. Enhanced fixation with hydroxyapatite coated pins. Clin Orthop 1998;346:171–159.

119. Moroni A, Toksvig-Larsen S, Maltarello MC, Orienti L, Stea S, Giannini S. A comparison of hydroxyapatite coated, titanium-coated and uncoated tapered external-fixation pins. An in vivo study in sheep. J Bone Joint Surg Am 1998;80:547–554.

120. Van Oosterwyck H, Duyck J, Vander Sloten J, Van der Perre G, De Cooman M, Lievens S. The influence of bone mechanical properties and implant fixation upon bone loading around oral implants. Clin Oral Implants Res 1998;9:407–418.

121. Misch CE. Implant design considerations for the posterior regions of the mouth. Implant Dent 1999;8:376–386.

122. Hansson S. The implant neck: Smooth or provided with retention elements. A biomechanical approach. Clin Oral Implants Res 1999;10:394–405.

123. Tada S, Stegaroiu R, Kitamura E, Miyakawa O, Kusakari H. Influence of implant design and bone quality on stress/strain distribution in bone around implants: A 3-dimensional finite element analysis. Int J Oral Maxillofac Implants 2003;18:357–368.

124. Lee JS. Contact Non-linear Finite Element Model Analysis of Immediately-Loaded Orthodontic Mini Implant [thesis]. Seoul, Korea: Yonsei University, 2005.

125. Johansson CB, Albrektsson T. A removal torque and histomorphometric study of commercially pure niobium and titanium implants in rabbit bone. Clin Oral Implants Res 1991;2:24–29.

126. Nedir R, Bischof M, Szmukler-Moncler S, Bernard JP, Samson J. Predicting osseointegration by means of implant primary stability. Clin Oral Implants Res 2004;15:520–528.

127. Deguchi T, Takano-Yamamoto T, Kanomi R, Hartsfield JK Jr, Roberts WE, Garetto LP. The use of small titanium screws for orthodontic anchorage. J Dent Res 2003;82:377–381.

DESIGN AND FUNCTION OF NEW, SCREW-TYPE ORTHODONTIC MINI-IMPLANTS

3

STABILITY OF ORTHODONTIC MINI-IMPLANTS

Failure of the mini-implant

Failure of the mini-implant can be divided into *early* (short-term) and *later* (long-term) *failure*; these categories can be further subdivided into *hard tissue–implant interface failure*, *soft tissue–implant interface failure*, *implant failure*, and *psychological failure*[1] (Fig 3-1).

Hard tissue–implant interface failure

Failure at the hard tissue–implant interface results in loosening of the implant.[1–5] According to studies of the success rate of orthodontic mini-implants, most failures result from the loosening of the implant shortly after implantation[1,3,4,6,7] (Park YC and Choi YJ, unpublished data, 2005) (Table 3-1). The time to failure was investigated in 66 cases of failure of the ORLUS mini-implant (Ortholution). Half of the failures occurred within the first month (Park YC and Choi YJ, unpublished data, 2005). To increase the success rate, stability[8–11] in the early stages must be enhanced.

Early failure at the hard tissue–implant interface is related to primary stability,[8–11] which is obtained from mechanical support from the surrounding bone tissue. In other words, primary stability is related to the thickness of the cortical bone at the implantation site, the amount of damage caused by surgical trauma, and the closeness of the contact between the bone and the implant.

Later failure at the hard tissue–implant interface is related to the type of interface formed through the healing process following implantation.[4,12] Long-term failure is also associated with the type of stress loaded on the implant. Formation of fibrous tissue at the bone-implant interface is regarded as the most important risk factor in the loosening of screws,[7] and shear stress is more detrimental to the bone-implant interface than compressive or tensile stress.[13] Primary stability, biocompatibility of the implant, and the trauma resulting from implantation all contribute to the type of interface that is formed.[9,11–13] Primary stability, which is the mechanical stability present immediately following implantation, has significant effects on both short-term and long-term stability.[13,14]

Soft tissue–implant interface failure

Plaque accumulation around the implant or persistent mechanical irritation can cause soft tissue interface problems, such as acute or chronic inflammation or infection. Epithelial hyperplasia or epithelial covering may also occur. In severe cases, infection can progress to abscesses. The potential for this kind of problem to develop is significantly increased when the implant is placed on movable tissue.[15]

Some investigators have suggested that chronic inflammation around implants is a risk factor for loosen-

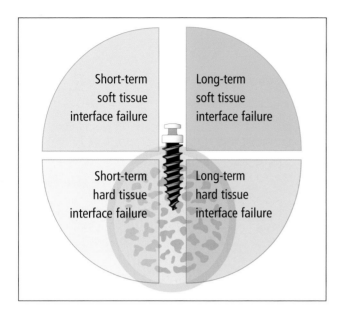

Fig 3-1 Types of failure in orthodontic implant applications.

Table 3-1	Time to failure of 66 failed orthodontic mini-implants*	
< 1 mo	**1–3 mo**	**> 3 mo**
35/66	13/66	18/66
53.0%	19.7%	27.3%

*Unpublished data from Park YC and Choi YJ, 2005.

ing,[2,3] but these reports have been disputed[1] (Park YC and Choi YJ, unpublished data, 2005). Inflammation around an implant could also be a sequela of loosening.

The orthodontic implant should be removed immediately from patients with infection plus any general symptoms such as fever or abscesses, sustained discomfort, and affected adjacent periodontal attachments.

Implant failure from fracture

Implant fracture may occur during surgical placement or removal[2,14,16] but will not occur during orthodontic force application. This will be covered in detail later in this chapter.

Psychological failure

Psychologically, implant placement is not always accepted by patients or the parents of patients. A cost-benefit analysis of implant placement should be thoroughly explained at the consultation.[17] For example, implant placement is one of several treatment options to relieve crowding. However, to achieve nonsurgical correction of a long face, placement of an implant is the only option.

Factors that influence stability

Host factors

General conditions

As described in chapter 2, bone is a dynamic tissue in which the modeling and remodeling processes are continual. Therefore, the general condition of the bone is relevant to stability.[18]

Local hard tissue conditions

The condition of the hard tissue depends on the age and sex of the patient and on the location of the implant placement site; the quantity and quality of the host bone bed at the implantation site also greatly influence primary stability. The quantity and quality of cortical bone are especially important for obtaining mechanical support (Fig 3-2).[19–21] The condition of the trabecular bone may also affect stability; dense trabecular bone is more favorable than low-density trabecular bone.

Extremely hard cortical bone is vulnerable to surgical trauma, because more frictional heat is produced during preparation and because cortical bone has lower healing potential as a result of its limited vascularity. Extremely dense cortical bone may also increase stress during placement, which results in degradation of bone tissue at the implant-bone interface.[5,22,23] Consequently, overall stability may be compromised.

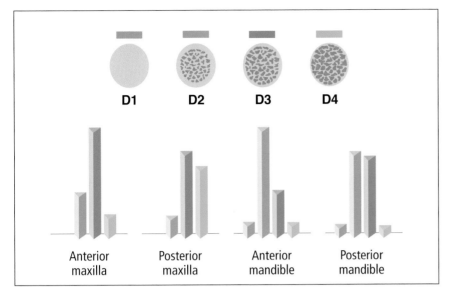

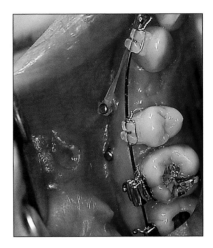

Fig 3-2 Misch[20] described four bone densities found in the edentulous regions of the maxilla and mandible: (D1) Primarily dense cortical bone; (D2) dense to thick porous cortical bone on the crest and coarse trabecular bone underneath; (D3) thinner porous cortical crest and fine trabecular bone within; (D4) almost no crestal cortical bone; the fine trabecular bone comprises almost all of the total bone volume. Bone classified as D4 is unfavorable for use in obtaining primary stability, but almost 40% of the posterior alveolus consists of D4 bone.

Fig 3-3 An implant located between the maxillary second premolar and first molar has loosened. Based on the ulceration and hyperactivity of the cheek, it appears that stress from the cheek muscle may have contributed to the loosening.

Local soft tissue conditions

The condition of the soft tissue is also important for maintenance. An implant placed in the attached gingiva has a more stable soft tissue–implant interface. Implants in the mucosa or movable soft tissue, however, have a less stable soft tissue–implant interface and are likely to cause soft tissue problems, such as infection.[15]

Local stress conditions

Stress from the surrounding regions may compromise the stability of implants (Fig 3-3). For example, excessive forces may occur during mastication in the area between the mandibular first and second molars.

Operator factors

In general, primary stability is also dependent on the dexterity of the operator. Primary stability is related to how much cortical bone support is obtained, but cortical bone may be damaged during any invasive procedure.

As mentioned previously, surgical trauma during implantation procedures also has an effect on stability[6,11] (Fig 3-4). Proper surgical protocols are very important in preventing unnecessary surgical trauma (Fig 3-5). For example, cortical bone is very hard; therefore, excessive vertical force can easily be delivered during the drilling procedure. These excessive forces can damage the cortical bone, leaving the implant in weaker trabecular bone. In other words, the initial mechanical stabilization obtained from the cortical bone may differ depending on the skill of the operator.

The creation of a flap to prevent soft tissue entrapment between bone and implants does not appear to guarantee more stability,[24] but, with a flap operation, the visual field for surgery can be improved through the exposure of the working field of cortical bone.

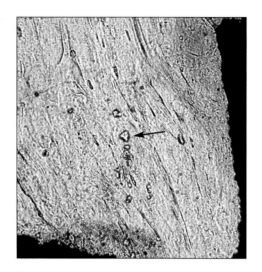

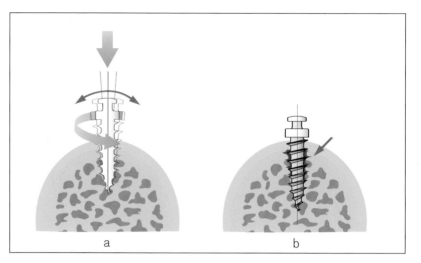

Fig 3-4 Histologic examination after implantation in a rabbit femur. Despite placement of the implant at 30 rpm under saline irrigation, empty lacunae *(arrow)* have resulted from necrosis of the adjacent bone cells. This necrosis was inevitable despite the efforts of the operator. (Hematoxylin-eosin; original magnification × 400.)

Fig 3-5 Eccentric insertion of the implant. *(a)* If excessive vertical force *(wide blue arrow)* is delivered during insertion of an implant in cortical bone, a lateral force *(red arrow)* is produced and the axis vibrates easily *(narrow blue arrow)*. If the axis vibrates during the insertion procedure, the cortical bone needed for support is injured. *(b)* As a result, support is provided only by weaker trabecular bone *(red arrow)*. Consequently, sufficient early stability cannot be obtained.

Implant factors

Biocompatibility

The physical properties of the implant materials, particularly those on the surface in direct contact with tissue, determine the adsorption of biomolecules or foreign materials and cell adhesion patterns.[9,25,26] Hence, these properties mediate the dominant biologic reactions to implants and influence interface formation between the implant and the bone. They also significantly influence the speed of the healing process.[9] Biocompatibility is related to the medium-term and long-term maintenance of the interface.[10]

Materials may be considered bioactive, bioinert, or biotolerant.[27] It has been reported that, when used in implants, bioactive materials such as hydroxyapatite or aluminum oxide can form chemical bonds with bone.

Additionally, an implant should have sufficient strength, meaning that mechanical failure and fatigue failure should be absent. Undesirable ional leakage and corrosion products should also be absent. Stainless steel and chrome-cobalt alloy are generally considered to be stable materials. Nevertheless, it has been reported that these materials are not inert for a long period in vivo.[10] Under such circumstances, corrosion products may be formed, leading to fibrous encapsulation and chronic inflammation.

Design

The implant design influences the distribution of stress to the adjacent bone tissues.[28–30] It has been reported that the cylinder-type or basket-type prosthodontic endosseous implant has a poor long-term prognosis because high levels of shear stress, to which bone is susceptible, are produced in vertical loading.[11]

Length

A nonlinear finite-element model analysis using two-dimensional models, which reflected the condition of the bone-implant interface immediately after implantation, was used to investigate which screw parameters affect early stability.[30] The length of the mini-implant was shown to have little effect on the distribution of stress,[1,30] but the thread design and the diameter had a significant effect on the distribution (Fig 3-6). Thus, the thread design and the diameter are important for initial stability.

To confirm the results of the study using two-dimensional models and to study the physiologic threshold, three-dimensional finite-element model analyses were performed.[1] The results indicated that stress was concentrated on the relatively narrow area, and the effects of screw design parameters on the stress distribution were almost the same as those shown in two-dimensional analyses (Fig 3-7).

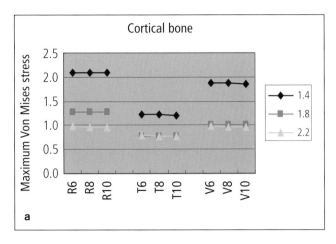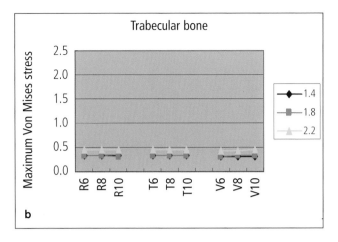

Figs 3-6a and 3-6b Maximum Von Mises stress in **(a)** cortical bone and **(b)** trabecular bone according to implant length (6.0, 8.0, or 10.0 mm), diameter (1.4, 1.8, or 2.2 mm), and thread design (reverse buttress [R], trapezoidal [T], or V-shaped [V]).

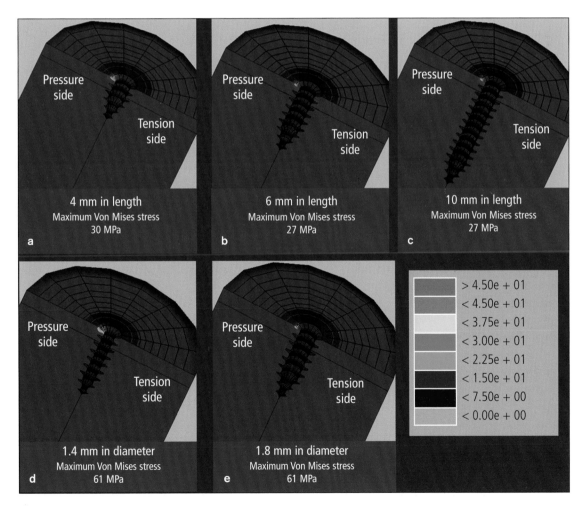

Fig 3-7 *(a to c)* Von Mises stress distribution according to implant length (1.2-mm cortical bone thickness, 1.8-mm implant diameter, trapezoidal thread, and 200-g orthodontic load). Cortical bone can tolerate 45 to 60 MPa of stress. *(d and e)* Von Mises stress distribution according to diameter (1.2-mm cortical bone thickness, 6.0-mm implant length, trapezoidal thread, and 200-g orthodontic load).

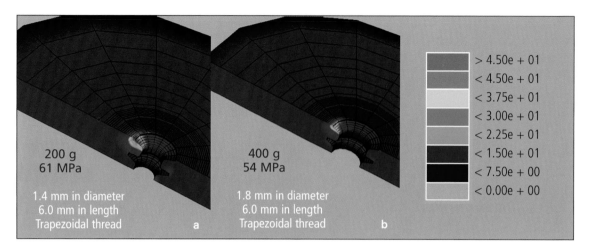

	> 4.50e + 01
	< 4.50e + 01
	< 3.75e + 01
	< 3.00e + 01
	< 2.25e + 01
	< 1.50e + 01
	< 7.50e + 00
	< 0.00e + 00

200 g
61 MPa

1.4 mm in diameter
6.0 mm in length
Trapezoidal thread   a

400 g
54 MPa

1.8 mm in diameter
6.0 mm in length
Trapezoidal thread   b

Fig 3-8 Stress distribution in cortical bone (1.2-mm cortical bone thickness, 6.0-mm implant length, and trapezoidal thread). *(a)* Maximum Von Mises stress with a 1.4-mm implant diameter and 200-g orthodontic load; *(b)* maximum Von Mises stress with a 1.8-mm implant diameter and 400-g orthodontic load. The physiologic threshold is 45 to 60 MPa.

According to finite-element studies, there is little difference between implants that extend 4.0 mm in bone and implants that extend 6.0 mm in bone.[1,30] The length implanted within the bone does not matter greatly because the length of the implant has little effect on the distribution of stress. However, a pilot study of mini-implants extending 4.0 mm in bone showed unsatisfactory success rates (Lee JS, unpublished data, 2005). The implants were placed after predrilling through cortical bone. The criterion for success was the absence of mobility after orthodontic forces had been applied for 3 months. Although the sample size of 30 implants was small, the results showed relatively low success rates. Only 8 of 14 maxillary implants (57%) and 9 of 16 mandibular implants (56%) were considered successful. The poor results may have been due to the insertion procedure. That is, the screw should "bite" bone and be engaged in bone for the final seating, and 4.0 mm does not seem to be sufficient length to ensure a stable insertion procedure.

Therefore, at least 5.0 mm of screw length engaged in bone seems to be needed for the insertion procedure, but increasing the length of implants beyond that is not an effective means of improving primary stability unless it is intended to have bicortical anchorage.[31]

Thread shape

The thread design, or cross-sectional shape of the thread, is related to both the stress distribution under loading and the implantation method[30] (see Fig 3-6). The reverse buttress thread provides the easiest insertion but is least advantageous in terms of stress distribution.[29] A trapezoidal or rectangular shape results in more difficult insertion but provides the most advantageous distribution of stress.

Diameter

The diameter mediates a significant effect on the stress distribution within the bone[30] (Figs 3-6 to 3-8). In cortical bone, the thicker the diameter, the more favorable the stress distribution.[30–33] According to three-dimensional finite-element model analyses, a 1.4-mm-diameter implant that is placed in 1.2-mm-thick cortical bone can tolerate 150 g of orthodontic forces, while a 1.8-mm-diameter implant can tolerate 350 g of orthodontic forces (Lee JS, unpublished data, 2005).

Placement method

In general, two types of trauma may be delivered during implantation.[34–36] Screwing into the bone produces physical pressure, which may cause trauma to the adjacent bone. Particularly in the case of a drill-free screw, the adjacent bone tissue is likely to be injured by the physical pressure and cutting action, which induces microfracture of the bone tissues, tearing of the periosteum or endosteum, and necrosis of bone cells.[5,9,23,34] The other type of trauma results from the heat generated by friction between the bone and implant during insertion.[35–37]

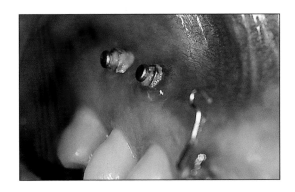

Fig 3-9 Inflammation induced by plaque does not seem to be a direct cause of loosening. As in the patient shown here, inflammation without mobility may not necessarily cause problems.

According to a morphologic study using scanning electron microscopy, a self-tapping screw seemed less traumatic than a self-drilling screw.[34] A functional study, on the contrary, indicated that the self-tapping screw caused more trauma than the self-drilling screw because of frictional heat produced throughout the predrilling procedure.[35,36]

Thus, because the drill has greater cutting efficiency, predrilling may decrease mechanical trauma to structures such as the periosteum and bone.[34] However, engine-driven drilling may cause more frictional heat, therefore causing more injuries to the bone tissue and cells.[35,36] Therefore, to minimize surgical trauma, cortical bone should be predrilled manually with a sharp drill of high cutting efficiency to minimize heat production. Copious irrigation with coolants is also necessary, especially where cortical bone is thick.[38,39]

Maintenance factors

Loading conditions

Overloading past the physiologic threshold may disintegrate the bone-implant interface,[12,13] but there are no exact guidelines as to how much force the mini-implant can withstand[1,40–43] (Lee JS, unpublished data, 2005).

According to a three-dimensional finite-element analysis (Lee JS, unpublished data, 2005), 400 g of orthodontic forces can be tolerated by the implant (see Fig 3-8). The threshold that can be tolerated by cortical bone is about 45 to 60 MPa. With implants that are 1.8 mm in diameter, 400 g of orthodontic loading produces 30 MPa of force. Clinically, 200 to 400 g of force can be withstood by a single mini-implant, but this is also dependent on the condition of the bone.[28]

In particular, bone has poor resistance to impact stress,[10,12,13] which is induced by chewing of hard food and oral habits. Therefore, clear instructions should be relayed to patients during the implantation process.

Oral hygiene

Chronic peri-implantitis may cause bone resorption.[3,4] However, there is no evidence that chronic inflammation is a risk factor for loosening of the implant without the jiggling force seen with occlusal trauma[1] (Park YC and Choi YJ, unpublished data, 2005) (Fig 3-9).

DESIGN OF A NEW SCREW-TYPE MINI-IMPLANT

When surgical bone screws were first used to provide orthodontic anchorage in earlier days, the focus was on how easily they could be used in orthodontic treatment (Fig 3-10). Since then, numerous screw-type micro-implants and mini-implants have been developed to increase clinical efficiency. However, all of these differ in the coronal structure rather than in the structure of the screw that is implanted in the bone, which is the part that directly relates to the stability of the implant. Although stability is the most important factor for orthodontic anchorage, there was little consideration for this fact in the designs of screw parts.

In cases in which the treatment plan is based on the orthodontic implant, particularly when the molars have to be distalized or intruded, dependency on the orthodontic implant is absolute. Therefore, it is of the utmost importance that the implant be reliable and stable (Fig 3-11).

From a biologic aspect, the mini-implant should not induce an unfavorable biologic reaction. From a mechanical aspect, the mini-implant must be a structure that will secure bone support and distribute orthodontic stress well. It must also minimize trauma during implantation. From a clinical aspect, the procedure of implantation should be simple, and the stability of screws should not be technique-dependent or site-dependent (Fig 3-12).

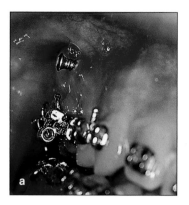 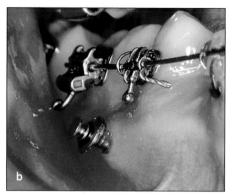

Fig 3-10a Surgical bone screw used for orthodontic anchorage.

Fig 3-10b Surgical screw used for orthodontic treatment after a sandblasting surface treatment of the head area and the attachment of a button.

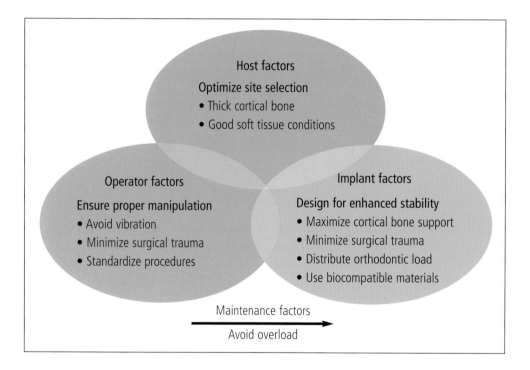

Fig 3-11 Causes of orthodontic mini-implant failure and ways to avoid them.

Host factors

Optimize site selection
- Thick cortical bone
- Good soft tissue conditions

Operator factors

Ensure proper manipulation
- Avoid vibration
- Minimize surgical trauma
- Standardize procedures

Implant factors

Design for enhanced stability
- Maximize cortical bone support
- Minimize surgical trauma
- Distribute orthodontic load
- Use biocompatible materials

Maintenance factors
→
Avoid overload

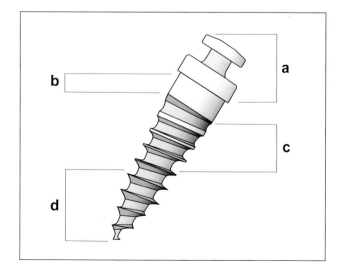

Fig 3-12 The newly developed ORLUS implant consists of four components: (a) the part designed for orthodontic treatment; (b) the part designed to encourage the interface between soft tissue and the implant; (c) the part designed to obtain support from cortical bone for primary stability; and (d) the part designed to facilitate insertion.

For enhanced stability

● No thread for soft tissue sealing

■ Wider diameter to increase cortical bone support

▲ Trapezoidal thread to maximize cortical bone support

○ Tapered core for bone-condensing effect

★ Sandblasted and acid-etched surface for biocompatibility

Fig 3-13 The newly developed screw-type orthodontic mini-implant has structures that can improve stability.

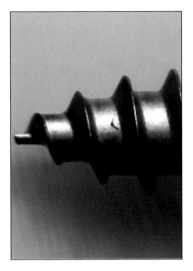

Fig 3-14a Apically, the new orthodontic mini-implant has a reverse buttress thread.

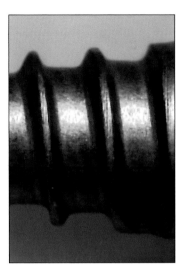

Fig 3-14b Coronally, the new implant has a trapezoidal thread.

Fig 3-15 *(a)* Dual threads and dual diameters decrease the chances of injury to cortical bone from vibration *(narrow blue arrow)* because this new design reduces the vertical *(wide blue arrow)* and lateral *(red arrow)* forces that can be exerted during insertion. *(b)* Therefore, the implant is designed to be less influenced by the dexterity of the operator and to maximize cortical bone support *(red arrow)*.

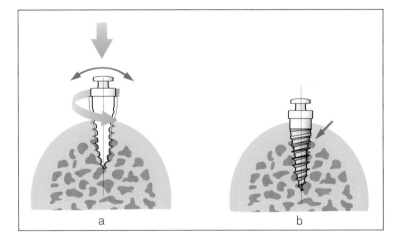

Design features that enhance stability

A newly developed screw-type orthodontic implant has been designed for enhanced stability based on biologic and mechanical principles.

Maximized primary stability

Primary stability (initial mechanical stabilization) not only is the most important factor for short-term stability but also is a prerequisite for healing with a stable osseous interface.[13] Such primary stability is closely related to cortical bone support.[12,13]

The newly developed implant has a structure that maximizes cortical bone support (Figs 3-13 to 3-15). The coronal part of the screw, which makes contact with cortical bone, has a wider diameter in the neck and trapezoidal threads, while the apical part has a narrower diameter and reverse buttress threads. A tapered core and dual threads can have a bone-condensing effect that improves the quality of bone[44] and prevents undesirable cortical bone damage caused by vibration (that is, eccen-

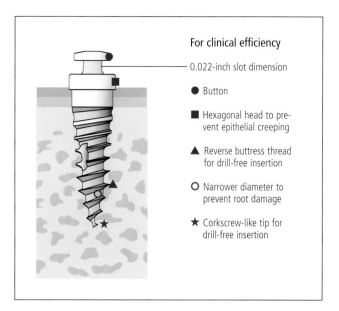

For clinical efficiency

— 0.022-inch slot dimension

● Button

■ Hexagonal head to prevent epithelial creeping

▲ Reverse buttress thread for drill-free insertion

○ Narrower diameter to prevent root damage

★ Corkscrew-like tip for drill-free insertion

Fig 3-16 The newly developed mini-implant has structures that can improve clinical efficiency.

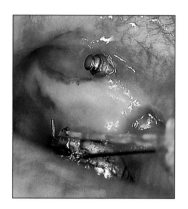

Fig 3-17 The implant can be stable not only in attached areas of the gingiva but also in the oral mucosal area.

tric insertion or shaking of the axis during insertion). They also offset inevitable cortical damage during implant insertion. Therefore, the stability of the implant will not be greatly influenced by the dexterity of the operator or the location of implant insertion.

Increased biocompatibility

The mini-implant is made of titanium alloy instead of pure titanium; pure titanium may be more biocompatible, but it has insufficient strength for use in a mini-implant.[16,27,45–48] To increase biocompatibility, the surface of the implant has been sandblasted and acid etched.[9,26,28]

Minimized surgical trauma

The apical end has a reverse buttress–type thread while the apex has a corkscrew-like tip. These features facilitate insertion and minimize surgical trauma.[35,36] Additionally, in the area in which the diameter begins to widen, there is a lateral groove to prevent the concentration of excess stress on the adjacent tissues.

Stress distribution

For stability, excessive stress should not be concentrated on the adjacent bone tissues.[12,49] The new implant is

structured to distribute stress through efficient orthodontic loading. Because most stress is concentrated at the cortical bone area,[1,30,32,33] the implant has a trapezoidal thread and a wider core in the coronal part that contacts the cortical bone.

Soft tissue sealing

A cylindrical neck has been designed for the implant–soft tissue interface, which facilitates soft tissue attachment and cleaning. The coronal area of the implant has a hexagonal head with a diameter larger than that of the cylindrical neck. These features prevent the soft tissue coverage that arises from epithelial creeping.

Increased mechanical strength

The mini-implant is made of titanium alloy of a higher strength than pure titanium,[45–48] but the diameter of the mini-implant is relatively narrow, so the risk of fracture remains. Because the torsional strength of the screw varies with the cube of the core diameter, only a small increase in diameter greatly increases the strength.[16,50] With the tapered core, the implant has a wider diameter in the neck area, so the risk of fracture is lowered. Nevertheless, even wider mini-implants have a small diameter, so very cautious handling is necessary.

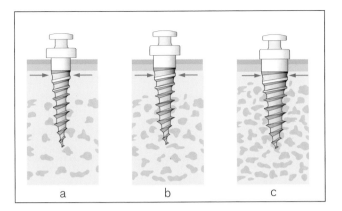

Fig 3-18 There are three mini-implant diameters *(arrows)*, each used for varying hard tissue conditions. *(a)* The mini-type implant diameter is used where space is not abundant, such as the anterior alveolus. *(b)* The regular-type diameter is used in general areas where the bone quality is adequate. *(c)* The wide-type diameter is useful in areas of inadequate bone quality.

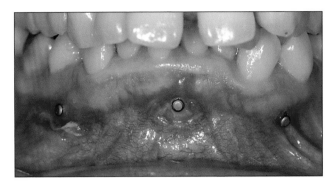

Fig 3-19 A mini-type diameter is useful where the interdental space is narrow, such as the mandibular anterior alveolus.

Design features that enhance clinical efficiency

The orthodontic implant should be fail-safe. The implant is easy to use and has a wide variety of applications (Figs 3-16 and 3-17).

Fail-safe

An orthodontic mini-implant should not cause irreversible tissue damage. The apical end of the implant has a narrower diameter to reduce the possibility of root damage. Additionally, a safe, manual drill system has been designed to eliminate the possibility of causing permanent damage to important anatomic structures such as the root.

Simplified procedures

The procedures for insertion and removal should be simple. Regular or wide mini-implants can be inserted without predrilling or preparation of a flap, because of the corkscrew-like tip and reverse buttress threads at the apical end. A hexagonal female driver tip makes the handling efficient and easy.

Easy and broad applications

The new type of orthodontic mini-implant has a button structure in its coronal portion to facilitate the use of elastic materials. There is also a 0.022-inch structure just apical to the button; this space can be used for placement of the orthodontic wire. Therefore, the implant can be used easily for both direct and indirect applications.

Specifications and system composition

The implants are available in mini, standard, and wide diameters. The new implants are also available in long and regular lengths. An appropriate implant should be selected according to the conditions of the hard tissues and soft tissues at the location of placement.

Diameter

There are three main types of implant diameter, differentiated by their appropriateness for certain hard tissue conditions (Fig 3-18).

Mini type

The mini-type implant is 1.4 mm in diameter at the center and 1.6 mm at the cervical area. It is used in places where abundant space is not available, such as the anterior alveolus (Fig 3-19).

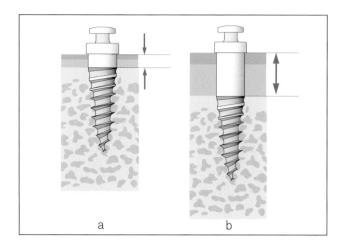

Fig 3-20 The two types of implant length, particularly at the cylindrical neck *(arrows)*, are useful for different soft tissue conditions. *(a)* The regular-type length, with a 1.0-mm length at the cylindrical neck, is normally selected for the buccal area of the maxilla and mandible. *(b)* The long-type implant, with a 2.0-mm cylindrical neck, is sometimes preferred for movable tissues.

Regular type

The regular-type implant is 1.6 mm in diameter at the center and 2.0 mm at the cervical area. This type is used in general areas where the bone quality is adequate.

Wide type

The wide-type implant is 1.8 mm in diameter at the center and 2.2 mm at the cervical area. This type is used in general areas and is useful in areas of inadequate bone quality.

Length

A screw length of 5.0 mm with predrilling and 6.0 mm without predrilling is usually sufficient for the bone contact. The length of the screw used for bone support is 5.0 to 7.0 mm and that used for soft tissue sealing is 1.0 to 4.0 mm at the cylindrical neck area (Fig 3-20).

Regular type

The length of the regular-type screw in the bone is 5.0 to 7.0 mm, and the length of the cylindrical neck is 1.0 mm (see Fig 3-20). For the cylindrical neck section at the soft tissue–implant interface, a length of 1.0 mm is normally selected for the buccal area of the maxilla and mandible.

Long type

The long implant is designed for various soft tissue conditions at the location of placement (see Fig 3-20). In long implants, the length of the screw in the bone is 5.0 to 6.0 mm, depending on the operator's personal preference, while the cylindrical neck is 2.0 to 4.0 mm long at the implant–soft tissue interface.

Implants with 2.0 mm of cylindrical neck are sometimes preferred for movable tissues; this prevents coverage by the epithelium. In the posterior palatal area and the retromolar area, the length of the cylindrical neck should be chosen by direct measurement with a periodontal probe, because the thickness of the soft tissues in the posterior palatal area and the retromolar area varies from about 3.0 to 6.0 mm.

Instruments

Instruments are designed for direct implantation (Fig 3-21) and for indirect implantation (Fig 3-22). To minimize surgical trauma during implantation and to prevent root damage, a manual predrilling system was developed (Fig 3-23). The length of the ORLUS drill (Ortholution) is limited to 4.0 mm; therefore, it can only bore into soft tissue and cortical bone. The drill is unable to reach root surfaces at the mucogingival junction.

Clinical applications

Orthodontic loading

The following should be considered when the timing of orthodontic loading is determined.

Orthodontic loading must not have adverse effects on the healing process. Although the load may be applied in the same manner, the stress delivered to bone tissue may differ, depending on bone conditions and other factors.

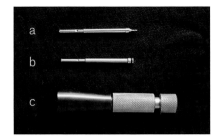

Fig 3-21 Instruments for the direct approach. *(a)* Manual ORLUS drill. *(b)* Driver tip. *(c)* Driver handle.

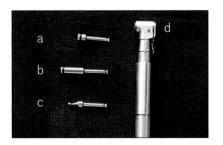

Fig 3-22 Instruments for the indirect approach. This is a dental latch type, which is inserted into a handpiece. *(a)* Standard driver tip. *(b)* Long driver tip. *(c)* ORLUS drill. *(d)* Handpiece.

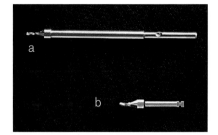

Fig 3-23 ORLUS predrilling system for safe implantation procedures. The ORLUS drill has been designed to perforate cortical bone efficiently and to prevent root injuries. *(a)* Hand-driver type. *(b)* Dental latch type, which is inserted into a handpiece.

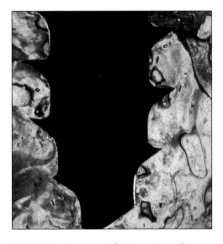

Fig 3-24a Low-magnification view of a section of an implant placed in a dog in the immediate-loading group (hematoxylin-eosin stain).

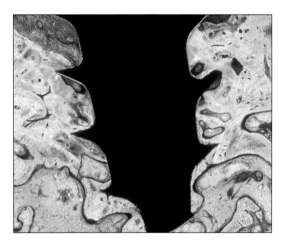

Fig 3-24b Low-magnification view of a section of an implant placed in a dog in the delayed-loading group. There was no significant difference between stability in the immediate-loading group (see Fig 3-24a) and the delayed-loading group (hematoxylin-eosin stain).

Theoretically, orthodontic loading within the physiologic range may stimulate bone formation.[28,40,51,52] However, optimal loading time and optimal amounts of loading are hard to estimate because they are complex functions of bone conditions, surgical trauma, and oral environment. Although many studies have been conducted,[51–57] there is no accurate clinical guideline for the timing of orthodontic loading in adults or growing patients.

When the bone quality is excellent and stress can be distributed appropriately, immediate loading is possible.[13,14,52–55,57] For example, splinted implants in the maxillary midpalatal suture area can be loaded immediately after insertion.[57]

It is generally possible to apply orthodontic forces immediately; however, a 4- to 6-week healing period may be advisable in a growing patient. There is a lag time for tooth movement immediately after orthodontic loading, so this lag time can be used as a healing period for the implant. However, even without orthodontic loading, other stress from the oral environment is immediately applied to mini-implants. If enough primary stability is obtained, immediate loading does not compromise stability.[13,14,53–55] One study found that there was no significant difference in the stability between an immediate-loading group and a delayed-loading group (ie, loading occurred 2 weeks after implant placement) when orthodontic mini-implants were placed in dogs[56] (Fig 3-24).

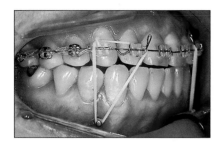

Fig 3-25 Intra-arch fixed appliances and inter-arch elastic applications are very practical.

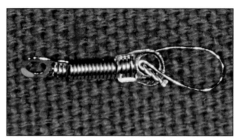

Fig 3-26a The mini-implant head is designed for elastic chains; for the use of a nickel-titanium coil spring, a metal ligature is necessary.

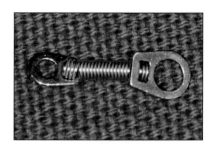

Fig 3-26b A nickel-titanium coil spring specially designed with a bigger hole for mini-implants can be used without a ligature.

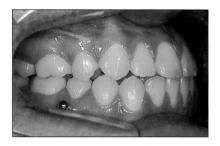

Fig 3-27a Anterior crossbite has been corrected by growth modification, but a slight relapse has occurred as a result of late mandibular growth.

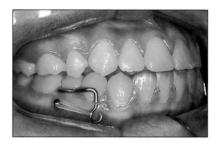

Fig 3-27b For active retention, implants were placed between the mandibular second premolar and first molar, and a clear aligner with a hook was used at night. Elastics were also attached to the implants.

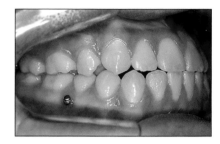

Fig 3-27c At the 1-year follow up, the occlusion is maintained.

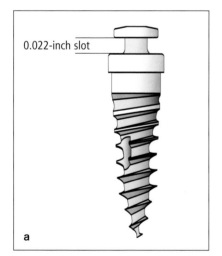

0.022-inch slot

a

Fig 3-28a The 0.022-inch structure just apical to the button can be used for placement of the orthodontic wire.

Figs 3-28b and 3-28c The wire can be attached to the implant and the tooth with flowable resins.

Fig 3-28d The orthodontic mini-implant has provided the individual tooth with three-dimensional anchorage.

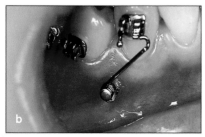

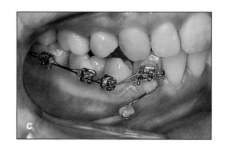

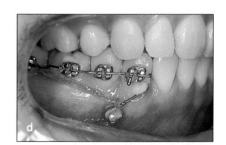

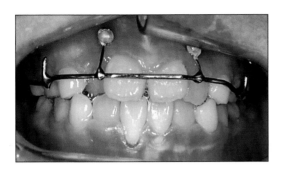

Fig 3-29 Implants can be attached to a labiolingual appliance to achieve maxillary protraction.

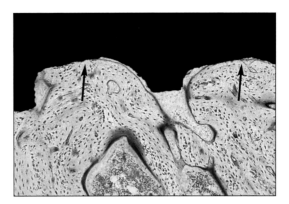

Fig 3-30 Cross-section of a mini-implant placed in the femur of a male rabbit after 8 weeks without loading. No unfavorable tissue responses were observed under histologic examination. Direct contacts with living bone tissue are observed at the interface *(arrows)* (hematoxylin-eosin stain; original magnification × 200).

Orthodontic applications

The mini-implant can be used in direct or indirect applications to apply continuous or intermittent force. Clinically, one implant can tolerate 200 to 400 g of orthodontic force[1] (Lee JS, unpublished data, 2005) (see Fig 3-8). The orthodontic mini-implant is generally used for retractive mechanics but can also be used for pulling mechanics.

Direct application

It is possible to hook an elastic chain or a nickel-titanium coil spring directly to the button in the coronal part of the implant (Figs 3-25 and 3-26). A nickel-titanium coil spring designed for mini-implants or a general nickel-titanium coil spring with metal ligature can be used. The mini-implant can also be used with removable appliances (Fig 3-27). However, the bone-implant interface is vulnerable to impact stress, so orthodontic force should first be applied to teeth or hooks, and the force can later be applied to the implant to avoid unnecessary stress to the implant.

Indirect application

If the coronal head part of an implant is used, splinting with teeth or an implant is possible, and various attachments can be bonded without surface treatment (Figs 3-28 and 3-29). In general, surface treatment of mini-implant heads is not necessary for bonding of attachments. However, a sandblasting surface treatment does increase bond strength[58] and is recommended where bonding stability is critical.

CLINICAL AND LABORATORY TRIALS OF THE NEW MINI-IMPLANTS

Clinical trials

The unique design of a new type of mini-implant was proven to be effective by animal studies (Lee JS, unpublished data, 2004), finite-element analyses (Lee JS, unpublished data, 2005), and 3 years of clinical trials[1] (Park YC and Choi YJ, unpublished data, 2005). In the animal study, ORLUS mini-implants (n = 30) were placed in the femurs of 3- to 6-month-old male rabbits to investigate tissue reactions to loaded mini-implants. After observation periods of 1 week to 6 months, the rabbits were killed. All mini-implants were stable (Fig 3-30).

In a blind clinical study, the screw-type mini-implants were inserted by one operator, and another investigator examined the success rate. The new type of implant showed a 95% success rate[1] (Fig 3-31).

Another study was performed to investigate the success rate obtained in the Department of Orthodontics at Yonsei University (Park YC and Choi YJ, unpublished data, 2005) (Table 3-2). The new type of mini-implants (ORLUS) showed a higher success rate than drill-free bone screws (KLS Martin).

The aforementioned blind study[1] also calculated the success rates based on the location of the implantation

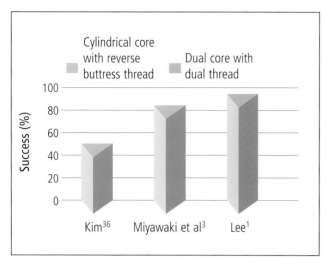

Fig 3-31 Success rates of two different screw-type mini-implants. The dual core–dual thread implant showed a 95% success rate.

Table 3-2	Success rates of drill-free bone screws (KLS Martin) and orthodontic mini-implants (ORLUS)*			
Implant	**Maxilla**	**Mandible**	**Midpalate**	**Total**
KLS Martin	153/205	145/167	94/101	392/473
	74.6%	86.8%	93.1%	82.9%
ORLUS	210/231	149/165	99/103	458/499
	90.9%	90.3%	96.1%	91.8%

*Unpublished data from Park YC and Choi YJ, 2005.

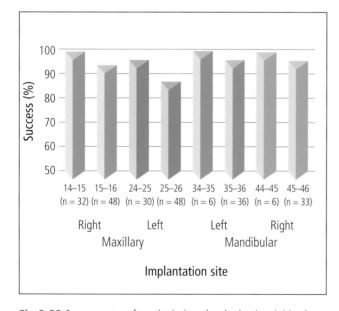

Fig 3-32 Success rates of newly designed orthodontic mini-implants placed buccally in various insertion sites (n = 239).[1] Although there is no statistically significant difference, the right side shows a higher success rate. FDI tooth-numbering system.

site (Fig 3-32). Although there was no statistically significant difference, the right side showed a higher success rate. This seemed to be due to differences in accessibility. The operator was right handed, so the operator had better accessibility on the right side. This indicates that even a skillful operator can be influenced by accessibility. In other words, the importance of using a standardized surgical protocol cannot be overemphasized.

There were no statistically significant differences in success rates based on the patient's anteroposterior or vertical skeletal relationships[1] (Fig 3-33).

Problems and solutions

After 3 years of clinical trials, some problems were reported, and the design was modified to solve these problems[1] (Park YC and Choi YJ, unpublished data, 2005; Lee JS, unpublished data, 2005).

Relatively low success rate in young patients

In the first system developed, the success rate for patients 15 years of age and younger was about 80% (Fig 3-34).[1] This was a statistically significant difference from the success rates found in older groups. The difference in success rates between more mature patients and

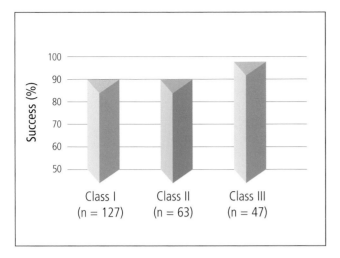

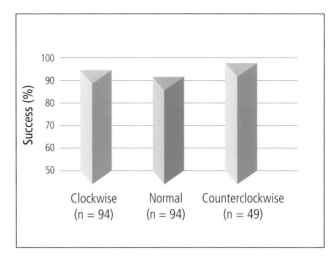

Fig 3-33a Success rates of newly designed orthodontic mini-implants according to the anteroposterior skeletal relationship (n = 237). The differences are not statistically significant.

Fig 3-33b Success rates of newly designed orthodontic mini-implants according to the vertical skeletal relationship (posterior facial height: anterior facial height) (n = 237). There is no statistically significant difference.

those aged 15 years and younger seems to be caused by the poor bone quantity and quality in the growing patients and their high bone turnover rates.[10,59,60] For clinical efficiency, the first system developed was inserted without predrilling.

To increase the success rate, the thread design of the implant was changed to maximize cutting efficiency, and the surface treatment of the implant was improved; the new thread design was also suited for softer bone. A manual predrilling system was introduced to minimize surgical trauma, and treatment protocols for growing patients were optimized (see chapter 5).

Implant fracture

An intrinsic limiting factor regarding implant fracture, the torsional strength of an implant depends on the physical properties of the material and is proportional to the cube of the diameter.[50] The best way to prevent fracture is to increase the diameter and to use stronger materials such as chrome-cobalt alloy[10,46,61]; however, both of these changes are impractical since a larger implant cannot be placed interproximally and stronger material has inferior biocompatibility (Figs 3-35 to 3-39).

The fracture site depends on the cause of fracture. The fracture of implants can be prevented by elimination of the possible causes of fracture. The design of the apical tip was altered to increase the mechanical strength of

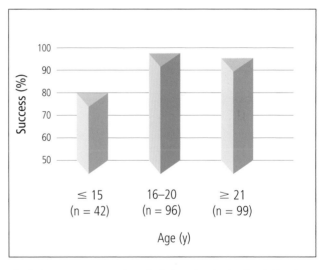

Fig 3-34 Success rates of newly designed orthodontic mini-implants according to the chronologic age of the patient (n = 237). The group of patients younger than 15 years showed a significantly lower success rate ($P < .05$).

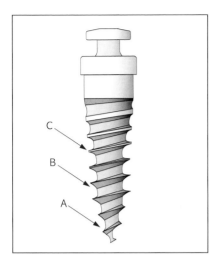

Fig 3-35 Causes according to fracture area. Fractures of area A or B may result from lateral forces produced by improper manipulations. Fracture of area C may result from the intrinsic limiting factor (ie, the torsional strength of the material).

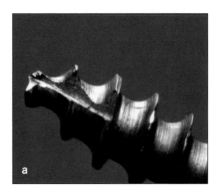

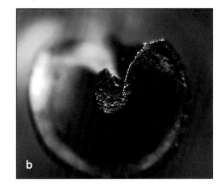

Figs 3-36a and 3-36b Area A shown in Fig 3-35 can be broken if the insertion angle is altered while the tip of the orthodontic implant is located in the cortical bone layer.

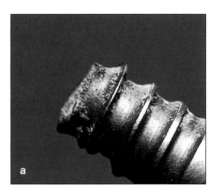

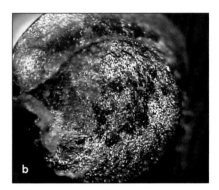

Figs 3-37a and 3-37b Area B in Fig 3-35 can be broken if the insertion angle is changed during implantation at an area where there is hard bone, such as the posterior mandible. It can also be broken by the leverage effect with a contra-angled long driver.

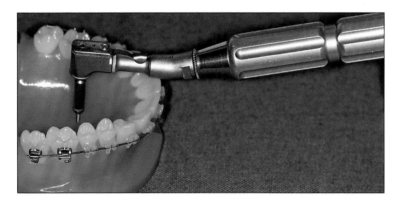

Fig 3-38 Particularly when a long driver is used, class I leverage occurs easily. Even a small lateral force can cause fractures at an area where there is hard bone.

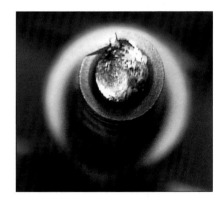

Fig 3-39 Area C in Fig 3-35 can be broken if torque beyond the torsional strength of the implant material itself is applied during insertion. This is the mini-type diameter, which was broken in the posterior mandible, where bone is very hard.

Figs 3-40a and 3-40b If the tip is off the axis *(b, arrow)*, it is easy to insert but also easily fractured.

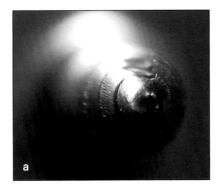

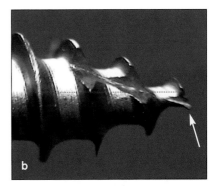

Figs 3-40c and 3-40d Positioning the tip at the center of axis *(d, arrow)* reduces the chances of fracture.

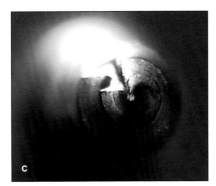

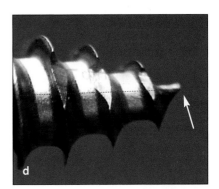

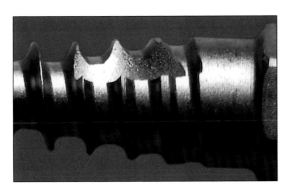

Fig 3-41 During insertion, stress is likely to be generated where the diameter starts to increase, so a lateral cutting groove has been incorporated to prevent concentration of stress.

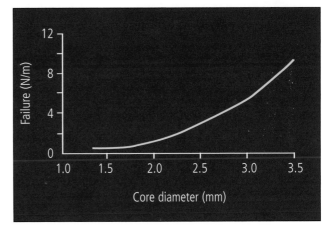

Fig 3-42 Torsional strength of a screw according to the diameter.[50]

the tip (Fig 3-40), and a lateral cutting groove was added to prevent stress concentration (Fig 3-41). Because the torsional strength is proportional to the cube of the core diameter (Fig 3-42), a very small enhancement of core diameter can greatly increase the strength of a screw. The mini-type diameter should not be used where cortical bone is comparatively thick (see Fig 3-39).

To prevent fractures, predrilling through cortical bone is obligatory, particularly in areas where accessibility is poor and cortical bone is very hard, such as the mandibular posterior buccal alveolar area, buccal shelf area, and midpalatal suture area. A short implant is recommended for these areas for prevention of fracture. Modifications of the design, proper manipulation, and use of the predrilling procedure can minimize implant fracture.

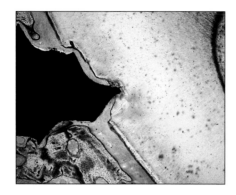

Fig 3-43 Minor injuries to the root surface, such as this one that occurred in a dog study, may be acceptable. The injuries generally heal with secondary cementum (hematoxylin-eosin stain; original magnification × 50). (Courtesy of Dr JH Cho, Seoul, Korea.)

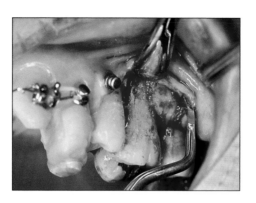

Fig 3-44a If a root has been split, the neighboring periodontal attachment apparatus becomes injured, and this leads to irreversible injuries. A flap operation was performed because of periodontal abscess. The periodontal injuries resulted from the splitting of a root and turned out to be irreversible.

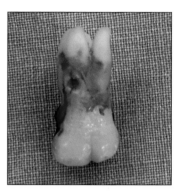

Fig 3-44b The tooth was extracted.

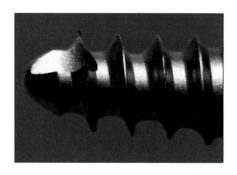

Fig 3-45 A blunt-tipped mini-implant that cannot penetrate the root was designed to prevent injury. However, a pilot study revealed that the success rate was unsatisfactory.

Iatrogenic root injury

Orthodontic implants are placed in interdental areas, and the procedure can bring about root injuries.[62,63] Root injuries are very rare but usually fatal to the tooth (Figs 3-43 and 3-44). Based on the finite-element model analyses and manual predrilling system, the ORLUS tip was developed to eliminate root injuries.[1] A pilot study showed very disappointing results, which may have been the result of the tip design[1] (Fig 3-45). That is, the blunt tip disturbs final seating of implants, and it compromises primary stability. Thirty-two mini-implants with a blunt tip (2.2 mm thick and 6.0 mm long in bone) were placed after predrilling through cortical bone. Nineteen (59%) of these modified implants failed to achieve the criterion for success, which was the absence of mobility after force had been applied for 3 months. That included 10 of 16 maxillary implants (63%) and 9 of 16 mandibular implants (56%).

Rather than modification of the design of the implant, establishment of proper treatment protocols and development of the ORLUS manual drill system can eliminate root injuries (see chapter 5).

SUMMARY

Failure of orthodontic mini-implants can arise from many factors, including host factors, such as bone and soft tissue conditions; operator factors, such as lack of experience or improper manipulation of the implant; implant factors, such as design or biocompatibility problems; and maintenance factors, such as overloading of the implant. A newly developed screw-type orthodontic implant has been designed to enhance the short- and long-term stability of orthodontic anchorage. The new design is intended to enhance biocompatibility, minimize trauma during implantation, secure bone support, and distribute orthodontic stress well. Finite-element analyses and clinical trials have indicated that the new type of implant can provide reliable orthodontic anchorage, if patients and implantation sites are selected carefully and recommended surgical protocols are followed scrupulously.

REFERENCES

1. Lee JS. Development of orthodontic mini implant anchorage system. Presented at Pre-Conference: Basic Researches on Implant Orthodontics, 4th Asian Implant Orthodontics Conference, Seoul, Korea, 3–4 Dec 2005.
2. Park HS, Jeong SH, Kwon OW. Factors affecting the clinical success of screw implants used as orthodontic anchorage. Am J Orthod Dentofacial Orthop 2006;130:18–25.
3. Miyawaki S, Koyama I, Inoue M, Mishima K, Sugahara T, Takano-Yamamoto T. Factors associated with the stability of titanium screws placed in the posterior region for orthodontic anchorage. Am J Orthod Dentofacial Orthop 2003;124: 373–378.
4. Cheng S-J, Tseng Y, Lee SS, Kok SH. A prospective study of the risk factor associated with failure of mini-implants used for orthodontic anchorage. Int J Oral Maxillofac Implants 2004;29: 100–106.
5. Motoyoshi M, Hirabayashi M, Uemura M, Shimizu N. Recommended placement torque when tightening an orthodontic mini-implant. Clin Oral Implants Res 2006;17:109–114.
6. Esposito M, Hirsch JM, Lekholm U, Thomsen P. Biological factors contributing to failures of osseointegrated oral implants. (I). Success criteria and epidemiology. Eur J Oral Sci 1998;106:527–551.
7. Moroni A, Vannini F, Mosca M, Giannini S. State of the art review: Techniques to avoid pin loosening and infection in external fixation. J Orthop Trauma 2002;16:189–195.
8. Franchi M, Fini M, Martini D, et al. Biological fixation of endosseous implants. Micron 2005;36: 665–671.
9. Brunski JB, Puleo DA, Nanci A. Biomaterials and biomechanics of oral and maxillofacial implants: Current status and future developments. Int J Oral Maxillofac Implants 2000;15:15–46.
10. Simon SR (ed). Orthopaedic Basic Science, ed 1. Rosemont, IL: American Academy of Orthopaedic Surgeons, 1994.
11. Albrektsson T, Albrektsson B. Osseointegration of bone implants. A review of an alternative mode of fixation. Acta Orthop Scand 1987;58:567–577.
12. Esposito M, Hirsch JM, Lekholm U, Thomsen P. Biological factors contributing to failures of osseointegrated oral implants. (II). Etiopathogenesis. Eur J Oral Sci 1998;106:721–764.
13. Gapski R, Wang HL, Mascarenhas P, Lang NP. Critical review of immediate implant loading. Clin Oral Implants Res 2003;14: 515–527.
14. Simon H, Caputo AA. Removal torque of immediately loaded transitional endosseous implants in human subjects. Int J Oral Maxillofac Implants 2002;17:839–845.
15. Choi BH, Zhu SJ, Kim YH. A clinical evaluation of titanium miniplates as anchors for orthodontic treatment. Am J Orthod Dentofacial Orthop 2005;128:382–384.
16. Carano A, Lonardo P, Velo S, Incorvati C. Mechanical properties of three different commercially available miniscrews for skeletal anchorage. Prog Orthod 2005;6(1):82.
17. Costa A, Maric M, Danesino P. Comparison between two orthodontic skeletal anchorage devices: Osseointegrated implants and miniscrews—Medical-legal considerations. Prog Orthod 2006; 7(1):24–31.
18. Bryant SR. The effects of age, jaw site, and bone condition on oral implant outcomes. Int J Prosthodont 1998;11:470–490.
19. Gedrange T, Hietschold V, Mai R, Wolf P, Nicklisch M, Harzer W. An evaluation of resonance frequency analysis for the determination of the primary stability of orthodontic palatal implants. A study in human cadavers. Clin Oral Implants Res 2005;16:425–431.
20. Misch CE. Bone character: Second vital implant criterion. Dent Today 1988;7(5):39–40.
21. Chen YJ, Chen YH, Lin LD, Yao CC. Removal torque of miniscrews used for orthodontic anchorage—A preliminary report. Int J Oral Maxillofac Implants 2006;21:283–289.
22. Albrektsson T. The healing of autologous bone grafts after varying degrees of surgical trauma. A microscopic and histochemical study in the rabbit. J Bone Joint Surg Br 1980;62:403–410.
23. Meredith N. Assessment of implant stability as a prognostic determinant. Int J Prosthodont 1998;11:491–501.
24. Campelo LD, Camara JR. Flapless implant surgery: A 10-year clinical retrospective analysis. Int J Oral Maxillofac Implants 2002; 17:271–276.
25. Davies JE. Mechanisms of endosseous integration. Int J Prosthodont 1998;11:391–401.
26. Hayakawa T, Kiba H, Yasuda S, Yamamoto H, Nemoto K. A histologic and histomorphometric evaluation of two types of retrieved human titanium implants. Int J Periodontics Restorative Dent 2002; 22:164–171.
27. Huang LH, Shotwell JL, Wang HL. Dental implants for orthodontic anchorage. Am J Orthod Dentofacial Orthop 2005;127:713–722.
28. Wiskott HW, Belser UC. Lack of integration of smooth titanium surfaces: A working hypothesis based on strains generated in the surrounding bone. Clin Oral Implants Res 1999;10:429–444.
29. Misch CE. Implant design considerations for the posterior regions of the mouth. Implant Dent 1999;8:376–386.
30. Lee JS. Contact Non-linear Finite Element Model Analysis of Immediately Loaded Orthodontic Mini Implant [thesis]. Seoul, Korea: Yonsei University, 2005.
31. Freudenthaler JW, Haas R, Bantleon HP. Bicortical titanium screws for critical orthodontic anchorage in the mandible: A preliminary report on clinical applications. Clin Oral Implants Res 2001;12:358–363.
32. Gallas MM, Abeleira MT, Fernandez JR, Burguera M. Three-dimensional numerical simulation of dental implants as orthodontic anchorage. Eur J Orthod 2005;27(1):12–16.
33. Chen F, Terada K, Hanada K, Saito I. Anchorage effect of osseointegrated vs nonosseointegrated palatal implants. Angle Orthod 2006;76:660–665.
34. Sowden D, Schmitz JP. AO self-drilling and self-tapping screws in rat calvarial bone: An ultrastructural study of the implant interface. J Oral Maxillofac Surg 2002;60:294–299.
35. Heidemann W, Terheyden H, Gerlach KL. Analysis of the osseous/metal interface of drill free screws and self-tapping screws. J Craniomaxillofac Surg 2001;29(2):69–74.
36. Kim JW, Ahn SJ, Chang YI. Histomorphometric and mechanical analyses of the drill-free screw as orthodontic anchorage. Am J Orthod Dentofacial Orthop 2005;128:190–194.

37. Eriksson AR, Albrektsson T. Temperature threshold levels for heat-induced bone tissue injury: A vital-microscopic study in the rabbit. J Prosthet Dent 1983;50:101–107.

38. Albrektsson T. Bone tissue response. In: Brånemark PI, Zarb GA, Albrektsson T (eds). Tissue-Integrated Prostheses: Osseointegration in Clinical Dentistry. Chicago: Quintessence, 1985:135–136.

39. Tehemar SH. Factors affecting heat generation during implant site preparation: A review of biologic observations and future considerations. Int J Oral Maxillofac Implants 1999;14:127–136.

40. Buchter A, Wiechmann D, Koerdt S, Wiesmann HP, Piffko J, Meyer U. Load-related implant reaction of mini-implants used for orthodontic anchorage. Clin Oral Implants Res 2005;16:473–479.

41. Akin-Nergiz N, Nergiz I, Schulz A, Arpak N, Niedermeier W. Reactions of peri-implant tissues to continuous loading of osseointegrated implants. Am J Orthod Dentofacial Orthop 1998;114:292–298.

42. Wehrbein H, Merz BR, Hammerle CH, Lang NP. Bone-to-implant contact of orthodontic implants in humans subjected to horizontal loading. Clin Oral Implants Res 1998;9:348–353.

43. De Pauw GA, Dermaut L, De Bruyn H, Johansson C. Stability of implants as anchorage for orthopedic traction. Angle Orthod 1999;69:401–407.

44. Abels N, Schiel HJ, Hery-Langer G, Neugebauer J, Engel M. Bone condensing in the placement of endosteal palatal implants: A case report. Int J Oral Maxillofac Implants 1999;14:849–852.

45. Disegi JA, Eschbach L. Stainless steel in bone surgery. Injury 2000;31(suppl 4):2–6.

46. Misch CE, Bidez MW, Sharawy M. A bioengineered implant for a predetermined bone cellular response to loading forces. A literature review and case report. J Periodontol 2001;72:1276–1286.

47. Misch CE. Contemporary Implant Dentistry. St Louis: Mosby, 1999.

48. Zardiackas LD, Disegi J, Givan D. Torsional properties of implant grade titanium. J Biomed Mater Res 1991;25:281–293.

49. Collinge CA, Stern S, Cordes S, Lautenschlager EP. Mechanical properties of small fragment screws. Clin Orthop Relat Res 2000;(373):277–284.

50. Perren SM. Force measurements in screw fixation. J Biomech 1976;9:669–675.

51. Romanos GE, Toh CG, Siar CH, Swaminathan D. Histologic and histomorphometric evaluation of peri-implant bone subjected to immediate loading: An experimental study with Macaca fascicularis. Int J Oral Maxillofac Implants 2002;17:44–51.

52. Trisi P, Rebaudi A. Peri-implant bone reaction to immediate, early, and delayed orthodontic loading in humans. Int J Periodontics Restorative Dent 2005;25:317–329.

53. Melsen B, Costa A. Immediate loading of implants used for orthodontic anchorage. Clin Orthod Res 2000;3:23–28.

54. Cho JH. Effects on Orthodontic Miniscrew Implants According to the Timing of Force Application [thesis]. Seoul, Korea: Yonsei University, 2004.

55. Crismani AG, Bernhart T, Schwarz K, Celar AG, Bantleon HP, Watzek G. Ninety percent success in palatal implants loaded 1 week after placement: A clinical evaluation by resonance frequency analysis. Clin Oral Implants Res 2006;17:445–450.

56. Ohashi E, Pecho OE, Moron M, Lagravere MO. Implant vs screw loading protocols in orthodontics. Angle Orthod 2006;76:721–727.

57. Tarnow DP, Eskow RN, Zamzok J. Aesthetics and implant dentistry. Periodontol 2000 1996;11:85–94.

58. Oesterle LJ, Shellhart WC, Henderson S. Enhancing wire-composite bond strength of bonded retainers with wire surface treatment. Am J Orthod Dentofacial Orthop 2001;119:625–631.

59. Szulc P, Delmas PD. Biochemical markers of bone turnover in men. Calcif Tissue Int 2001;69:229–234.

60. Rauch F, Schoenau E. Changes in bone density during childhood and adolescence: An approach based on bone's biological organization. J Bone Miner Res 2001;16:597–604.

61. Marti A. Cobalt-base alloys used in bone surgery. Injury 2000;31(suppl 4):18–21.

62. Roberts WE, Helm FR, Marshall KJ, Gongloff RK. Rigid endosseous implants for orthodontic and orthopedic anchorage. Angle Orthod 1989;59:247–256.

63. Asscherickx K, Vannet BV, Wehrbein H, Sabzevar MM. Root repair after injury from mini-screw. Clin Oral Implants Res 2005;16:575–578.

TREATMENT PLANNING

4

SEQUENCE OF TREATMENT

Problem-oriented diagnosis and treatment planning

Orthodontic mini-implants make it possible to move teeth beyond the classic envelope of discrepancy and to do so in a more accurate manner. Treatment planning is essential to a successful outcome. Spending time with the patient in discussion and direct clinical examination has also become more important than ever. Problem-oriented diagnosis and treatment planning is the standard approach for orthodontic treatment using mini-implants. The problem-oriented diagnostic and treatment planning approach has been well documented by Proffit et al[1] (Box 4-1).

In recent years, treatment with orthodontic mini-implants has been added to the existing options for orthodontic therapy. As Proffit and colleagues[1] indicate, an organized diagnosis and treatment planning process minimizes the chance that a clinician's preferred treatment approach will distort the diagnosis. The first standard of decision making becomes the question of what would be best for a given patient.

The process of planning for orthodontic treatment with implants is similar to the process of planning for surgical orthodontics. Orthodontic treatment with implants can change the relationship between basal bones; in contrast, surgical orthodontics can change the shape of basal bones as well as the relationship between basal bones.

The treatment plan should be determined after the problems, priorities, treatment objectives, and cost-benefit analyses have been considered; this analysis should include the number of implants needed and the insertion sites. The assessment should also include examination for conditions that are detrimental to bone quality and quantity, because these conditions are risk factors in implant orthodontics (Box 4-2).

Informed consent

If orthodontic mini-implants are deemed necessary for treatment, the available implant placement site should be examined to determine if implant insertion is possible. An adequate amount of information should be provided to the patient concerning treatment.[1] The available options, including the use of mini-implants, should be presented. A cost-benefit analysis of implant use, pain and discomfort from implants, possible side effects, and unwanted sequelae should also be presented as objectively as possible (Box 4-3).

It is crucial that the patient make his or her own choice, and informed consent is required for the purpose of risk management in the event that unwanted results, such as loosening, occur. Orthodontic mini-implants do not have a success rate of 100%. The success rate of these procedures is greater than 95%, indicating nearly a 5% failure rate.[3]

| Box 4-1 | Problem-oriented diagnosis and treatment planning[1] |

Collect an adequate database of information about the patient

Create a problem list to establish a diagnosis
- Diagnose the pathologic conditions
- Define the orthodontic problem, treatment priority, and possible solutions

Establish a treatment plan with several treatment options
- Determine insertion site and number of implants after consideration of accessibility, stability, and applicability, if needed

Confirm the treatment plan
- Consult with the patient and parent
- Obtain informed consent

Outline the treatment plan concept

Clarify treatment plan details using a "visual treatment objective"

| Box 4-2 | High-risk groups for placement of orthodontic mini-implants |

General conditions[2]
- Patients with artificial organs or artificial valves, considering the high risk for infections
- Patients with metabolic bone diseases or endocrine problems (ie, diabetes)
- Patients with uncontrolled cardiovascular problems, considering the stress involved in surgery
- Patients with psychological problems

Local conditions
- Sites with significant anatomic structures that interfere with implant placement
- Sites without space for implant insertion (eg, because of root proximity)
- Sites with an excessively developed torus
- Sites with mechanical irritation, such as areas near the vestibular fornix
- Sites with strong occlusal forces
- Sites without an opposing tooth

| Box 4-3 | Unwanted sequelae of orthodontic implantation |

- In patients 15 years and older, approximately 5% to 10% of implants may loosen[3]; this loosening necessitates reimplantation.
- In patients younger than 15 years, approximately 10% to 20% of implants may loosen.[3]
- Abnormal bone conditions adversely affect the stability of implants.
- It is possible for implants to fracture during insertion in sites where bone is extraordinarily hard or accessibility is poor, although this rarely occurs.
- In case of fracture, additional surgical procedures may be needed, or the broken tip may be left in the mouth; this decision is determined by specific conditions. The surgical procedure of tip removal should be performed by an oral surgeon or periodontist.
- Although the occurrence is very rare, roots of the adjacent teeth can be injured during surgical placement of orthodontic implants.
- Although it has never been reported, nerve injury is theoretically possible.
- Inflammation, infection, and gingival overgrowth can result if oral hygiene around the implant is not maintained. In the case of gingival overgrowth, an implant seems to be "driven into the gingiva," and a simple operation to expose the head of the implant may be needed.
- Oral ulceration can result from the stress of surgery or mechanical irritation.

| Box 4-4 | Preoperative information for patients |

- It takes about 10 minutes to place one implant; this does not include administration of anesthetic.
- During surgical placement, a feeling of stiffness may occur in spite of local anesthesia.
- The teeth may be sore even though they are not touched during the procedure.
- Soft tissue surgery, such as frenectomy, may be indicated in certain patients.
- The position of implant placement can be modified during the process of surgery, depending on the soft tissue and hard tissue conditions.

Specific treatment plan

The goal of treatment planning is to develop a plan that will maximize the benefit to the patient.[1] Through patient-parent consultation, the treatment plan concept is established. The detailed treatment plan is then finalized to include where implants are placed, which implants are used, how many implants are used, and how implants are incorporated in mechanotherapy. Additionally, because patient responses are not uniform, patients should be informed that the treatment plan may have to be reevaluated and modified depending on the individual response to treatment (Box 4-4).

Table 4-1	Selection of implantation sites in the maxilla and mandible							
Site	Fail-safe	Accessibility	Hard tissue	Soft tissue	Usability	Discomfort	Irritation	Total grade
Maxilla								
Buccal alveolus	A	A	B	A	A	A	Cheek	A
Edentulous area	A	A	B	A	A	A		A
Posterior palatal alveolus	A	B	B	A	A	A	Tongue	A
Midpalatal suture	A	B	A	A	C	C	Tongue	B
Anterior alveolus	B	A	A	B	A	B	Lip	B
Anterior rugae	A	B	A	A	A	B	Tongue	B
Infrazygomatic crest	B	A	A	C	A	C	Cheek	C
Maxillary tuberosity	B	C	B	A	A	A		C
Mandible								
Buccal alveolus	A	A	A	A	A	A	Cheek	A
Edentulous area	A	A	A	A	A	A		A
Retromolar area	C	C	A	B	A	B	Muscle	B
Buccal shelf	A	B	A	C	A	C	Cheek	B
Anterior alveolus	B	A	A	B	A	B	Lip	B
Lingual alveolus	A	C	A	A	A	C	Tongue	C

(A) Favorable; (B) acceptable; (C) unfavorable.

SELECTION OF THE INSERTION SITE

When choosing a site for the placement of an orthodontic mini-implant, the clinician should consider the following factors (Table 4-1 and Figs 4-1 and 4-2):

1. Fail-safe: Areas in which the potential for irreversible injury to important anatomic structures is high should be avoided whenever possible.
2. Accessibility: Good accessibility will allow proper surgical procedures and therefore will lead to adequate stability.
3. Hard tissue conditions (quality and quantity of cortical bone): The cortical bone must be thick enough to provide sufficient primary stability (mechanical stabilization immediately after implantation).[4,5] Sufficient primary stability is required for early stability and favorable healing. Bone structure in individuals younger than 15 years of age may be relatively softer[6–9] and thus offer less favorable primary stability.[3]

4. Soft tissue conditions: Attached gingiva is advantageous for proper soft tissue sealing. If there is excessive movement of soft tissues, continuous irritation may be directed toward the mini-implant, leading to difficulty in maintenance as well as persistent peri-implantitis.
5. Usability: An implant should be placed in a biomechanically favorable position to allow application of the necessary orthodontic force. The implant should also be in a position that allows the orthodontic force system to be adjusted easily according to the progression of treatment.
6. Discomfort: Implants should be placed in areas that result in minimal discomfort for the patient.

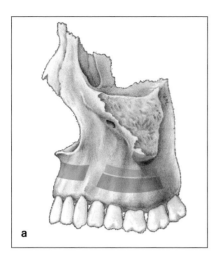

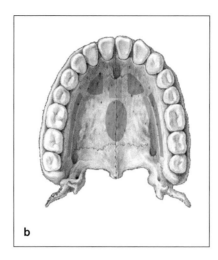

Figs 4-1a and 4-1b Selection of an implantation site in the maxilla. The safe zones are indicated in blue, while the danger zones are indicated in red. (Courtesy of Prof HJ Kim, Seoul, Korea.)

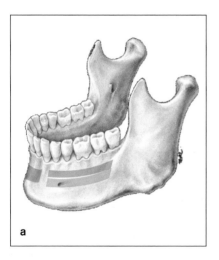

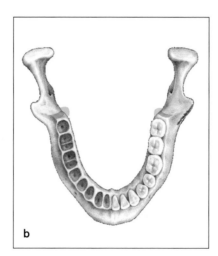

Figs 4-2a and 4-2b Selection of an implantation site in the mandible. The safe zones are indicated in blue, while the danger zones are indicated in red. (Courtesy of Prof HJ Kim, Seoul, Korea.)

7. Irritation caused by the surrounding tissue: Areas that are irritated by the perioral muscles, such as the canine area, or areas that are irritated by food during mastication, such as the area between the mandibular first and second molars, should be avoided when possible.

8. Necessity: The necessity for an implant should be greater than the risks involved and the patient discomfort that it will cause. In cases in which implants are necessary for treatment, such as for occlusal plane control or molar distalization, proper numbers of implants should be placed.

Nongrowing patients

Although the cortical bone of the maxilla is considered a thin bone in the body, it is thick enough to provide sufficient primary stability in orthodontic anchorage; thus, the buccal alveolus can be considered the best site for insertion because of its favorable accessibility. For cases in which greater biomechanical efficacy is required, such as molar intrusion, implantation on the palatal side (the posterior palatal alveolus or the midpalatal suture area) should be considered.

The cortical bone of the mandible is thicker than that of the maxilla[10–13] and is thus advantageous for obtaining primary stability. However, possible irritation by food during mastication serves as a disadvantage. Furthermore, the mandibular lingual area is not feasible for the placement of an implant because the tongue is located in this area and this could lead to patient discomfort. The tongue may also compromise the overall accessibility.

In most patients, the maxillary buccal alveolus, the posterior palatal alveolus, and the mandibular buccal alveolus provide a reasonable number of insertion sites for orthodontic mini-implant anchorage.

Fig 4-3 Research regarding injuries to successor tooth buds or dental follicles is lacking; therefore, a conservative approach is advisable. Areas in which a successor tooth bud exists should be avoided whenever possible.

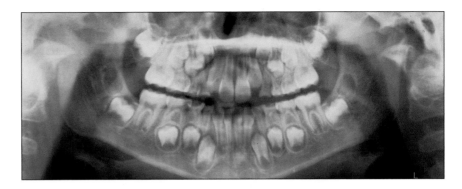

Fig 4-4 When the buccal cortical bone of **(a)** adults is compared with that of **(b)** patients younger than 15 years old, younger bone shows comparatively poor bone quality and quantity. Therefore, it is hard to obtain primary stability in younger patients.

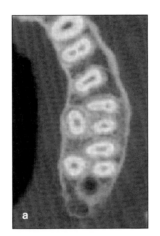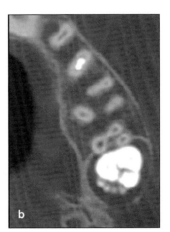

Fig 4-5 When the cortical bone in the midpalatal suture and infrazygomatic area of **(a)** adults is compared with that of **(b)** patients younger than 15 years old, younger bone again shows comparatively poor bone quality and quantity.

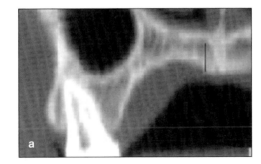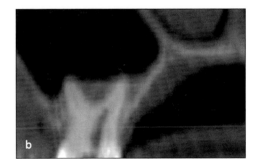

Growing patients

Selection of an implant site in growing patients requires special consideration. Permanent tooth buds are present in the alveolar bone of a growing patient (Fig 4-3). In addition, the bone quality and quantity are relatively poor in young teenage patients, compromising primary stability (Figs 4-4 and 4-5). Moreover, sutural growth is still occurring in the midpalatal suture of young patients. Therefore, the clinician should consider the following recommendations:

1. To prevent injury to successor tooth buds, areas in which permanent teeth have not yet erupted should be avoided whenever possible.
2. The success rates in individuals younger than 15 years of age is relatively low; in particular, stability in the maxillary buccal area may be relatively poor.
3. Predrilling through cortical bone is recommended to minimize surgical trauma.
4. The area between the first and second premolars provides more favorable accessibility as well as slightly superior bone quality.[13] Thus, this area should be

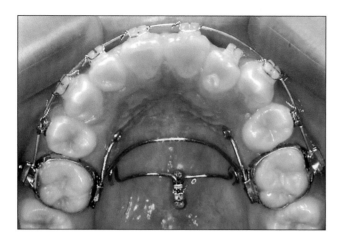

Fig 4-6 Implantation in the parasagittal area of the mid-palate is recommended in growing patients to prevent injury at growing sites. (Courtesy of Dr TK Kim, Bun-dang, Korea.)

chosen in preference to the area between the second premolar and first molar.

5. Implants should be inserted deeper to minimize stress from the oral environment during the healing and treatment periods.
6. The use of light continuous force is preferable to the use of heavy intermittent force. In other words, nickel-titanium coil springs should be used instead of elastomeric chains. The applied force should not exceed 150 g.
7. In the case of repeated failure, use of the midpalatal suture area should be considered because it has better bone quality and quantity than do other areas. If growth occurs in the suture, then the parasagittal area may be considered (Fig 4-6).

SELECTION OF THE ORTHODONTIC MINI-IMPLANT

The diameter should be determined according to the condition of the hard tissue (see Fig 3-18). Briefly, the mini-type diameter is used where space is limited, the regular-type diameter is used where the bone quality is adequate, and the wide-type diameter is useful in areas of poor bone quality.

The length should be determined according to the condition of the soft tissue (see Fig 3-20). The regular-type length is normally selected for the buccal area of the maxilla and mandible, while the long-type implant is normally selected for areas with thick soft tissue and sometimes preferred for movable tissues.

DETERMINATION OF INSERTION DEPTH

As the amount of implant exposure increases, the discomfort of the patient and stress from the oral environment also increase. This can have adverse effects on the healing process and maintenance of the implant. However, if the exposure is inadequate, particularly in the oral mucosa or areas in which the soft tissue moves a great deal, soft tissue covering, persistent inflammation, or the development of abscesses may occur. Therefore, exposure of the mini-implants should be adequate.

An adequate exposure level of the mini-implant is determined by the condition of the soft and hard tissues and the surrounding environment within the oral cavity (Figs 4-7 and 4-8).

When poor bone quality or insufficient primary stability is an issue, it is better to place the implant deeper, even though soft tissue problems are likely to occur. Deeper placement of the implant decreases the stress to the implant from the oral environment and, hence, produces more favorable conditions for the healing process. Furthermore, when placed deeper, the tapered core of an implant increases the bone-condensing effect, which then improves the quality of bone so as to enhance primary stability.

In the palatal interdental area, it is best that the implant be inserted at a sufficient depth, because the palatal gingiva is keratinized[14] thickly and is specialized mucosa; therefore, soft tissue problems do not occur frequently. When tissue problems do occur, they rarely progress to infection. Deep placement increases stability while maintaining a minimal area of exposure, which consequently reduces irritation from the tongue.

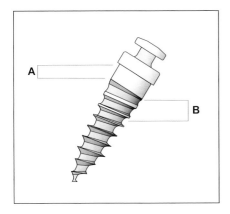

Fig 4-7 The area without threads (A) is designed for contact with the soft tissue, while the area with trapezoidal threads (B) is designed for contact with cortical bone to obtain primary stability. In every case, area B should remain in contact with cortical bone for stability. In areas with thick soft tissue, area A of an implant should be of appropriate length to accommodate the thickness of the soft tissue.

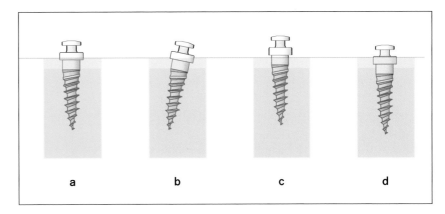

Fig 4-8 The insertion depth of the implant is determined by the condition of the soft tissues, the condition of the hard tissues, and stress from the surrounding tissues. To prevent soft tissue coverage, (c) areas in which the soft tissue is very mobile need greater exposure than do (a and b) areas with general conditions. (d) In thick keratinized tissue, such as the palatal interdental area, minimum exposure is acceptable. Implants that will be used for indirect anchorage or bonding of the attachment must have sufficient head exposure to allow adequate moisture control during the placement of resin materials.

When an implant is placed in the mucosa, adequate exposure is needed to ensure that the implant does not become covered. However, it should be kept in mind that the greater the exposure, the more negative the effect on the healing process, which, in turn, could adversely affect the stability of the implant. Covering the implant head with an elastic, light-curing provisional filling material such as Fermit (Ivoclar Vivadent) can prevent soft tissue coverage to some extent.[15]

PRECAUTIONS IN THE MAXILLA

Buccal alveolus

For implantation in the maxillary buccal alveolus, precautions must be taken to prevent injury not only to the teeth[12,16] but also to the maxillary sinus[17] (Figs 4-9 to 4-14). Even in the case of sinus invasion, as long as the maxillary sinus is not severely inflamed, there are no unfavorable sequelae if the implant is removed.

The greatest advantage of this area is the superior accessibility for placement and utilization of the implant. Although cortical bone is relatively thin compared to other insertion sites (Fig 4-15), it is able to provide enough primary stability for orthodontic anchorage in adult patients, and the cortical thickness of the maxilla does not seem to affect the success rate. Although the success rate is relatively low in younger patients, it is clinically acceptable under the proper surgical protocol. The soft tissue conditions are also appropriate for treatment (Fig 4-16).

Two major problems are associated with the use of buccal alveolar implants. The first is the risk of root injury. Irreversible root injury is very rare,[3,18] but these injuries are critical. However, proper treatment protocols, such as predrilling through cortical bone with a manual drill, accurate positioning, and oblique insertion, can reduce or eliminate the risk of root injury.

The second problem is that implants placed in an interdental area may impede mesiodistal movement of the adjacent teeth. Even with proper treatment protocols, including off-center and oblique insertion at the area between the second premolar and the first molar, 3 mm of mesiodistal tooth movement is not feasible. If more than 3 mm of movement is needed, placement of another implant may be useful after the teeth have moved 3 mm mesiodistally.

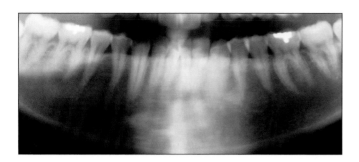

Fig 4-9 Because the shape of the root is conical, more space is available toward the apex than coronally.

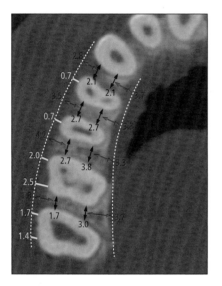

Fig 4-10a Distances (mm) between the maxillary teeth 4 mm apical to the cemento-enamel junction.

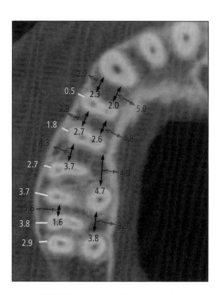

Fig 4-10b Distances (mm) between the maxillary teeth 8 mm apical to the cemento-enamel junction. (Figs 4-10a and 4-10b courtesy of Prof KJ Lee, Seoul, Korea.)

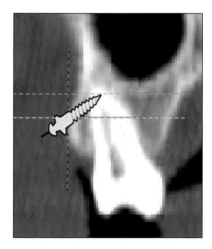

Fig 4-11 When the implant is inserted obliquely, the apex of the implant is more apical and buccal. As a result, more space can be used with oblique insertion than with perpendicular insertion.

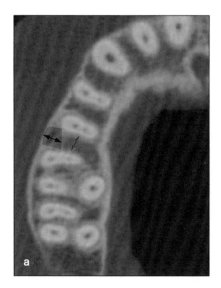

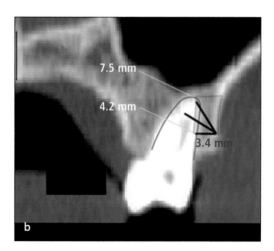

Figs 4-12a and 4-12b (a) Because the buccal space *(blue arrow)* is wider than the interdental space *(red arrow)*, especially in molar areas, the space of the buccal alveolus is used for orthodontic mini-implants instead of the interdental space. (b) Oblique insertion causes the implant apex to be more apical and buccal to secure more space.

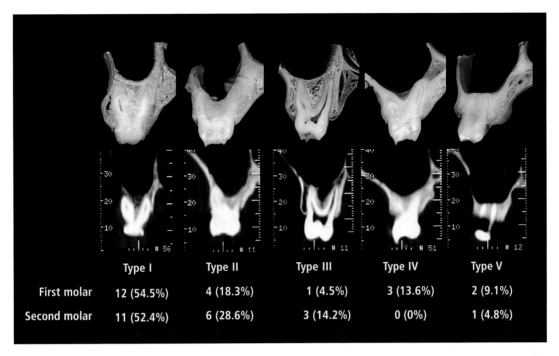

	Type I	Type II	Type III	Type IV	Type V
First molar	12 (54.5%)	4 (18.3%)	1 (4.5%)	3 (13.6%)	2 (9.1%)
Second molar	11 (52.4%)	6 (28.6%)	3 (14.2%)	0 (0%)	1 (4.8%)

Fig 4-13 Classification of vertical relationships between the inferior wall of the maxillary sinus and the roots of the maxillary molars.[17] The numbers represent the number of specimens observed. In any type, there is little risk of injuring the maxillary sinus if the apex of an implant is located below the level of the root apex. (Courtesy of Prof HJ Kim, Seoul, Korea.)

Fig 4-14 Panoramic radiograph of a 22-year-old woman in whom implants were to be placed between the maxillary second premolar and first molar. Advanced pneumatization is revealed over that area *(arrows)*, so the implant placement site was changed to the mesial side of the second premolar. Pneumatization of the maxillary sinus may occur irrespective of the patient's age or the presence of teeth, so the shape of the sinus should be assessed with panoramic radiography.

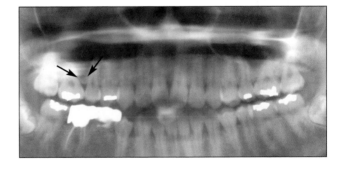

In fact, both the distance between the roots and the buccolingual space are correlated with the risk of root injury and the amount of possible tooth movement. The buccolingual space is particularly important in securing available space. That is, there is less available space where the buccolingual dimension is narrow, such as at the anterior alveolar area, premolar area, and areas where expansion has been accomplished previously with expansion appliances. The clinician should use caution when placing implants in these areas and remember that the mesiodistal movement of the adjacent tooth is more likely to be limited.

Implant size

Generally, the regular- or wide-diameter implant is chosen. When an acceptable level of primary stability is difficult to obtain, the wide-diameter implant should be used. The regular-type length can be used for the mucosa. However, if an area demonstrates substantial soft tissue movement, the implant head should be exposed more; thus, the long-type implant might be more appropriate for an open method. When the exposure level of the implant head is increased, the amount of stress placed on the implant head also increases; therefore, use of the wide type may be advisable in these situations.

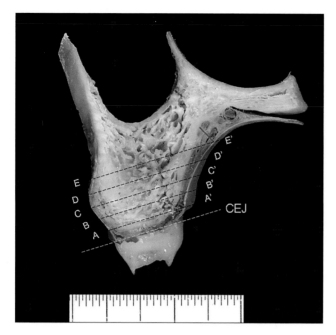

Fig 4-15a The thicknesses of the cortical bone and soft tissue were measured on lines drawn parallel to the buccolingual cementoenamel junction (CEJ) line.[13]

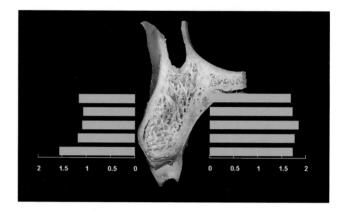

Fig 4-15b Thickness (mm) of the cortical bone between the premolars.[13]

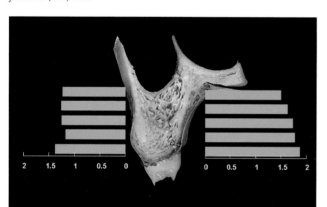

Fig 4-15c Thickness (mm) of the cortical bone between the second premolar and first molar.[13]

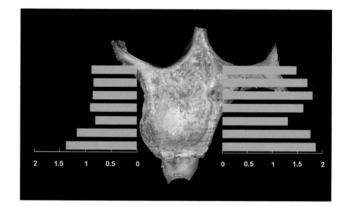

Fig 4-15d Thickness (mm) of the cortical bone between the molars. The cortical bone of the premolar region (see Fig 4-15b) is thicker than that of the molar region.[13]

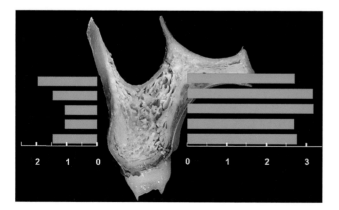

Fig 4-16a Thickness (mm) of the gingiva between the second premolar and the first molar.[13]

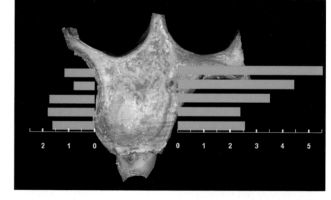

Fig 4-16b Thickness (mm) of the gingiva between the molars. Palatal gingiva, especially near the root apex, was comparatively thick at both sites.[13]

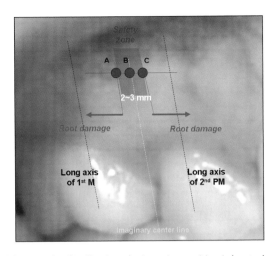

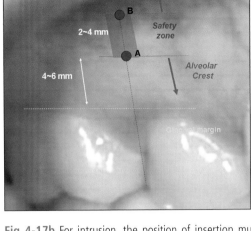

Fig 4-17a (A) For molar distalization, the insertion position is located 1 to 2 mm distal to the imaginary central line between the two teeth. (C) For molar protraction, the insertion position is placed 1 to 2 mm mesial to the imaginary central line. (B) If there is to be no mesiodistal movement of the adjacent teeth, the insertion position is located on the central line. (A, B, C represent insertion sites.) (M) Molar; (PM) premolar.

Fig 4-17b For intrusion, the position of insertion must be located sufficiently apical; otherwise the implants will restrict further movement as the teeth are intruded. (A, B represent insertion sites.) (Mx) Maxillary.

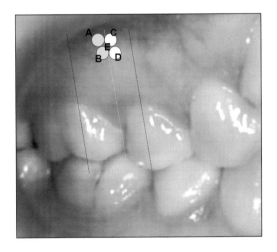

Fig 4-17c The insertion position is determined according to the anteroposterior and vertical tooth movement required. (A, B, C, D, E represent insertion sites.)

Insertion site and angle

When an orthodontic implant is inserted in the maxillary buccal area, slight adjustments in anteroposterior positioning may be needed, depending on the plan for anteroposterior movement of adjacent teeth (Fig 4-17). Generally, a mini-implant should be inserted near the mucogingival junction (Fig 4-18).

The vertical positioning of the implant should generally be slightly closer to the root apex than to the mucogingival junction (see Fig 4-17b). The closer the implant is positioned to the root apex, the greater the intrusive forces that can be obtained and the greater the space

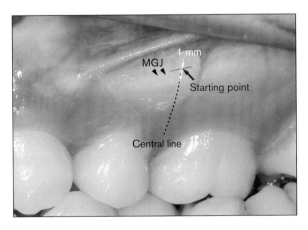

Fig 4-18 Generally, a mini-implant should be inserted near the mucogingival junction (MGJ). For this reason, at the start, the tip of the implant should be placed about 1 mm apically from the mucogingival junction, depending on the diameter of the implant.

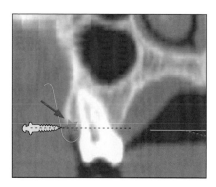

Fig 4-19a The alveolar crest *(arrow)* is located apical to the gingival margins.

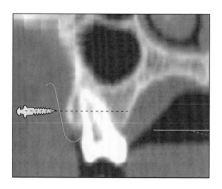

Fig 4-19b The vertical position of the implant should be located sufficiently apical to the alveolar crest to avoid injury of the crest.

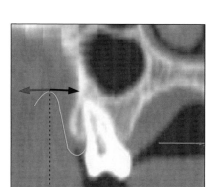

Fig 4-20 An implant head or an extension wire should not be located lateral to the mucobuccal fold *(red arrow)* because of excessive stress from facial muscles, such as the cheeks. The implant should be positioned medial to the mucobuccal fold *(blue arrow)*.

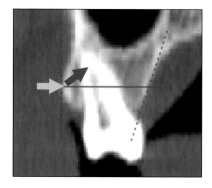

Fig 4-21 An oblique insertion *(blue arrow)* is recommended in cases in which an adjacent tooth moves mesiodistally, because it provides more space. However, it is preferable that the implant be inserted perpendicularly *(yellow arrow)* when cortical bone will be perforated. Therefore, the working angle for insertion changes during the procedure.

that can be utilized for mesiodistal movement. Alveolar structure underneath the gingiva must be considered during positioning (Fig 4-19). When the attached gingiva is narrow or the sulcus is shallow, insertion toward the root apex is restricted. The implant head should never be exposed more laterally than the vestibular fornix (Fig 4-20).

Insertion at an oblique angle allows for the use of more space, reduces the possibility of root injury, and increases the surface in contact with the cortical bone (Fig 4-21). If obliquely inserted, implants may not be supported by the surrounding cortical bone in certain areas because of the inclination of the buccal surface (Figs 4-22 to 4-26). The implant should be supported by enough volume of surrounding cortical bone.

Precautions

1. As with other sites, proper surgical protocol should be followed, especially to obtain reliable stability and to prevent iatrogenic root injury.
2. Proper positioning according to a treatment plan is important. Improper positioning may lead to irreversible injury; for example, insertion in the alveolar crest may cause permanent loss of periodontal attachments (see Fig 4-19a).
3. A horizontal incision should be made where the frenum passes the insertion site. When the implant is to be inserted in the area of the frenum, a frenectomy should be performed to prevent possible mechanical irritation around the implant during function (see Fig 5-20).
4. Because of perioral muscle tonicity, an indirect approach using contra-angled instruments may be preferred in the area between the first and second molars.

Figs 4-22a and 4-22b A sufficient quantity of cortical bone should sustain the implants even with oblique implantation. It does not matter if an implant is inserted more obliquely, as shown in Fig 4-22b. (*Arrows* indicate insertion site, and *dotted lines* indicate direction.)

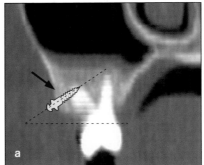
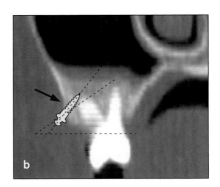

Figs 4-22c and 4-22d The quantity of bone that holds an implant may not be adequate because of the surface topography, as shown in Fig 4-22c. Oblique implantation may be problematic in such cases. The angle of insertion should be determined by the surface topography. *(blue arrow)* Sufficient quantity of bone; *(red arrow)* insufficient quantity of bone.

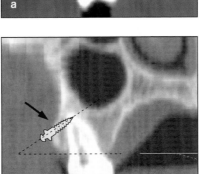
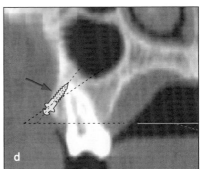

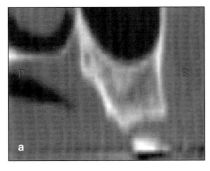
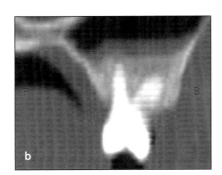
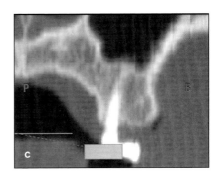

Figs 4-23a to 4-23c The surface topography of cortical bone is diverse in different patients. Hence, it is not appropriate to uniformly base the insertion angle on the occlusal plane. The surface topography should be examined by palpation prior to a procedure. First, it is efficient to implant perpendicular to the cortical bone because it prevents slippage on the surface. After cortical bone is perforated, the angle of insertion can be changed. An angle of approximately 30 to 45 degrees to the occlusal plane is recommended to minimize the risk of root injury and to maximize the available space. (P) Palatal; (B) buccal.

Posterior palatal alveolus

Caution must be taken to prevent injury to the greater palatine neurovascular bundle and maxillary sinus[3,17,18] (Figs 4-13 and 4-27).

For intrusion of the maxillary molar segment and arch constriction, posterior palatal implants are necessary for biomechanical efficiency. Additionally, because palatal space is abundant, various attachments can be utilized to change the line of action (Fig 4-28).[19] Cortical bone is thicker here than in the buccal area, and the keratinized gingiva is thicker. As a result, the incidence of soft tissue problems is very low. There is more mesiodistal space available palatally than there is buccally. Furthermore, because transpalatal attachment is not necessary for treatment, the posterior palatal alveolar area provides an easier application point of palatal force and results in less patient discomfort than does the midpalatal area.

The main disadvantage of this site is related to the condition of the soft tissue. Gingiva of the posterior palatal

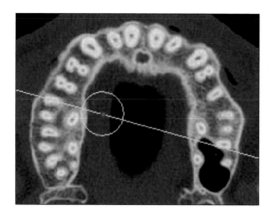

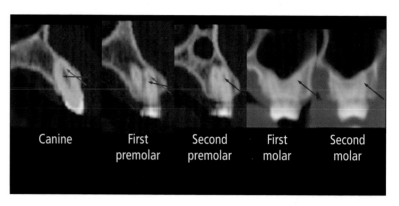

Fig 4-24 Differences in the buccal alveolar bone volume and surface topography of cortical bone in the same individual depend on the areas.

Fig 4-25 In buccolingual cross section, the inclination of the labial and buccal alveolar surface increases from the posterior to the anterior area. Oblique implantation is not favorable *(red arrows)* in the regions of the anterior teeth, canines, and first premolars, for the same reasons noted in Figs 4-22c and 4-22d.

Canine | First premolar | Second premolar | First molar | Second molar

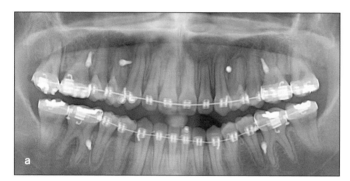

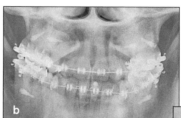

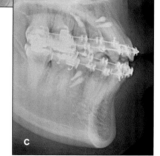

Figs 4-26a to 4-26c In consideration of the surface topography of cortical bone, the angle of insertion of anterior and posterior implants should differ. In this patient, the implant between the canine and the first premolar is inserted almost parallel to the occlusal plane with regard to the slope of the cortical bone surface. The implant between the second premolar and the first molar is inserted obliquely at 45 degrees to the occlusal plane. Less space is available when an implant is inserted parallel to the occlusal plane because of the location of the tip of the implant.

alveolar area has a thick submucosal layer containing glandular tissue, so it is relatively thick and may vary widely in individuals.[14]

There is also less accessibility to the palatal area than the buccal area. Hence, the posterior palatal area is not suitable for direct implantation. Because accessibility is lower, comparatively more skill may be required of the clinician.

Implant size

Following administration of anesthetic, the thickness of the soft tissue at the insertion site is measured with a periodontal probe (Fig 4-29). Ideally, the soft tissue contact area of an implant should be 0.5 to 1.0 mm shorter than the measured soft tissue thickness at the insertion site considering the insertion depth (Fig 4-30).

In most cases, regular-type implants with a 2.0-mm-long cylindrical neck are used, because the thickness of the gingiva is usually about 2.0 to 3.0 mm. For patients with poor bone quality or thick soft tissue, a wide-type implant is recommended. An insertion depth of 6.0 mm in the bone seems to be sufficient. Areas where the soft tissue is thicker than 4.0 mm are unfavorable from a biomechanical point of view. Therefore, a change in insertion site should be considered.

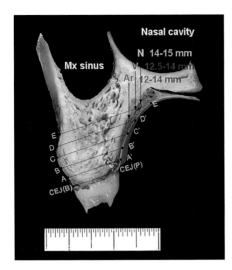

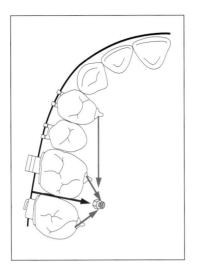

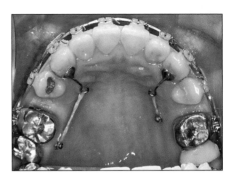

Fig 4-27 The neurovascular bundle passes through the greater palatine foramen and near the palatal vault.[13] Because it is located 12 mm above the palatal cementoenamel junction (CEJ), the risk of causing injury to the neurovascular bundle is usually quite low unless the implant is inserted superior to the root apex. Moreover, damage to the neurovascular bundle can be prevented if the area is examined preoperatively with a periodontal probe. (Mx) Maxillary; (B) buccal; (P) palatal; (N) nerve; (V) vein; (Ar) artery.

Fig 4-28a A maxillary palatal alveolar implant is useful for molar intrusion, arch constriction, and anterior retraction. *(blue arrow)* Constriction; *(green arrow)* intrusion; *(red arrow)* retraction.

Fig 4-28b By controlling the line of action using the palatal space, maxillary palatal alveolar implants can create a force system suited to the treatment objective. (Courtesy of Dr BS Yoon, Seoul, Korea.)

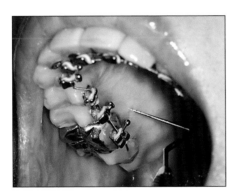

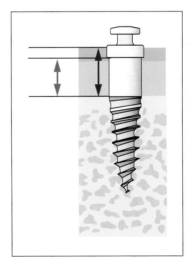

Fig 4-29 The thickness of soft tissue at the insertion point should be measured with a periodontal probe before implantation. The size of the implant should be chosen according to the thickness of the soft tissue. If the gingiva at the planned position is too thick, the insertion position should be changed.

Fig 4-30 An implant can be deeply inserted in the maxillary palatal alveolus, because the palatal gingiva is thick keratinized epithelium. Therefore, the length of the soft tissue contact area *(green arrow)* is selected to be slightly shorter than the thickness of the soft tissue *(blue arrow)*.

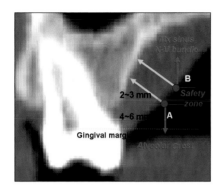

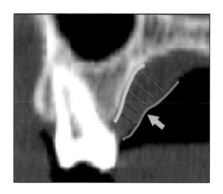

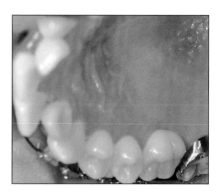

Fig 4-31 Determination of the implant site and insertion angle. It is very dangerous for the implant to be placed close to the root apex. The apical end of an implant should not extend beyond the root apex because this will increase the risk of injury to both the maxillary (Mx) sinus and the neurovascular (N-V) bundle. The gingiva in this area is also very thick and is not suitable for implant placement.

Fig 4-32 The thickness of the soft tissue has an influence on the determination of the vertical position of an implant. It is not efficient to insert an implant superior to the breakpoint *(arrow)* where the gingiva begins to thicken. The gingiva thickens rapidly around the parts in which the submucosal layer starts.

Fig 4-33 The area in which the gingiva begins to thicken appears dark.

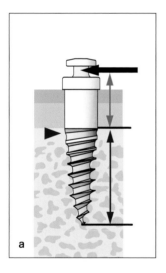

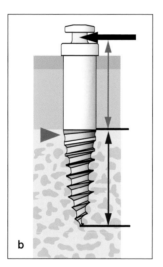

Figs 4-34a and 4-34b The further away from bone support that the orthodontic force is applied, the longer the lever becomes. Therefore, even with the same orthodontic force applied, **(a)** an implant in thinner gingiva is subjected to a lighter load than **(b)** an implant in thicker gingiva. *(red arrowhead)* Greater stress potential; *(blue arrowhead)* less stress potential.

Insertion site and angle

Insertion with a direct view is impossible, so delicate anteroposterior positioning for procedures such as buccal insertion is difficult. The shape of a palatal root is also checked with a panoramic radiograph before positioning of the implant.

For posterior intrusion, insertion between the first and second molars is recommended. For lingual orthodontic treatment, insertion between the second premolar and first molar or between the molars is recommended.

The implant should be placed in the apical area, one third to one half the distance between the alveolar bone crest and root apex. The vertical positioning can then be adjusted according to the amount of vertical force and

vertical tooth movement needed (Fig 4-31). It is preferable that the implant not be placed apical to the area where the soft tissue begins to thicken (Figs 4-32 to 4-34), and it is safer if the end of the implant does not exceed the root apex.

The implant should be placed at an angle of 30 to 45 degrees to the occlusal plane, but, because of the slope of the palatal alveolus, the palatal alveolar implant is placed perpendicular to the cortical bone in most cases (Fig 4-35). Furthermore, the implant should be placed perpendicular mesiodistally. A direct approach to the maxillary palatal alveolus is not recommended because the insertion angle is horizontally slanted, increasing the risk of root injury (Fig 4-36). Hence, an indirect approach with

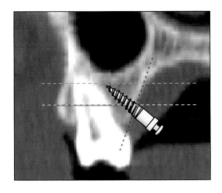

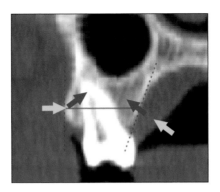

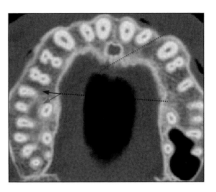

Fig 4-35a The principle for palatal alveolar implants is the same as that for buccal implants: Oblique insertion is recommended to decrease the risk of root injury and to attain more available space.

Fig 4-35b Unlike buccal implants *(left arrows)*, palatal alveolar implants should be inserted perpendicular to the cortical bone from beginning to end, without a change in the insertion angle *(right arrows)*, because the slope of cortical bone is different palatally than it is buccally. Buccally, the approach initially is perpendicular and then changed to 45 degrees.

Fig 4-36 A direct approach *(red arrow)* to the maxillary palatal alveolus is not recommended because the risk of root injury may increase since the angle of implantation is horizontally slanted. The indirect approach *(blue arrow)* with contra-angled instruments is recommended for insertion at a right angle.

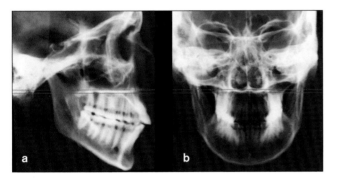

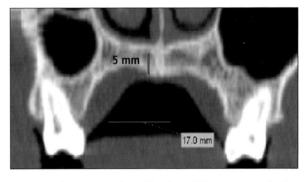

Figs 4-37a and 4-37b (a) Little information can be obtained from lateral cephalometric radiography because the amount of available bone in the midpalate is often underestimated. Lateral cephalometry reveals the bone quantity of the parasagittal plane instead of the bone quantity of the midsagittal plane, as shown in the frontal radiograph **(b)**. (*Red lines* denote the thickness of bone, as revealed radiographically.) (From Miyashita.[26] Reprinted with permission.)

Fig 4-38 The portion indicated by the *red line* appears in the lateral cephalogram. In general, the available bone quantity is sufficient because the bone in the midsagittal plane is used.

contra-angled instruments is recommended for insertion at a right angle (see Fig 5-28).

Precautions

1. The thickness of soft tissue varies widely.[13] Therefore, the thickness of the soft tissue should be measured with a periodontal probe prior to implantation (see Fig 4-29). If the soft tissue is thicker than 4.0 mm, implantation in another area should be considered (see Fig 4-34). The reason for this site change should be explained to the patient beforehand. This precaution also minimizes the risk of damage to the greater palatine vessels.

2. Patients should be instructed not to place their tongue over the implant after insertion, because this could lead to loosening of the implant as a result of continuous irritation from the tongue.

Midpalatal suture

Precautions should be taken to prevent injury to the nasopalatine canal or nasal cavity[20–25] (Figs 4-37 to 4-46).

The thick cortical bone provides excellent primary stability, and the risk of irreversible injury to anatomic structures is relatively low.[22,24,27] In this area, there are no

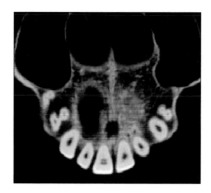

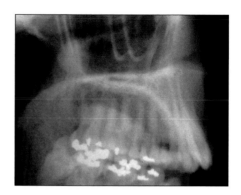

Fig 4-39 The nasopalatine canal passes through the anterior portion of the maxilla, and the nasopalatine foramen opens behind the lingual side of the central incisors. The neurovascular bundle also passes through the nasopalatine canal, so caution must be taken to prevent injury to these structures.

Fig 4-40 The path of the nasopalatine canal may be visible on the lateral cephalometric radiograph.

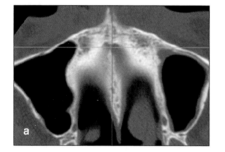

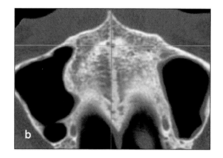

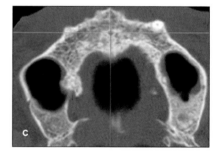

Figs 4-41a to 4-41c The nasopalatine canal **(a)** starts in the nasal cavity on both sides, **(b)** merges inside the maxilla, and **(c)** opens in the lingual area of the maxillary central incisors.

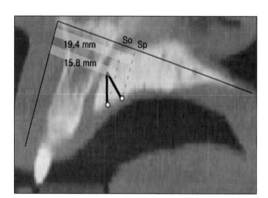

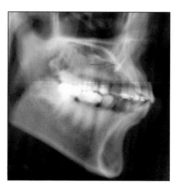

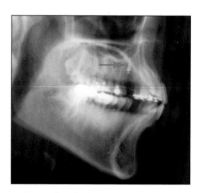

Fig 4-42 A safety zone was measured on three-dimensional computed tomograms when a 6-mm-long implant was placed in the midpalatal suture area.[24] On average, with implantation perpendicular to the occlusal plane and to the palatal bone surface, there is little possibility of damage to the nasopalatine canal when an implant is inserted at points 15.8 mm and 19.4 mm, respectively, posterior to the anterior nasal spine on the anterior nasal spine–posterior nasal spine line. It may not be safe to insert an implant in the anterior 30% to 40% portion of the anterior nasal spine–posterior nasal spine line from the midsagittal plane. (So) Safe point from occlusal plane; (Sp) safe point from palatal plane.

Fig 4-43a The nasopalatine canal may be damaged if an anterior part of the midpalatal suture area in the midsagittal plane is used for implantation *(red arrow)*. When an implant is inserted perpendicular to the cortical surface, there is an especially high risk of damage.

Fig 4-43b Insertion of the implant perpendicular to the occlusal plane is recommended *(red arrow)*. (Figs 4-43a and 4-43b courtesy of Dr JK Lim, Seoul, Korea.)

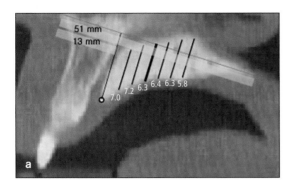

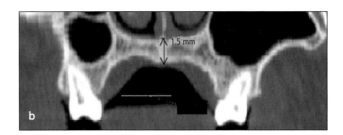

Figs 4-44a and 4-44b Vertical bone quantity available for inserting a cylindrical implant of 1.5 mm in diameter in the midsagittal plane. Normally, there is enough bone for implantation.

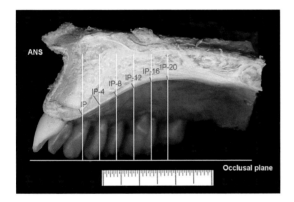

Fig 4-45a The thickness of the soft tissue was measured in a sectioned specimen of the midsagittal plane. (ANS) Anterior nasal spine; (IP) incisive papilla.

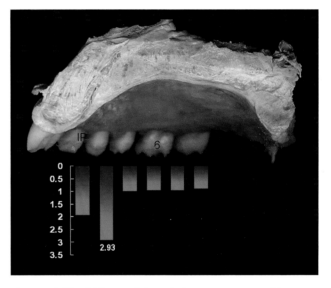

Fig 4-45b The thickness of the soft tissue was measured in a sectioned specimen of the midpalatal suture area. (IP) Incisive papilla.

Fig 4-46 Anteroposterior positioning of implant insertion in the maxillary midpalatal suture area: The anterior 40% of the midsagittal plane is a dangerous area. The middle 40% on the anterior nasal spine–posterior nasal spine line is a safe area. The lateral cephalogram reveals which part is appropriate for implantation on the basis of tooth position. (From Miyashita.[26] Reprinted with permission.)

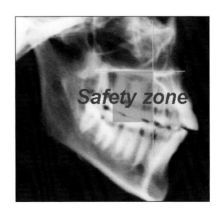

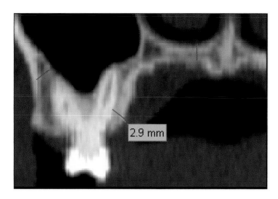

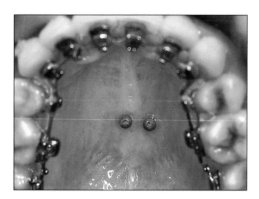

Fig 4-47a In general, the farther away laterally from the midsagittal plane, the smaller the bone quantity. Therefore, it is desirable that an implant be placed in the midsagittal plane whenever possible to maximize the amount of available bone. To minimize the risk of implant fracture, the implant should be placed slightly away from the midsagittal plane or in the parasagittal plane.

Fig 4-47b Two implants inserted in the parasagittal plane and attached for use in treatment.

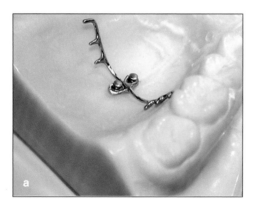

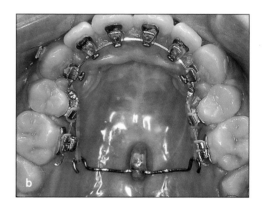

Figs 4-48a and 4-48b An attachment is needed to use midpalatal implants.

structures that will interfere with orthodontic tooth movement. Additionally, the palatal side provides enough space to allow the use of lever arms to control the line of action.[19] The condition of the soft tissue is also suitable for implantation because the soft tissue in this area is the mucoperiosteum (Fig 4-47).

However, accessibility is poor; for implants in this area to be used for treatment, construction of additional transpalatal attachments may be required. Consequently, the use of transpalatal appliances tends to increase patient discomfort (Fig 4-48). Furthermore, the risk of surgical trauma during implantation is high because of the thick cortical bone, and, because the blood supply is poor, the healing potential is low. Additionally, hard bone renders a high risk of implant fracture during the insertion procedure. In growing patients, this is an area of sutural growth; thus, special consideration should be taken. Placing the implant off center from the midpalatal suture area is an option for solving these problems (see Fig 4-46).

Usually, direct application with midpalatal implants is not possible because of patient discomfort. Indirect application with bonded attachments, such as implant-supported transpalatal attachments, is preferable. Usually, with two implants, an attachment is designed according to the purpose of treatment. The attachment is then bonded to implants for orthodontic applications (Fig 4-49).

With the use of midpalatal implants and attachments, the line of action can be formulated according to its biomechanical purposes.

Implant size

Generally, a regular-size implant is sufficient. If the bone is suspected to be especially hard, as found in men with low mandibular angles, either the implant should be placed away from the suture, or a special type of fracture-resistant implant should be used.

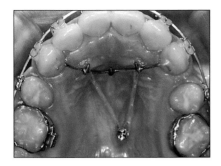

Fig 4-49a Depending on the treatment objective, the line of action can be controlled by various palatal attachments. Midpalatal implants can be used for anterior bodily retraction.

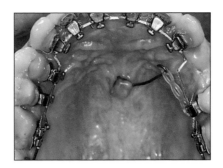

Fig 4-49b Midpalatal implants also can be used for molar protraction, as well as for other methods.

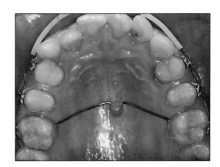

Fig 4-49c Midpalatal implants can be also used as indirect anchorage by connecting implants to teeth with a transpalatal appliance. (Figs 4-49a to 4-49c courtesy of Dr BS Yoon, Seoul, Korea.)

Insertion site and angle

To avoid injury to the nasopalatine canal and nasal cavity,[25] a lateral cephalogram should be used to guide anteroposterior positioning. An implant should not be placed in the area 40% anterior to the midsagittal plane. Placement in the middle 40% is recommended for safety considerations (see Figs 4-45a and 4-45b), although there may be individual variations.

The midpalatal area is the place where cortical bone meets (see Fig 4-46); thus, the bone quantity is excellent. In terms of the quantity of bone, implantation on the midpalatal suture is desirable.

However, from the perspective of bone quality, the results may or may not be desirable. If the bone quality of the buccal area is inadequate, midpalatal suture areas, where cortical bone meets, are good for obtaining primary stability. However, the bone in the midpalatal suture area may be extremely hard, especially in male patients with low mandibular angles. The stability in these patients would be rather low because of surgical trauma induced by frictional heat and physical pressure during drilling of the hard cortical bone. The risk of implant fracture also increases. Therefore, the implant should be placed slightly away from the midsagittal plane or in the parasagittal plane where hard bone is expected.

Insertion of an implant slightly away from the midsagittal plane is also preferred when sutural growth is still occurring in growing patients.

The implant should generally be inserted perpendicular to the bone surface to secure the needed quantity of available bone. When direct insertion is performed, there is a tendency to place the implant tilted forward because of limitations in mouth opening, yet slight anterior tilting does not seem to present any clinical problems.

When one implant is used with an attachment, it may be inserted with an anteroposterior angulation or with a lateral angulation for higher resistance to orthodontic forces (Figs 4-50 and 4-51).

Precautions

1. Direct implantation is not recommended. For direct implantation, the patient has to open the mouth widely for a long period of time, which may overstress the temporomandibular joint. Direct implantation is impossible in patients with a high palatal vault.
2. When the indirect approach with contra-angled instruments is used, a long neck driver and a long neck drill should be used to prevent premature blockage by the anterior teeth (Fig 4-52).
3. The patient will feel "pressure" under the nose during or after insertion.
4. The risk of surgical trauma to the tissue or fracture of the implant during implantation is increased because the midpalatal suture area is composed of thick cortical bone. Poor accessibility makes matters worse. Implantation away from the midline may help to reduce such risks.
5. Special attention is required for surgical placement, because it is difficult to assess the available bone quality using conventional radiography.[25]
6. The effects on the growth site are not yet well established, but attention must be given to possible irreversible injury to the growth site of the midpalatal suture in growing patients.

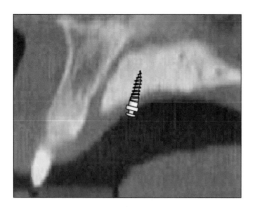

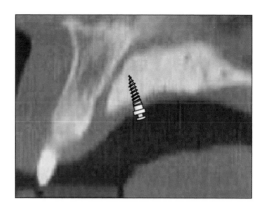

Fig 4-50a A direct approach to the midpalatal suture may be possible if the patient's mouth is held wide open. The insertion angle would be tilted forward, but this is not clinically significant.

Fig 4-50b In patients with deep palatal vaults, a direct approach may not be possible. With an indirect approach, it is recommended that the implant be inserted perpendicular to the surface of the bone.

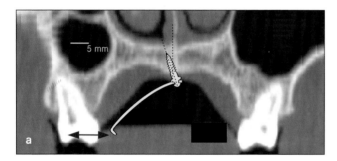

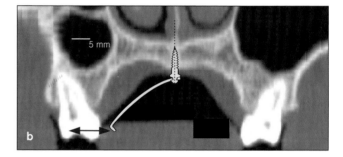

Figs 4-51a and 4-51b Depending on the design of the attachment and the amount of orthodontic force needed, it may be better **(a)** to place the implant obliquely slightly to the left and right sides than **(b)** to place the implant vertically. (*Arrows* indicate direction of force.)

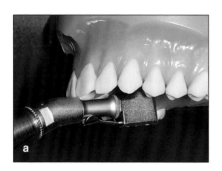

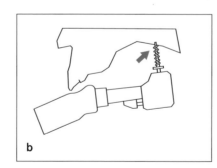

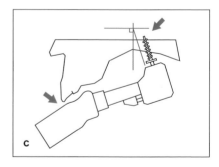

Figs 4-52a to 4-52c When a short driver tip is used, vibration is likely because the handpiece is caught on the maxillary central incisor edge. In addition, the path of insertion changes when the implant contra-angle driver is caught in the maxillary central incisor; this damages cortical bone, which provides primary stability.

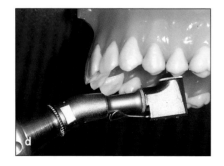

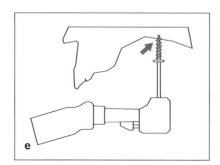

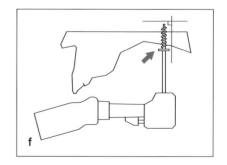

Figs 4-52d to 4-52f The neck of the driver tip should be of an appropriate length to prevent catching in the maxillary central incisor and subsequent vibration.

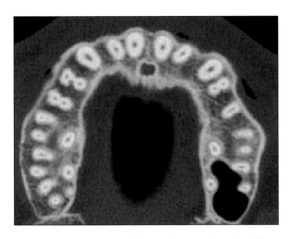

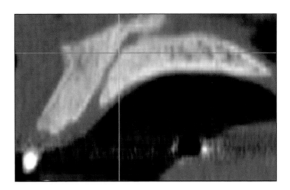

Fig 4-53 The anterior teeth have less interdental and buccolingual space available than do the posterior teeth.

Fig 4-54 Because the nasopalatine canal is located at the lingual side of the central incisors, there is almost no risk of injury to the neurovascular bundle when implants are placed in the anterior alveolus; however, the labial slope of the anterior alveolus makes oblique insertion impossible. The available space is therefore decreased, necessitating apical (ie, vertical) insertion of the implant, which may increase its risk of being covered by the mucosa.

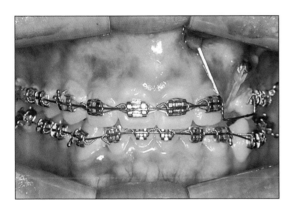

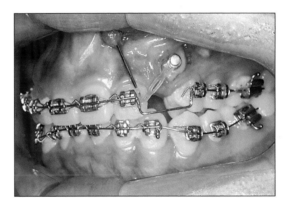

Fig 4-55a The lips and the mucosa tend to move extensively, so the soft tissues may easily impinge on implants in the anterior area.

Fig 4-55b In indirect application, the head is fixed with resin, which reduces irritation to the lips and prevents epithelial covering.

Anterior nasal spine and anterior alveolus

In the anterior alveolus, there is comparatively limited available space because of narrow interdental and labiolingual dimensions (Figs 4-53 and 4-54). Patient discomfort from the implant and stress from the surrounding tissues may be relatively high because of perioral muscle activity. The steep slope of the labial side of the anterior alveolar bone may lead to impingement of soft tissue (Fig 4-55).

However, the bone quality in this area is favorable and is able to provide good primary stability,[28] and the location is also ideal for delivering intrusive forces to the anterior teeth with a labioversion vector. This is useful in the case of Class II division 2 malocclusion.

Depending on the condition of the frenum, the open method (Fig 4-56) or the closed method (Fig 4-57) should be chosen. In the closed method, the implant head is not exposed; instead, only the wire extension is exposed.

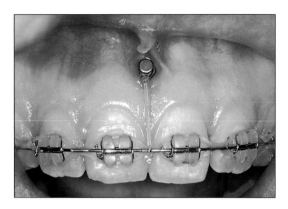

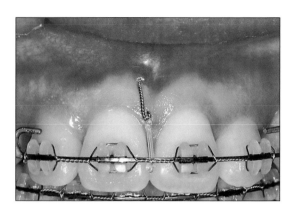

Fig 4-56 If the frenum is low, the implant can get buried if a frenectomy is not accomplished. When the anterior teeth are intruded and retracted with the assistance of anterior interdental implants, the elastic chains and implant may be buried in the soft tissue as teeth move. Therefore, a closed method using an extension wire might be advisable in those cases. (Courtesy of Dr JK Lim, Seoul, Korea.)

Fig 4-57 Even in the anterior alveolar area, there are few problems with soft tissue if the frenum is high. In these cases, the patient feels relatively little discomfort. (Courtesy of Dr JK Lim, Seoul, Korea.)

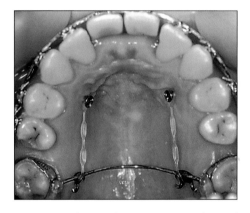

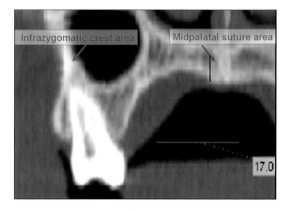

Fig 4-58 Implants in the rugae area may be used for molar protraction. This can reduce the tendency for mesial tipping by lowering the line of action. (Courtesy of Dr BS Yoon, Seoul, Korea.)

Fig 4-59 The quality of bone in the infrazygomatic crest area is superior because the cortical bone is thick, but the volume of bone may be insufficient because it is close to the maxillary sinus.

Anterior rugae

The quality and quantity of bone in this area are good for implants.[29,30] Although the soft tissue is thick, it is keratinized and of good condition.[14] Nevertheless, the tongue is located in this position, so discomfort to the patient or stability during the initial healing period may be affected. Implants in the rugae area can be utilized for mesial movement of molars in adult patients, for orthopedic applications, and for molar distalization in growing patients. Like any palatal implants, it is advantageous to control the line of action by changing the point of force application (Fig 4-58).

In the rugae area, the midsagittal plane should be avoided so as not to injure the nasopalatine neurovascular bundle.

Infrazygomatic crest

Although a low success rate was observed in the maxillary buccal alveolar area in the early days of mini-implants, much attention was drawn to the infrazygomatic crest area because of its superior cortical bone quality, which provides greater primary stability (Fig 4-59). Moreover,

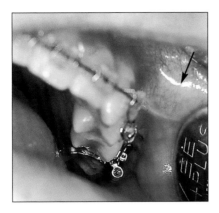

Fig 4-60a An implant in the infrazygomatic crest area has caused an abscess *(arrow)*. In the infrazygomatic crest area, soft tissue moves a great deal, which increases the risk that the implant will be buried by the mucosa and cause soft tissue problems.

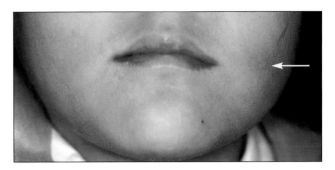

Fig 4-60b The abscess in the area of the implant has caused the cheek to swell *(arrow)*. The implant was removed and general antibiotics were prescribed.

the fact that the location of the implant is much higher is advantageous. This is favorable for the application of intrusive forces and does not cause any interference to the movement of adjacent teeth.

However, because the infrazygomatic crest is in the vestibular area, there is considerable movement of soft tissue, and the implant may readily be covered. Not only does this make the open method difficult to apply, but there is also a relatively high risk of the development of soft tissue problems (Fig 4-60). Because the implant is inserted in a higher position, bone quantity may be insufficient, thus increasing the risk of maxillary sinus injury.

Maxillary tuberosity

Although this is a favorable position for the delivery of distalizing forces, accessibility is poor, and implantation may be inaccurate. Furthermore, the bone quality may not be sufficient because of pneumatization of the maxillary sinus, especially in edentulous areas. Presurgical examination with panoramic radiography is necessary.

PRECAUTIONS IN THE MANDIBLE

Buccal alveolus

Extra caution is necessary in the mandible because it houses the mandibular canal, an important anatomic structure (Figs 4-61 to 4-63). The risk of injury is quite low provided the implant tip does not surpass the tooth apex, but the course of the canal must always be checked with panoramic radiography prior to an insertion procedure. The cortical bone of the mandible is thicker than that of the maxilla (Figs 4-64 and 4-65) and provides better primary stability.

However, in cases of thick and hard cortical bone, minimizing surgical trauma may be difficult because of frictional heat. Additional irritation by food during mastication may compromise stability. Aside from these differences, implantation in the mandibular alveolus is quite similar to implantation in the maxillary buccal area.

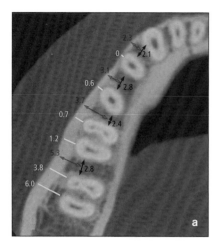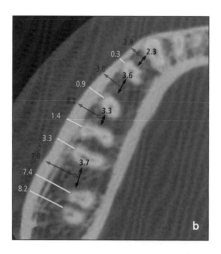

Fig 4-61a Distances (mm) between the mandibular teeth 4 mm apical to the cementoenamel junction. As was the case in the maxilla, the available buccolingual space is quite narrow in the anterior and premolar areas.

Fig 4-61b Distances (mm) between the mandibular teeth 8 mm apical to the cementoenamel junction. (Figs 4-61a and 4-61b courtesy of Prof KJ Lee, Seoul, Korea.)

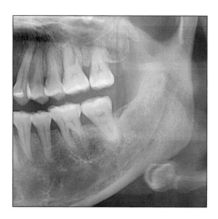

Fig 4-62a The pathway of the mandibular canal can be observed on the panoramic radiograph.

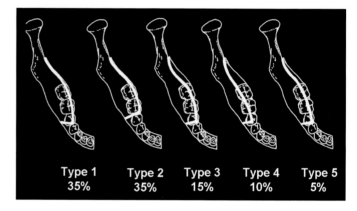

Fig 4-62b In the buccolingual dimension, the mandibular canal is generally located to the lingual side. However, there is little possibility that the canal will be damaged unless implants are inserted below the level of the root apex.

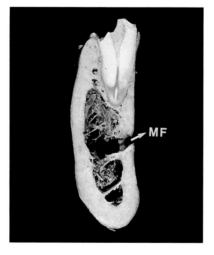

Fig 4-63 The mental foramen (MF) opens toward the occlusal plane, so it may be located at a point superior to that visible in the radiograph. However, this does not matter greatly if the apical end of an implant is located above the level of the root apex. (Courtesy of Prof HJ Kim, Seoul, Korea.)

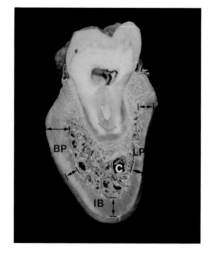

Fig 4-64 The cortical bone of the mandible is thicker than that of the maxilla. (BP) Buccal plate; (LP) lingual plate; (IB) inferior border. (Courtesy of Prof HJ Kim, Seoul, Korea.)

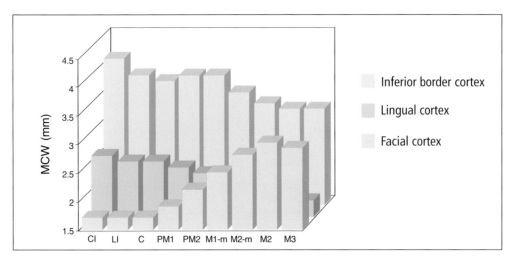

Fig 4-65 Cortical bone thickness according to the area in the mandible. (MCW) Mandibular cortical width; (CI) central incisor; (LI) lateral incisor; (C) canine; (PM1) first premolar; (PM2) second premolar; (M1-m) mesial root of first molar; (M2-m) distal root of first molar; (M2) second molar; (M3) third molar. (From Kim.[10] Reprinted with permission.)

Implant size

Implantation is similar to that in the maxillary buccal area. However, special care should be taken in harder bone to prevent implant fracture and to minimize surgical trauma. In most cases, a regular-width implant is chosen, but a wide type may be used in growing patients or when sufficient primary stability is not indicated during the implantation of a regular implant.

Insertion site and angle

Determination of insertion site and angle is similar to that in the maxilla (Fig 4-66). However, when the implant is placed between the mandibular first and second molars, the occlusion and vestibular space should be checked. The implant position should be determined with the consideration of possible stress from mastication and from the buccinator muscle.

Oblique implantation may allow the use of more buccal and interdental space and may also reduce the possibility of root injury while increasing the contact area with cortical bone. However, depending on the buccal slope of the cortical bone, oblique implantation may be impossible (Fig 4-67), as in the maxilla.

Precautions

1. Because cortical bone in molar areas may be hard, the risk of surgical trauma because of frictional heat or excessive pressure during implantation increases. The risk of implant fracture also increases, and poor accessibility makes matters worse. If contra-angled instruments are used for insertion, the risk of implant fracture is also increased by the leverage effect. The excessively high insertion torque indicates that strong pressure is delivered to the adjacent bone structure, and this means that the risk of implant fracture is also drastically increased. The high torque may also be a sign that excessive stress is being directed to adjacent bone tissue, so reverse rotation should be performed to relieve stress on adjacent bone during the guiding stage. However, reverse rotation should never be used during the finishing stage.
2. Stability may especially be decreased in the areas between the mandibular first and second molars because of irritation from food during mastication and pressure from the cheek muscles. Centric occlusion in the molar area must be checked; if possible, the implant should be placed at a point where the stress from mastication can be minimized.
3. The remaining precautions are similar to those for implantation in the maxillary buccal area (see page 62).

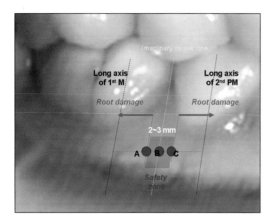

Fig 4-66a For mandibular molar distalization, an insertion position 1.5 mm distal to an imaginary central line between two teeth should be selected. For molar protraction, an insertion position 1.5 mm mesial to an imaginary central line should be selected. If there is to be no mesiodistal movement of adjacent teeth, an insertion position on the central line should be selected. (A, B, C represent implant insertion sites.) (M) molar; (PM) premolar.

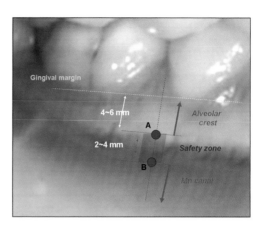

Fig 4-66b For intrusion, the insertion position should include sufficient depth apically. Otherwise, the implants will restrict further intrusion. (A, B represent implant insertion sites.) (Mn) Mandibular.

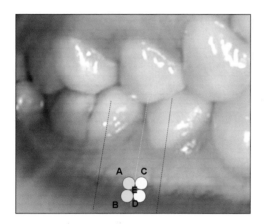

Fig 4-66c The insertion position should be determined based on the anteroposterior and vertical tooth movements required. (A, B, C, D, E represent implant insertion sites.)

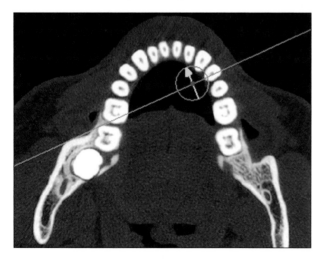

Fig 4-67a As in the maxillary buccal site, the surface topography of cortical bone in the mandibular buccal site differs among various areas and within each individual.

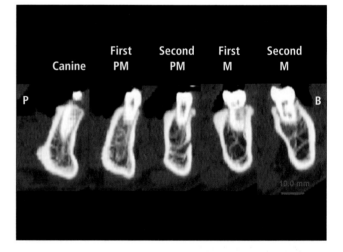

Fig 4-67b The buccolingual section reveals that the closer to the anterior teeth, the more inclined the implant is to the labial side. The working angle during insertion should be determined according to the surface topography of the cortical bone, as in the maxilla. (PM) Premolar; (M) molar.

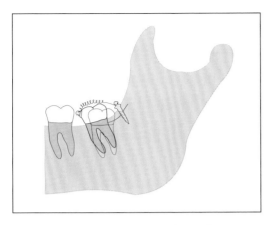

Fig 4-68a Biomechanically, an implant in the retromolar area is good for uprighting through the application of a single force, but uprighting is not a very difficult tooth movement.

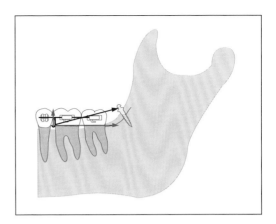

Fig 4-68b One of the most attractive advantages of the retromolar area implant is that extrusive forces can be applied along with distalizing forces. Most implants are likely to have an intrusive force vector, but it is a great advantage to have an extrusive force vector as well.

Edentulous area

The edentulous area is available for implant insertion, but bone resorption is present and the compact bone quality is poor; as a result, there is a greater chance of inadequate primary stability.

Retromolar area

A retromolar implant is advantageous for a distalizing force and as a single force for molar uprighting, and it can produce an extrusive force vector with distalization (Figs 4-68 and 4-69). Additionally, this implant does not interfere with tooth movement.

However, the mandibular canal is close to the retromolar area, and many important anatomic structures that require special attention during implantation are present in this area as well (Fig 4-70). Although the possibility of injuring the mandibular canal may be low, the outcome of any such injury can be disastrous. Before implantation, the passage of the mandibular canal should be assessed through panoramic views, and the bone bed should be ensured through palpation (Fig 4-71). During implantation, if any doubt exists, a periapical radiograph should be taken and safety should be reassessed.

One other disadvantage is the excessively hard bone. Hard and rich cortical bone can provide good primary stability, but it may also increase the surgical trauma and the risk of implant fracture. It is mandatory that predrilling be performed through the cortical bone at all times in the retromolar area. Because the associated soft tissue is thick and very mobile, maintenance is difficult and may render the open method difficult. Opposing teeth or the maxillary tuberosity can restrict the vertical space, so the opposing relationship of the usable space should be assessed in advance.

Implant size

Before insertion of the implant, the thickness and condition of the soft tissue in the insertion site should be examined with a periodontal probe. The available vertical space with opposing teeth or the maxillary tuberosity should also be assessed. Then, whether the open method or the closed method will be used should be determined according to the soft tissue condition and available vertical space. For an open method to be used, the implant head should be sufficiently exposed. For patients with insufficient interocclusal space or thick and movable soft tissue, a closed technique may be considered.

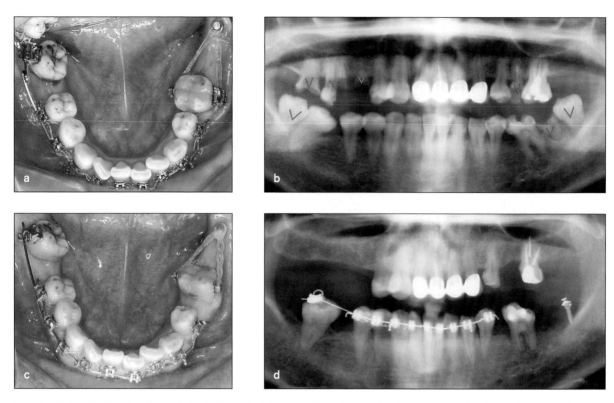

Figs 4-69a to 4-69d When the posterior teeth are lost, there is sufficient space for placement of an implant at the retromolar area. In this patient, the mesially angulated molar was uprighted using the single force from the mini-implant.

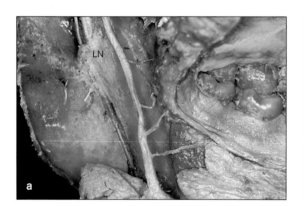

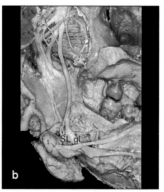

Figs 4-70a and 4-70b Many important anatomic structures are located in the retromolar area, especially on the inner side of the ramus. The lingual nerve (LN) travels near the retromolar area, and the mandibular canal is also close to the retromolar area. Therefore, much attention is needed to prevent injury to significant structures. (SL gl) Sublingual gland. (Courtesy of Prof HJ Kim, Seoul, Korea.)

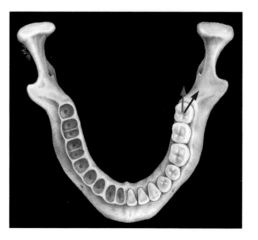

Fig 4-71 The mandible appears to be shaped much like a combination of the letters U and V, so the retromolar area is lateral to the most posterior molar. Before an implant is placed in the retromolar area, the bone bed should be confirmed through palpation to prevent insertion in the soft tissue. (*Red arrow* indicates the lack of bone distal to the molar; *blue arrow* indicates the direction of bone.) (Courtesy of Prof HJ Kim, Seoul, Korea.)

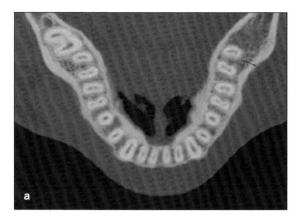

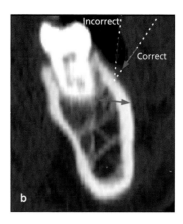

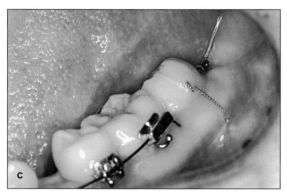

Fig 4-72a Biomechanically, the retromolar area is a good place to apply a single force for correction of second molar scissor bite. (*Green arrow* denotes the thinness of the cortical and trabecular bone.)

Fig 4-72b During the procedure, it is important to insert the implant in the proper direction and angle to prevent damage to the roots.

Fig 4-72c There is sufficient space on the buccal side of the second molar so that a scissor bite can be corrected with a closed technique. (Courtesy of Prof JK Lim, Seoul, Korea.)

Precautions

1. The tissue condition of the retromolar area varies among individuals. For example, in patients with a developing third molar tooth bud, insufficient space on the distal side of the molar or narrow interocclusal space may restrict implantation.

2. The risk of injury during implantation is relatively high because of the extremely hard bone and the presence of several significant anatomic structures (see Fig 4-70). The bone of the retromolar area is the hardest of all of the areas where orthodontic implants are placed. Because of the shape of the mandible itself, caution should be taken to prevent injury to the inner side of the ramus and the canal.

3. Because of the aforementioned factors, special precautions should be taken for implantation. Presurgical examination and a proper mechanical treatment plan are of the utmost importance. The thickness and mobility of the soft tissue and the relationship with opposing maxillary teeth should be assessed before implantation. Flap surgery is helpful to increase visibility and accessibility to prevent iatrogenic injury. If surgical removal of an impacted third molar is planned, it is

preferable that extraction and implantation be performed together. Predrilling through cortical bone with palpation of the implantation site should always be performed in advance to confirm the position of the bone bed. Predrilling can reduce surgical trauma and the risk of implant fracture.

Buccal shelf

Precautions are needed to prevent injury to the teeth and the mandibular canals. The advantages of the buccal shelf include thick cortical bone and an abundant mesiodistal space,[11,13] which does not restrict tooth movement. Additionally, the buccal shelf is in a good position to deliver intrusive forces, distalizing forces, and expansion forces to correct scissor bites (Fig 4-72). However, being in the vestibule area with excessive soft tissue movement, a buccal shelf implant can be irritated by the cheek muscles, which may lead to loosening and maintenance problems. The accessibility is low in this area.

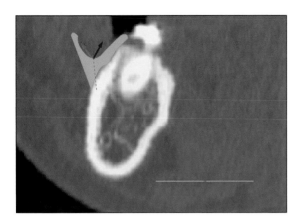

Fig 4-73 An implant head or an extension wire should not be located lateral to the mucobuccal fold *(red arrow)* because of the excessive stress from facial muscles, such as the cheeks. The implant should be positioned medial to the mucobuccal fold *(blue arrow)*.

Implant size

An implant is selected according to the tissue conditions of the implantation site and the desired application method. For an open method to expose the head of the implant, an implant with soft tissue contact of more than 2.0 mm may occasionally be needed, but when there seems to be a great chance of irritation from the cheek muscle, the closed method is preferable, especially for correction of a scissor bite.

Precautions

1. Because cortical bone in this area is very hard, pre-drilling is necessary.
2. The slope of the buccal area may vary, so the surface topography should be assessed by palpation to determine the implantation angle.
3. The implant should be placed a certain distance from the vestibular fornix (mucobuccal fold). The implant head should never be placed more buccal across the vestibular fornix (Fig 4-73).

Anterior alveolus

Although available space is limited because of the narrow labiolingual dimensions and interdental space (Fig 4-74), the bone quality of the anterior alveolus is superior[31] (Fig 4-75). This is an ideal position at which to provide intrusive force to the anterior teeth (Figs 4-76 and 4-77). Continuous irritation from lip muscles may cause a problem (Fig 4-78).

Lingual alveolus

The lingually placed implant has a biomechanical advantage (Fig 4-79). It is in a good position to provide intrusive lingual forces as well as constriction forces for posterior teeth (Fig 4-80). Thin soft tissue and good cortical bone in this area provide adequate primary stability, but poor accessibility and continuous tongue irritation may compromise this stability.

The greatest disadvantage is the patient discomfort caused by the tongue. Important anatomic structures are present in the floor of the mouth[32]; thus, the implant should not be placed inferior to the floor of the mouth (Fig 4-81).

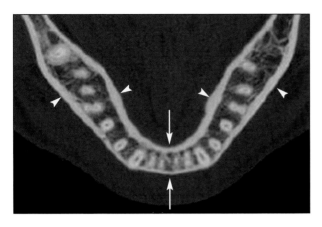

Fig 4-74 The mini-type implant is recommended for the anterior alveolus because of the narrowness of the available space *(arrows)*. The anterior teeth have less buccolingual and interdental space available than do the molars *(arrowheads)*.

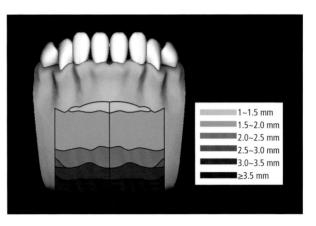

Fig 4-75 Cortical bone thickness in the mandibular symphysis area. The bone quality is very good for achieving primary stability. (Courtesy of Prof HJ Kim, Seoul, Korea.)

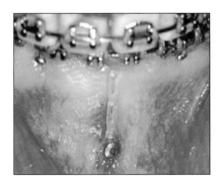

Fig 4-76a An implant is apically positioned in the mandibular area.

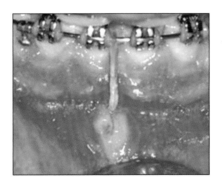

Fig 4-76b Apically positioned mandibular implants are easily buried because the lips and the mucosa move a great deal.

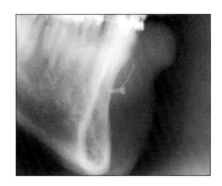

Fig 4-76c In such cases, the closed technique is used.

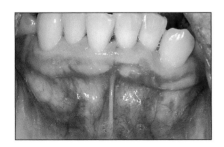

Fig 4-77a The frenum located near the insertion sites calls for a frenectomy to be performed simultaneously with the implant insertions, so that the implants can be used in the open method without any further problems.

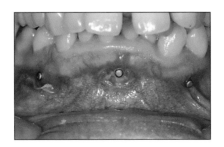

Fig 4-77b Appearance 1 week after the frenectomy and insertion of the mini-implants.

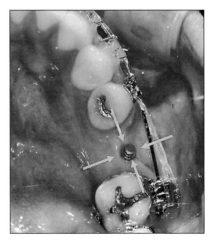

Fig 4-78 Distalization, protraction, constriction, and expansion forces are used by implants placed in the edentulous area. (Courtesy of Dr BS Yoon, Seoul, Korea.)

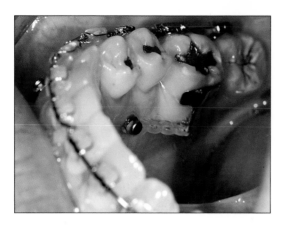

Fig 4-79 On the lingual side, there is a biomechanical advantage to changing the direction of force. (Courtesy of Dr BS Yoon, Seoul, Korea.)

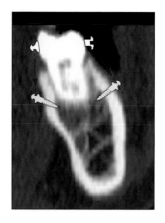

Fig 4-80 A lingual implant is very useful for controlling torque and arch form during mandibular molar intrusion. However, it may cause significant patient discomfort.

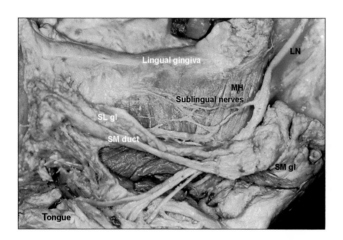

Fig 4-81 The implant should not be inserted below the floor of the mouth because of the presence of important anatomic structures, such as the mylohyoid muscle, glands, and nerves. (SL gl) Sublingual gland; (SM) submandibular; (MH) mylohyoid muscle; (LN) lingual nerve; (SM gl) submandibular gland. (Courtesy of Prof HJ Kim, Seoul, Korea.)

SUMMARY

A problem-oriented diagnosis and treatment planning process ensures that the diagnosis will be based on the patient's individual needs and not on the clinician's preferred mode of treatment. The benefits, risks, and limitations of the proposed treatment plan must be clearly explained to the patient. After it has been determined that the use of an orthodontic mini-implant is both safe and necessary, the clinician should select the implantation site on the basis of accessibility, the condition of the hard and soft tissues, the ability to use the site orthodontically, the comfort of the patient, and the possibility of irritation from surrounding oral tissues. Each potential site has its own advantages and disadvantages, which must be assessed within the context of the treatment goals.

REFERENCES

1. Proffit WR, White RP, Sarver DM. Contemporary Treatment of Dentofacial Deformity in Orthodontics. St Louis: Mosby, 2003: 127–145.
2. Sugerman PB, Barber MT. Patient selection for endosseous dental implants: Oral and systemic considerations. Int J Oral Maxillofac Implants 2002;17:191–201.
3. Lee JS. Development of orthodontic mini-implant anchorage system. Pre-Conference: Basic Researches on Implant Orthodontics. The 4th Asian Implant Orthodontics Conference, Seoul, Korea, December 3–4, 2005.
4. Bischof M, Nedir R, Szmukler-Moncler S, Bernard JP, Samson J. Implant stability measurement of delayed and immediately loaded implants during healing. Clin Oral Implants Res 2004;15: 529–539.
5. Gedrange T, Hietschold V, Mai R, Wolf P, Nicklisch M, Harzer W. An evaluation of resonance frequency analysis for the determination of the primary stability of orthodontic palatal implants. A study in human cadavers. Clin Oral Implants Res 2005;16:425–431.

6. Esposito M, Hirsch JM, Lekholm U, Thomsen P. Biological factors contributing to failures of osseointegrated oral implants. (II). Etiopathogenesis. Eur J Oral Sci 1998;106:721–764.

7. Gilsanz V, Gibbens DT, Roe TF, et al. Vertebral bone density in children: Effect of puberty. Radiology 1988;166:847–850.

8. Zamberlan N, Radetti G, Paganini C, et al. Evaluation of cortical thickness and bone density by roentgen microdensitometry in growing males and females. Eur J Pediatr 1996;155:377–382.

9. Fujita T, Fujii Y, Goto B. Measurement of forearm bone in children by peripheral computed tomography. Calcif Tissue Int 1999;64: 34–39.

10. Kim HJ. Morphology of the Mandibular Canal and the Structure of the Compact and Sponge Bone in Korean Adult Mandibles [thesis]. Seoul: Yonsei University, 1993.

11. Masumoto T, Hayashi I, Kawamura A, Tanaka K, Kasai K. Relationships among facial type, buccolingual molar inclination, and cortical bone thickness of the mandible. Eur J Orthod 2001;23:15–23.

12. Park HS. Anatomical study using CT image for the implantation of micro-implants. Kor J Orthod 2002;32:435–441.

13. Yoon HS. Thickness of the Maxillary Soft Tissue and Cortical Bone Related with an Orthodontic Implantation [thesis]. Seoul: Yonsei University, 2002.

14. Ten Cate AR. Oral Histology: Development, Structure, and Function, ed 4. St Louis: Mosby, 1994:389–395.

15. Kim TK, Park SH. Relief of soft-tissue irritation from orthodontic appliances. J Clin Orthod 2002;36:509.

16. Joo E, Yu HS, Lee KJ. Radiologic Evaluation of Interdental Distance for Application of Orthodontic Mini-Implant [thesis], 2004. Yonsei University, Seoul, Korea.

17. Kwak HH, Park HD, Yoon HR, Kang MK, Koh KS, Kim HJ. Topographic anatomy of the inferior wall of the maxillary sinus in Koreans. Int J Oral Maxillofac Surg 2004;33:382–388.

18. Reiser GM, Bruno JF, Mahan PE, Larkin LH. The subepithelial connective tissue graft palatal donor site: Anatomic considerations for surgeons. Int J Periodontics Restorative Dent 1996;16:131–137.

19. Park YC, Choy K, Lee JS, Kim TK. Lever-arm mechanics in lingual orthodontics. J Clin Orthod 2000;34:601–605.

20. Wehrbein H, Merz BR, Diedrich P. Palatal bone support for orthodontic implant anchorage–A clinical and radiological study. Eur J Orthod 1999;21:65–70.

21. Bernhart T, Vollgruber A, Gahleitner A, Dörtbudak O, Haas R. Alternative to the median region of the palate for placement of an orthodontic implant. Clin Oral Implants Res 2000;11:595–601.

22. Kyung SH. A study on the bone thickness of midpalatal suture area for miniscrew insertion. Korean J Orthod 2004;34:63–70.

23. Mraiwa N, Jacobs R, Van Cleynenbreugel J, et al. The nasopalatine canal revisited using 2D and 3D CT imaging. Dentomaxillofac Radiol 2004;33:396–402.

24. Park YC, Lee JS, Kim DH. Anatomical characteristics of the midpalatal suture area for miniscrew implantation using CT image. Korean J Orthod 2005;35:35–42.

25. Crismani AG, Bernhart T, Tangl S, Bantleon HP, Watzek G. Nasal cavity perforation by palatal implants: False-positive records on the lateral cephalogram. Int J Oral Maxillofac Implants 2005;20:267–273.

26. Miyashita K. Contemporary Cephalometric Radiography. Tokyo: Quintessence, 1996.

27. Kyung SH, Hong SG, Park YC. Distalization of maxillary molars with a midpalatal miniscrew. J Clin Orthod 2003;37:22–26.

28. Misch CE. Bone character: Second vital implant criterion. Dent Today 1988;7:39–40.

29. Bernhart T, Freudenthaler J, Dörtbudak O, Bantleon HP, Watzek G. Short epithetic implants for orthodontic anchorage in the paramedian region of the palate. A clinical study. Clin Oral Implants Res 2001;12;624–631.

30. Tosun T, Keles A, Erverdi N. Method for the placement of palatal implants. Int J Oral Maxillofac Implants 2002;17:95–100.

31. Park HD, Min CK, Kwak HH, Youn KH, Choi SH, Kim HJ. Topography of the outer mandibular symphyseal region with reference to the autogenous bone graft. Int J Oral Maxillofac Surg 2004;33: 781–785.

32. Kim SY, Hu KS, Chung IH, Lee EW, Kim HJ. Topographic anatomy of the lingual nerve and variations in communication pattern of the mandibular nerve branches. Surg Radiol Anat 2004;26:128–135.

SURGICAL PROCEDURES 5

SURGICAL PRINCIPLES

Surgical procedures for implantation of orthodontic mini-implants should be based on the following principles:

1. Aseptic principle
2. Atraumatic procedures
3. Thorough preoperative examination and precise implant positioning
4. Premedication for pain control
5. Standardized procedures

Aseptic principle

Implants and instruments should be used under aseptic conditions. The driver tip is a female type, so blood and saliva can gather easily in the driver tip. The driver tip should be cleaned with a smooth brush and a neutral detergent as soon as possible following the conclusion of the procedure.

Recycling of implants is prohibited by law and is also unfavorable from the viewpoint of stability, because the surfaces of implants are treated to increase biocompatibility; when in contact with body fluid, the surface changes continuously from the initial state. If there is even a small amount of surface contamination, the implant can be used after cleaning with an ultrasonic cleaner and autoclaving. However, repeated autoclaving has adverse effects on the biocompatibility of the surface.

Atraumatic procedures

As stated in chapters 2 and 3, necrotic bone tissue should be removed to promote healing of bone tissue. This removal process proceeds very slowly.[1] Therefore, it is essential to minimize surgical trauma during implant placement to allow favorable healing, because the necrosis of osseous tissue is inevitable.

To minimize surgical trauma, the surgical procedure should be performed with well-sharpened drills used at an appropriate speed under flowing saline coolant.[2-5] Appropriate cooling is needed to minimize damage from the heat generated during the insertion procedure.

If insertional torque seems to increase abruptly, further attempts at insertion are undesirable because increased torque may be a sign that adjacent bone tissue is over-stressed. Thus, reverse rotation should be used to relieve stress on the adjacent bone. However, reverse rotation should never be used during insertion of the last 2.0 mm of an implant, because, otherwise, sufficient primary stability cannot be obtained.

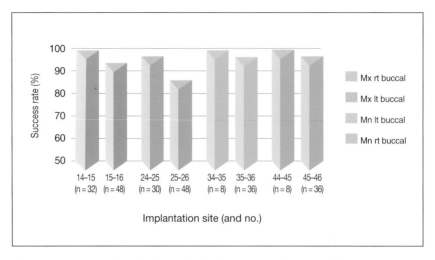

Fig 5-1 Success rates of newly designed orthodontic mini-implants according to insertion site (n = 246).[6] No statistically significant difference was observed, but the success rate tends to be higher on the right side than on the left side. This may be a result of a difference in accessibility, because the right side is easier for a right-handed operator to work on. (Mx) Maxillary; (rt) right; (lt) left; (Mn) mandibular; FDI tooth-numbering system.

Thorough preoperative examination and precise implant positioning

The clinician should minimize unnecessary injuries to the anatomic structures by attaining a full awareness of the anatomy of the insertion area. More specifically, if the movement of teeth adjacent to an implant is planned, precise positioning of implants should be performed to ensure enough available space.

Premedication for pain control

Pain control is very important to secure the patient's compliance. If the implant loosens, reinsertion is necessary, but the patient's experience with the first surgical placement of implants can greatly influence compliance with the second placement. For efficient pain control, premedication with analgesics 1 hour prior to or at surgery is recommended. In general, the prescription of systemic antibiotics, either preventatively before surgery or after surgery, is not necessary.

Standardized procedures

Although the new type of implant has a structure designed to minimize the influence of the operator's dexterity, the abilities and experience of the operator may still influence the success rate[6] (Fig 5-1). In other words, improper and inaccurate procedures cause failures, and stability can be improved by the standardization of procedures and greater accessibility.

To promote a standardized process, the surgical procedure is divided into five major stages:

1. Preoperative examination stage
2. Marking stage
3. Perforating stage
4. Guiding stage
5. Finishing stage

Specific goals for each stage of the procedure should be achieved before the next stage is initiated.

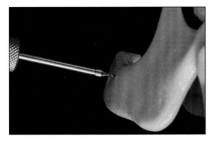

Fig 5-2a If possible, it is beneficial to use a perpendicular approach to perforation of the cortical bone.

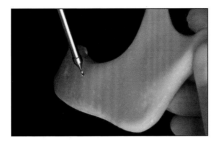

Fig 5-2b With the oblique approach, resistance from the cortical bone is strong.

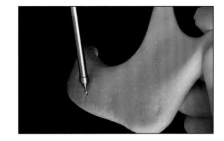

Fig 5-2c Because of the bone resistance during the oblique approach, there is a greater potential for slippage.

Preoperative examination stage

Selecting the site, administering anesthetic, and performing preoperative examinations

The insertion site is selected according to the anatomic conditions and biomechanical requirements. The implant placement site is confirmed by clinical and radiographic examinations. The anatomy of the insertion site should be checked; soft tissue conditions, such as the thickness of the attached gingiva, and the frenum attachment should also be checked. Abnormalities of root shape, pneumatization of a maxillary sinus, abnormal localization of the accessory canal, or other issues may be present. The intended location of the implant should also be palpated to confirm the topography of the bony tissue and to determine the initial insertion angle.

Local anesthesia is obtained through infiltration anesthetic. After the administration of anesthetic, the cortical bone surface should be examined with a periodontal probe.

Marking stage

Marking of the insertion position on the gingiva

The insertion site should be cleaned with povidone-iodine solution. After a periodontal probe is used to mark the horizontal and vertical reference lines on the gingiva, the gingiva should be perforated with a periodontal probe at the correct insertion point according to the treatment plan. At this time, the thickness of the soft tissue is also measured with the periodontal probe. If a frenum is present near the planned position of insertion, a frenectomy should always accompany the procedure.

Perforating stage

Perforating cortical bone

The perforating stage is important because cortical bone is the component most resistant to implant insertion and the most critical to primary stability.[7] Therefore, the main goals of this stage are to allow implantation to proceed easily and to protect cortical bone against unnecessary surgical trauma by cortical bone punching (Fig 5-2).

There are two ways to perforate cortical bone: use of the ORLUS surgical drill (Ortholution) and use of an implant (Fig 5-3; see also Fig 3-22). The former method is advisable because a drill is superior to a screw in cutting efficiency, and predrilling can increase the operator's tactile sensation during the procedure, so root touching can be recognized. For the first time, a new type of implant has been designed for drill-free insertion to minimize surgical trauma from the frictional heat generated by engine-driven drilling and to increase clinical efficiency.[8–10] However, the ORLUS surgical drill was designed and introduced to eliminate the chance of root injury and to reduce surgical trauma by increasing cutting efficiency.

With any method, perforation should be accomplished by virtue of screw mechanics, which can change rotational motion into translational motion.[11] A drill is also a kind of screw with long pitches.

Guiding stage

Bone grip and determining the implantation angle

During this stage, the screw should be engaged with the bone and inserted at a planned angle. With any type of insertion method, an implant should be inserted through

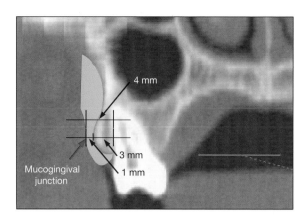

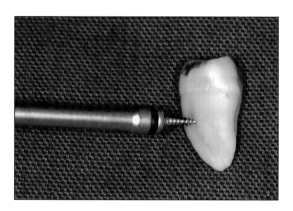

Fig 5-3 The ORLUS surgical drill, designed to prevent root injury, is 4.0 mm long so that the drill cannot reach root surfaces at the mucogingival junction.

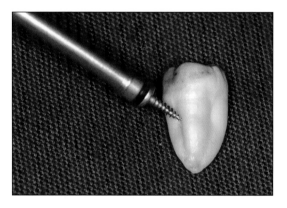

Fig 5-4a With an oblique insertion, more available space can be obtained for movement of adjacent teeth. Additionally, there is little chance of root injury. With an oblique insertion, slippage is likely to occur instead of penetration into the root.

Fig 5-4b Root penetration is more likely with a perpendicular insertion.

rotation of the screw with minimal vertical force, only enough to maintain the insertional angle. A pin or a nail is inserted by vertical force, or pushing, while a screw is inserted by means of rotation. Excessive vertical forces should never be applied, because they increase the chance of vibration and root injuries.

Finishing stage

Finishing and obtaining mechanical stabilization from cortical bone

Primary stability is obtained from cortical bone during this stage, meaning that this stage is the most important in terms of short-term stability. The implant should be inserted to the planned depth, and the implant head should be exposed to an adequate extent depending on the condition of the host bed.

This process can be finished only by rotation; this is made possible by the engagement of the screw threads with the bone during the guiding stage. Finishing solely

with rotational force is crucial to maximize contact with the cortical bone and to prevent vibration. Even a small vertical force may cause vibration, which causes critical damage to cortical bone and compromises primary stability.

Protocols for prevention of root injuries

Root injuries are rare, but fatal to the tooth. Therefore, protocols for prevention of root injuries cannot be overemphasized. Use of the ORLUS surgical drill, predrilling through cortical bone, and oblique insertion can all help to prevent root injuries (Figs 5-3 and 5-4a). The ORLUS surgical drill is 4.0 mm long, so it can perforate cortical bone but can drill only to a limited depth and cannot touch the root at the mucogingival junction. Predrilling through cortical bone makes the insertion process easier by allowing the implant to be placed with minimal vertical force and by improving the operator's tactile sensation

Fig 5-5 The new type of mini-implant has a unique structure; it can be inserted to a greater depth, and more support can be obtained from cortical bone because it has a tapered core that widens with height (a) and a dual thread (b), which consists of trapezoidal threads in the cervical area and reverse buttress threads in the apical area.

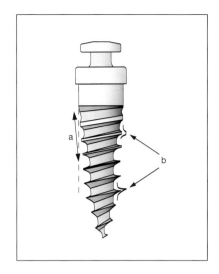

during the procedure. Placed with a limited vertical force, the mini-implant cannot perforate or split the root.

After cortical bone is perforated, strong resistance that blocks deeper insertion indicates that the implant has touched the root. Predrilling through cortical bone can also prevent implant fracture by reducing resistance to insertion.

To prevent unnecessary injuries to anatomic structures such as the roots, the following principles should be respected at each stage of implant placement:

1. Preoperative examination stage: The anatomic structure should be examined thoroughly.
2. Marking stage: The position of insertion must be marked accurately on the gingiva with the periodontal probe.
3. Perforating stage: Cortical bone should be predrilled with the ORLUS surgical drill. This is key to preventing root injury.
4. Guiding stage: The implant should be inserted obliquely with rotational motion and a minimal pressing force to maintain the insertion angle. The root may be perforated or split by an implant inserted at a perpendicular angulation but not at an oblique angulation (see Figs 5-4a and 5-4b). In an oblique angulation, slippage may occur instead of perforation. With oblique insertion, available space also is increased. The use of only a small amount of vertical force is ample for insertion because cortical bone is perforated and cancellous bone shows little resistance to insertion. Vertical force must not be exerted, particularly in the indirect approach, because tactile sensation may be compromised. If additional advancement is not possible with rotational motion, and strong resistance is felt, it is

highly possible that the implant is touching the root. Therefore, the placement position should be confirmed again, and the placement site should be changed if necessary. If the first and second stages are performed properly, such a situation will rarely occur.
5. Finishing stage: Implantation should be finished with rotational motion only. If further advancement is limited even with rotational motion, this normally indicates that the root is being touched.

SURGICAL PROCEDURES

As noted previously, the clinician should perform this surgical procedure with a full understanding of the rationale of the design of the mini-implant, the biologic mechanism, and the surgical principles (Fig 5-5).

Scheduling

In general, maxillary mini-implants cause less pain and discomfort and therefore are placed first; mandibular mini-implants are placed afterward. From the patient's point of view, placement of all implants at the same time with the aid of strong analgesics may be more convenient. However, in this case there may be a greater burden on the operator, which may affect the stability of the implant. The surgical procedure should always be

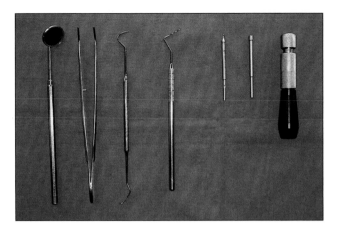

Fig 5-6a Required instruments for the direct approach *(left to right)*: dental mirror, tweezer, explorer, periodontal probe, manual ORLUS surgical drill, standard hand-driver tip, and standard hand-driver handle.

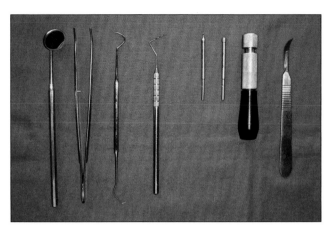

Fig 5-6b If a frenectomy is necessary, the following instruments are required *(left to right)*: dental mirror, tweezer, explorer, periodontal probe, manual ORLUS surgical drill, standard hand-driver tip, standard hand-driver handle, and blade holder with no. 12 blade.

performed in a comfortable situation, because it requires a high degree of concentration from the operator.

If implants are placed before tooth extraction, care should be taken not to damage the bone-implant interface at the moment of extraction. Injury to cortical bone may compromise the stability of implants. Any dental procedure that could damage the bone-implant interface should be performed cautiously.

Placement in conjunction with simple extraction

If tooth extraction is needed, simple extraction and surgical placement can be done simultaneously in the same quadrant; this will reduce the number of times that local anesthetic must be administered and will limit the overall pain experienced by the patient. For instance, an implant can be placed on the right side during the extraction of the right premolar.

However, during the extraction procedure, luxation of a tooth may injure cortical bone. Therefore, an implant should be placed after extraction to prevent damage to the bone-implant interface. Clinically, to control bleeding, the implant should be placed after full luxation of a tooth and a minor amount of extraction from a socket. The tooth can then be removed from the socket.

Placement in conjunction with mandibular third molar extraction

If plans for extraction of the mandibular third molar will include flap operation and implant placement in the retromolar area, simultaneous procedures are advantageous. It is advantageous to form the flap in the retromolar area where soft tissue is thick, because the bone is very difficult to deal with in terms of hardness and accessibility. The presence of adjacent anatomic structures also is an issue. Predrilling through cortical bone is strongly recommended for insertion of implants in the retromolar area.

Separate surgical placement

A schedule should be created during treatment planning to account for the required period of healing. If surgical placement is completed prior to full bonding of orthodontic brackets, an adequate healing period can be planned.

Direct approach

If accessibility is adequate, a direct approach with a hand driver is recommended.

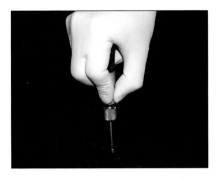

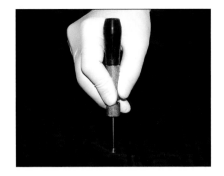

Fig 5-7a The palm grip is recommended for the perforating stage and the guiding stage because of its superior stability in handling.

Fig 5-7b The pen grip is not recommended because it allows unwanted lateral movement.

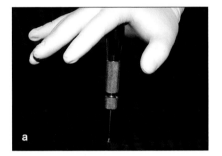

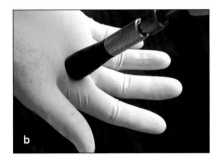

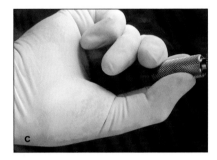

Figs 5-8a to 5-8c Palm grip: The driver is grasped slightly while the head is covered with the palm. The driver handle is located on the palm below the index finger.

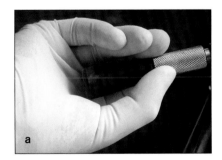

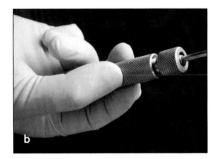

Figs 5-9a and 5-9b For the finishing stage, it is better to use the finger grip because rotation should be applied very cautiously. The handle should be grasped gently with only three fingers.

Required instruments or armamentaria

A periodontal probe is essential for marking the insertion point on soft tissue and for bone probing (Fig 5-6).

Proper grip

The driver handle should be gripped properly according to the stage of surgical procedure and the purpose of the procedure (Figs 5-7 to 5-9).

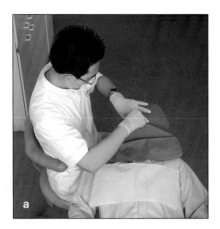

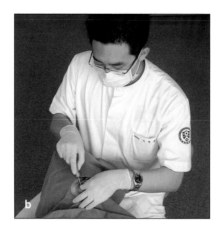

Figs 5-10a and 5-10b In general, the ideal operator position would be from **(a)** the 9 o'clock position to **(b)** the 1 o'clock position. For access to the left side, the 3 o'clock position may be better for right-handed operators. The operator should change working positions as the approach for perpendicular insertion progresses to the approach for oblique insertion. Throughout the procedure, no tension or stress should be placed on the wrist, the shoulder, or the neck. For example, for right-handed operators, the 12 o'clock position is preferable during perpendicular insertion at the right premolar area. In oblique insertion at the right premolar area, the 9 to 10 o'clock position is better.

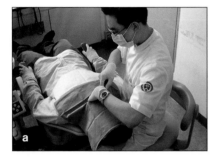

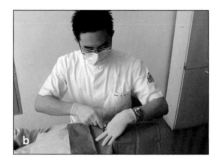

Figs 5-11a and 5-11b The posture of an operator should be natural and unstrained for better accessibility and results.

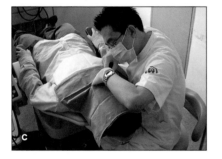

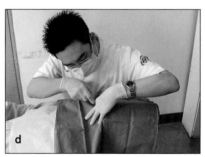

Figs 5-11c and 5-11d If the unit chair is not lowered to an appropriate height, the posture of the operator may be unnatural; unnatural posture decreases accessibility.

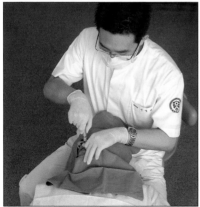

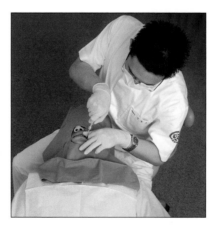

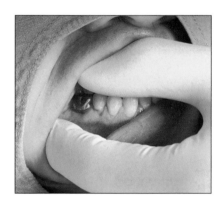

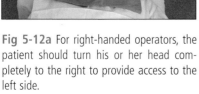

Fig 5-12a For right-handed operators, the patient should turn his or her head completely to the right to provide access to the left side.

Fig 5-12b If the head of the patient is not in the appropriate position, the visual field may be inadequate and the posture of the operator may be unnatural.

Fig 5-13 The operator must secure the visual field and accessibility by means of sufficient retraction of the soft tissue using the hand that does not handle the driver.

Fig 5-14 Pneumatization of the maxillary sinus has progressed significantly *(arrows)*, although the patient is only 21 years old.

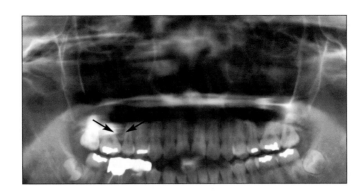

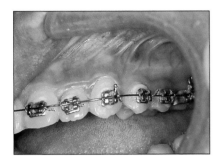

Fig 5-15 Operators should examine the width of the attached gingiva, the shape of the frenum, and the attachment position.

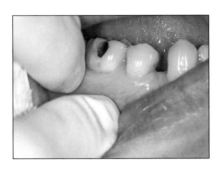

Fig 5-16a Because of individual variations, it is important for the operator to palpate the buccal slope to determine the insertion angle.

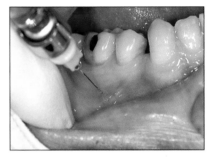

Fig 5-16b To reduce the pain from injection, infiltration anesthetic is administered on the mucosa, not on the attached gingiva, after full retraction of the soft tissue.

Figs 5-17a and 5-17b After infiltration anesthetic is administered, a longitudinal indentation between the two teeth and parallel to the long axis is made on the soft tissue with the periodontal probe. This line can be used as the vertical reference.

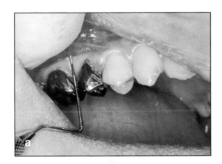

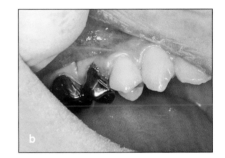

Posture

To ensure proper surgical placement, an adequate visual field and proper accessibility are very important. In other words, it is important that the implant always be inserted while the operator is in a natural posture without unnecessary tension (Figs 5-10 to 5-13).

Surgical procedures

Preoperative examination stage

The insertion site should be examined thoroughly through inspection, palpation, and panoramic radiography (Figs 5-14 and 5-15). The surface topography should be established by palpation to determine the insertion angle (Fig 5-16a). With full retraction of the soft tissue, infiltration anesthetic is administered on the mucosa (Fig 5-16b). After anesthesia is obtained, the bone quality is evaluated with a periodontal probe. If the bone appears to be soft and is easily penetrated with a probe, the site of insertion should be changed.

Marking stage

After the placement area is cleaned with povidone-iodine, the insertion site should be marked with the periodontal probe. The vertical reference line that bisects the interdental area parallel to the axes of the proximal teeth should be marked (Fig 5-17). The horizontal reference line should then be marked according to the position of

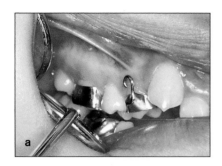

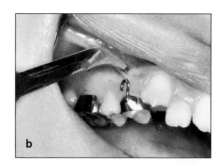

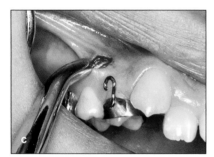

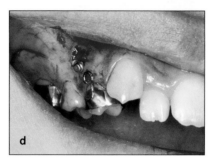

Figs 5-18a to 5-18d Frenectomy for implant placement. **(a)** After infiltration anesthetic, **(b and c)** a horizontal incision of about 3.0 mm up to the periosteum is made with a no. 12 blade. Bleeding should be controlled by the application of pressure using wet gauze for 5 minutes. **(d)** The implant should then be placed in the same way as in a normal case. After implantation, the patient should hold the wet gauze for approximately 15 to 30 minutes to control bleeding. Additional suturing is not necessary.

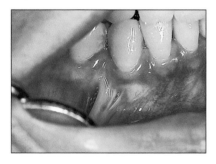

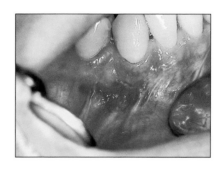

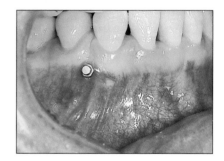

Fig 5-19a A frenum is present at the site where implant placement is planned.

Fig 5-19b A frenectomy is performed prior to implantation.

Fig 5-19c A stable soft tissue interface is observed 1 week after implantation.

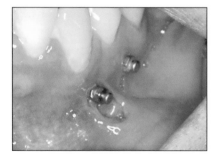

Fig 5-20 If the frenectomy is omitted, ulceration of the soft tissue appears as the movement of the frenum continually irritates surrounding tissue.

the alveolar crest and the required amount of vertical force.

A separate incision usually is not required. However, when the implant is to be inserted in the area of a frenum, a frenectomy should accompany the procedure to prevent possible mechanical irritation around the implant during function (Figs 5-18 to 5-21). Frenectomies can be performed before or after implantation. It can be advantageous to perform the procedure before implantation because it eliminates extra soft tissue, although the disadvantage of that sequence is that it requires bleeding control before implant placement.

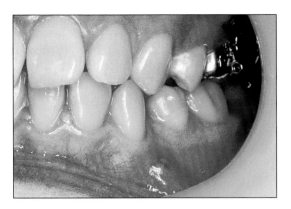

Fig 5-21a Inflammation has occurred after an implant was placed without frenectomy.

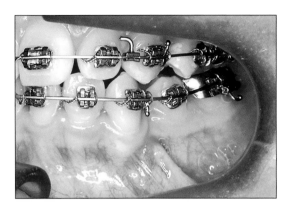

Fig 5-21b The implant is covered with soft tissue.

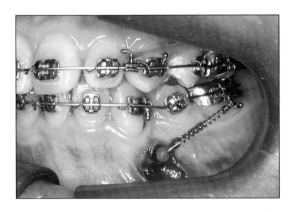

Fig 5-21c After administration of anesthetic, the head is uncovered and a nickel-titanium coil spring is used instead of the elastic chain. A ball of resin has been placed on the implant head to prevent it from being covered again. A frenectomy has been performed at the same time.

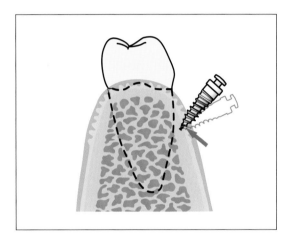

Fig 5-22 The operator should be careful not to break the tip when changing the insertion angle. The tip can be broken if the insertion angle is changed while the tip is in the osseous tissue. Hence, in the case of insertion without predrilling, the implant should be removed completely and then inserted again at the correct angulation.

For implantation on unattached gingiva, minimal retraction of soft tissue is generally adequate. If soft tissue gets entangled during insertion, it should be loosened through counterrotation of the driver, after which the procedure can continue. Depending on the preference of the operator, 3.0 mm of stab incision may be performed on the mucosa.

Perforating stage

There are two ways by which to perforate through cortical bone: use of the ORLUS surgical drill and use of an implant. As mentioned previously, selection of the former option is advisable. In the perforating stage, insertion perpendicular to the surface is recommended to prevent slippage on the surface. The slope of osseous tissue should be determined by palpation at an earlier stage.

To perforate cortical bone, an adequate amount of vertical force should be applied and a palm rest should be used to firmly establish the path and to turn the screw. At this time, lateral force should be avoided to prevent fracture (Fig 5-22). Operations should be performed by virtue of the function of the screw rather than by vertical force. The cortical bone should be perforated with the use of a turning motion. To reduce the risk of root injury and to minimize surgical trauma, it is desirable that a manual drill system be used.

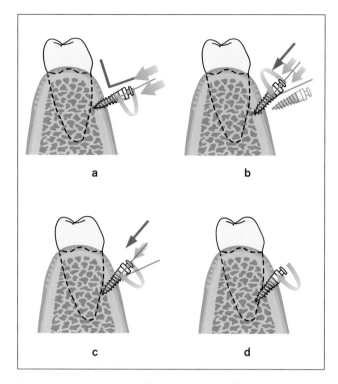

Fig 5-23 Surgical procedure for the placement of mini-implants without predrilling. *(a)* Perforating stage: The operator should approach perpendicular to the cortical bone to avoid slippage when perforating cortical bone to a depth of 1.0 to 1.5 mm. *(b)* Guiding stage I: The implant is withdrawn fully to change the insertion angle. *(c)* Guiding stage II: The implant is inserted according to the planned insertion angle. *(d)* Finishing stage: Finishing rotation should be applied without any vertical force to maximize cortical bone support.

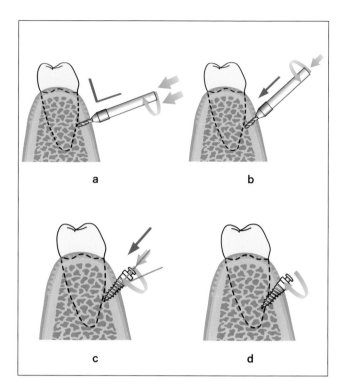

Fig 5-24 Surgical procedure for the placement of mini-implants with predrilling. *(a)* Perforating stage I: The operator should approach perpendicular to the cortical bone to avoid slippage during cortical bone perforation. *(b)* Perforating stage II (recapitulation): The drill is withdrawn fully and reinserted at the proper insertion angle. *(c)* Guiding stage: The implant is inserted according to the planned insertion angle to about two thirds of the full length. *(d)* Finishing stage: Finishing rotation should be applied without any vertical force to maximize cortical bone support.

Without predrilling. The new type of mini-implant has a screw that penetrates cortical bone without predrilling (Fig 5-23). To avoid slippage of the implant, the operator should make an approach perpendicular to the surface of cortical bone from the beginning of insertion to a depth of 1.0 to 1.5 mm in cortical bone.

After the implant is placed to a depth of approximately 1.0 mm into the cortical bone, the driver should be turned counterclockwise and the screw should be fully withdrawn.

Because of the risk of implant fracture, use of a narrower implant with a center diameter of less than 1.6 mm is not recommended for placement without predrilling, particularly in the mandible. Operators should be very careful not to break the tip of the implant; breakage usually results from a change in the angle of insertion while the tip of the implant is in the cortical bone.

With predrilling. The ORLUS surgical drill is designed to perforate cortical bone (Fig 5-24). To avoid slippage, the operator should work perpendicular to cortical bone to perforate it. The moment of perforation can be felt when resistance drastically decreases. After perforation, the drill should be fully withdrawn and the insertion site should be drilled again with the planned angle of insertion.

Guiding stage

After perforation of cortical bone, an implant should be inserted up to about two thirds of the full length according to the planned angle of insertion. During this stage, minimal vertical force should be applied as long as the insertion angle is maintained, and a palm rest should be used once again to provide a firm basis for securing the path. To avoid root structures and to increase the cortical bone contact area, the insertion angle against the surface of the cortical bone should be approximately 30 degrees.

As in the perforating stage, the implant should be inserted by virtue of the screw function, not by vertical force. That is, it should be inserted by the turning of the driver handle. Slight vibration may be allowed.

Without predrilling. An implant should be fully withdrawn and then reinserted according to the planned angle of insertion. The insertion angle should not be changed as long as the tip is in cortical bone. Otherwise, the risk of tip fracture is high.

With predrilling. The implant can be inserted according to the planned insertion angle from the beginning.

Finishing stage

The placement is finished with maximal support from cortical bone, because the insertion path is established through the recapitulation procedure. After approximately two thirds of the full length of the screw is inserted and its bone engagement is secured, implant placement should be finished with only rotational motion by a finger grip to maximize support from cortical bone. When the screw has engaged bone, rotational motion is enough to finish the procedure, because the screw will transform this rotation into the required translational movement. Forces in any direction can cause vibration and compromise intimate contact between bone and implant.

Prognosis

A tight fit should be felt during the final two or three turns of the implant. If not, the implant is likely to fail because of a lack of cortical bone support, excessive trauma, or vibration during insertion.

Indirect approach

Required instruments or armamentaria

An indirect approach is needed for sites in which a direct approach is impossible; these sites include the palatal area and areas between molars. To use an indirect approach, the operator requires a contra-angled instrument with the following properties (Figs 5-25 and 5-26):

1. Sufficient torque can be generated for implant placement.

2. Insertion speed can be controlled. To minimize surgical trauma, the number of rotations for insertion should not exceed 60 rpm. For perforating cortical bone, approximately 1,000 rpm is appropriate[5]; for insertion of mini-implants, approximately 30 to 60 rpm is adequate.
3. Tactile sensation is adequate during implant insertion. This is very helpful for preventing root injury.
4. The instrument is simple and easy to use, because accessibility is poor in an indirect approach.

For this purpose, an engine for prosthodontic implants, a 256:1 deceleration handpiece for a low-speed engine, and a contra-angled hand driver are appropriate. The engine type has the advantage that it requires very little effort for implantation, but it also carries disadvantages, such as decreased tactile sensation and difficulty in controlling the implanting speed in a delicate manner. The hand-driver type has the opposite advantages and disadvantages. From the viewpoint of workability, the engine type may be better.

An endodontic engine may be used, but this instrument can rarely generate sufficient torque. A 64:1 or 128:1 deceleration handpiece for a low-speed engine has excessive rpm and does an inadequate job of minimizing surgical trauma.

Posture

The basic posture for the indirect approach is almost the same as that used in the direct approach; however, the position should ensure a good direct and indirect view.

Surgical procedures

The surgical principles of the indirect approach are almost the same as those of the direct approach, and the procedure comprises the basic four stages (see Figs 5-23 and 5-24). The following are special considerations for the indirect approach:

1. It is strongly recommended that the operator place implants using a predrilling procedure because tactile sensation is diminished in the indirect approach.
2. The point and angle of insertion must be verified from various angles to ensure that the procedure takes place according to the plan (Figs 5-27 and 5-28). The direct view is impossible; therefore, the mirror should be used in the indirect approach.
3. Accessibility is relatively poor compared to that of the buccal approach, so it is probable that accessibility will

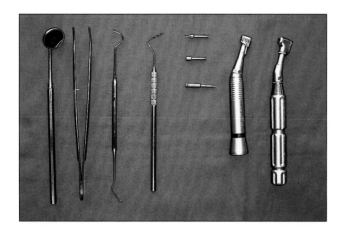

Fig 5-25 Required instruments for the indirect approach *(left to right)*: dental mirror, tweezer, explorer, periodontal probe, driver tips, deceleration handpiece, and manual contra-angled driver. For implantation in the palatal alveolus, a short driver tip is required. For implantation in the midpalatal suture area, a long driver tip is required.

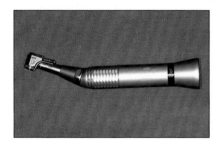

Fig 5-26a Contra-angled 256:1 deceleration handpiece for a low-speed engine.

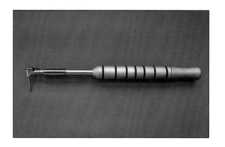

Fig 5-26b Contra-angled hand driver.

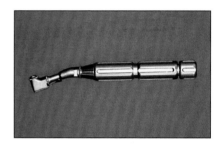

Fig 5-26c A short contra-angled hand driver is suitable to remove implants that were inserted by the indirect approach.

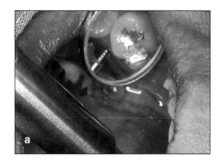

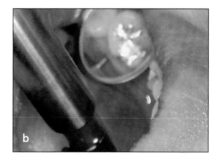

Figs 5-27a and 5-27b A mirror should be used because the indirect approach does not enable the operator to obtain a direct visual field. Accurate positioning of the mirror is crucial, because the position of the implant seems different, depending on the direction of the mirror.

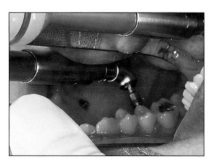

Fig 5-28a A side mirror designed for photography may be helpful.

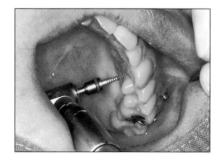

Fig 5-28b The operator must check and confirm the insertion angle from various angles by looking in the mirror at each stage and from a direct view.

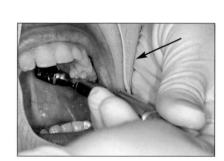

Fig 5-29 A firm rest utilizing the patient's face *(arrow)* should be secured when a manual contra-angled long driver is used. This rest allows the operator to apply rotational force only, especially in the final stage of the insertion, to prevent vibration.

| Box 5-1 | Postoperative instructions for patients |

General

- Any kind of mechanical irritation can cause loosening of an implant.
- Use prescribed mouth rinses for 2 to 4 days after the operation, and then brush the area gently.
- Brushing of the implant is also necessary. The soft bristles of a toothbrush should be used to brush as gently as possible, taking care that the head of the toothbrush does not touch the implant. Sonic brushes are not appropriate for cleaning around implants.
- Never touch an implant with a finger or with the tongue. Never rest the tongue on the implant.
- When eating a meal, hard food may cause mechanical irritation, which then leads to loosening.
- An oral irrigator and Rotadent are good for oral hygiene control.
- An implant is very weak to mechanical impact or stress, and thus the following precautions should be taken.
  - Lying on the side of the mini-implant is not recommended.
  - Resting the chin on the hands and habitual movement of the cheek are also not desirable.
  - Chewing hard foods should be avoided.
- (Other instructions for patients are the same as those given following periodontal surgery or minor surgery.)

Emergency situations

The following situations are considered emergencies. In the event of an emergency, an immediate visit to the dental office is recommended.

- Marked mobility of an implant means failure.
- An implant can be extruded unexpectedly because of loosening, but this does not cause severe problems. In general, reimplantation is required.
- Continuous pain over an implant may be a clinical sign indicating latent problems.
- Swelling over an implant or drainage of pus may be a clinical sign of infection.

| Box 5-2 | Information for patients regarding postoperative pain |

- There may be pain as the anesthetic wears off. This pain may last for 2 or 3 days.
- There are many differences among individuals in terms of the perception of pain, because pain is highly subjective. Generally, pain from surgical placement of implants can be similar to or less than the pain felt after premolar extraction.
- Pain can be significantly reduced by the use of appropriate analgesic agents.
- After implant placement, foreign-body sensation from the implant head may result but will likely diminish in 5 to 7 days.
- Ulceration may occur because of mechanical irritation or stress from the surgical procedure. This will generally improve in 5 to 9 days. In the case of ulceration, use of pain-relieving ointments or ointments containing steroids may be helpful.

Postoperative care

Postoperative instructions should be given to patients and parents of patients after the operation, and information on medication should be provided if necessary (Box 5-1). In general, the prescription of systemic antibiotics is not necessary.

Periodontal packing is not usually necessary, but it can be performed to reduce foreign-body sensation, to aid in favorable mucosal healing, and to ensure the sedative effect from the drugs in the pack. At removal, the periodontal pack should be removed completely. Because a mini-implant is small, the possibility that a remnant of the pack will remain is relatively high, particularly in the mucosa. Even a small remnant in the subgingival area is likely to cause an abscess.

The day after the procedure, a follow-up examination and dressing with povidone-iodine may be helpful. At this appointment, primary stability should be confirmed. If mobility is present, this should be considered a procedural failure. Treatment for such failure is described in detail later in this chapter.

The patient is likely to experience initial mouth soreness after orthodontic implantation (Box 5-2). Foreign-body sensation can be reduced by using a dressing or wax.

Education for oral hygiene maintenance is important. Brushing around implants is necessary; the single turf brush, oral irrigator, and Rotadent can be used for brushing. A sonic brush, however, may not be appropriate.

be affected by the operator's technique or proficiency to a certain degree.

4. Implant placement should be finished only with rotational motion. To increase primary stability (Fig 5-29) and to prevent implant fractures and iatrogenic root injuries, neither vertical nor lateral force should ever be applied.

5. The longer the driver is, the greater the risk of implant fracture becomes, because the leverage effect increases (see Fig 3-38). Therefore, special attention should be paid when an implant is placed in hard bone, such as at the midpalate or retromolar area.

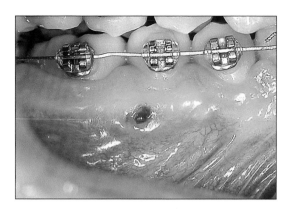

Fig 5-30 Immediately after implant removal, the bleeding is not serious.

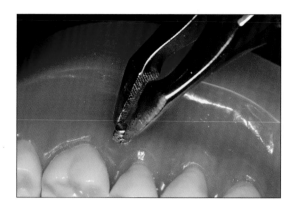

Fig 5-31 If an implant is inserted deep or is covered by soft tissue, infiltration anesthetic may be necessary. If the circumstances dictate, utility pliers can also be used to remove an implant, but this should be done carefully to prevent fracture.

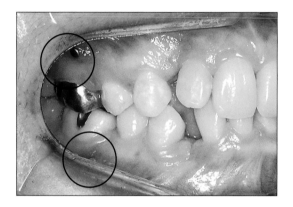

Fig 5-32a Extraction wounds tend to heal quickly without scars. *(insets)* Implants in place.

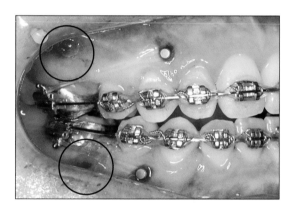

Fig 5-32b *(insets)* Appearance immediately after implant removal.

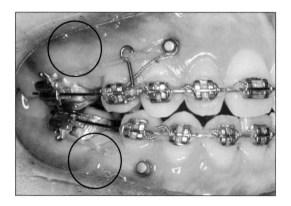

Fig 5-32c *(insets)* Healing after 3 weeks.

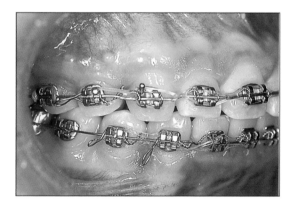

Fig 5-33 After implant removal, bony spicules or soft tissue scars may remain. As time goes on, these are remodeled.

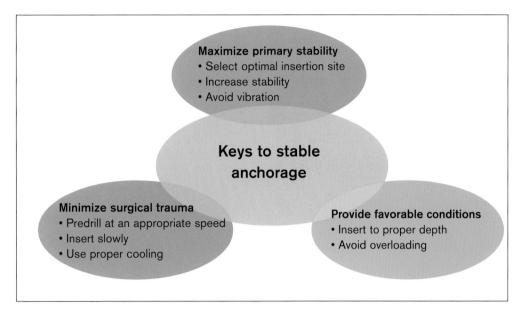

Fig 5-34 Keys to obtaining stable anchorage.

Removal

In case of removal, deep anesthesia is generally unnecessary. According to the preference of the individual patient, topical anesthetic or infiltration anesthetic may be administered. In most cases, simple topical anesthetic is adequate. There is no serious difficulty in bleeding control (Fig 5-30), and wet gauze held by the patient is normally sufficient. However, if the implant head is covered with soft tissue or an implant has been inserted deeply, infiltration anesthetic is needed (Fig 5-31).

Patients should avoid eating hot and salty foods for 2 to 3 days to prevent pain or aggravation of the wound. Generally, extraction wounds tend to heal quickly without any unwanted sequelae (Figs 5-32 and 5-33).

PROBLEMS AND SOLUTIONS

The use of orthodontic implants to facilitate orthodontic treatment is becoming universal. However, the occurrence of problems from orthodontic implants is also increasing.

Loosening of the orthodontic implant

The most common problem associated with orthodontic implants is loosening.[6,12,13] Although the success rate of orthodontic implants may have increased, loosening of the orthodontic implant may also occur; this situation is distressing for the clinician and the patient. Epidemiologic studies[6,12,13] have indicated the following: Most failures arise from the bone-implant interface, and most failures occur shortly after implantation. The failures of the bone-implant interface result from inadequate primary stability, excessive surgical trauma, and unfavorable healing conditions. During treatment, impact stress or irritation from surrounding tissues may also cause loosening.

For orthodontic implants that have an improved structure for enhanced stability, the use of a standardized procedure with full understanding of the mechanism of action can increase the rate of success (Fig 5-34). Additionally, the operator must also focus on the procedure.

The patient must be informed that there is a possibility of loosening of implants and a subsequent need for reimplantation before the surgical procedure is performed (Fig 5-35). Patients should be instructed that this procedure is not to be feared.

Premedication for pain control is very important and is also effective in decreasing anxiety in the event that reimplantation is necessary after initial failure.

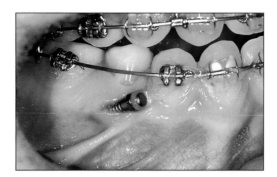

Fig 5-35 The implant has loosened and is partially extruded.

When a tight fit is not felt during the final stage, this indicates that sufficient primary stability cannot be obtained and that the implant will probably fail.[14,15] This is caused by poor bone quality, vibration, or unintentional excessive surgical trauma during insertion. If this situation occurs, the following steps may be helpful:

1. The presence of poor bone quality or poor primary stability should be noted to the patient or parents of the patient, because the patient may be surprised at unexpected implant loss.
2. A change to orthodontic implants with wider diameter and deeper insertion should be considered.
3. Placement of additional implants at another site should be considered.
4. Use of a nickel-titanium coil spring with a light force of no more than 100 g is also recommended. After confirmation of implant stability, orthodontic force may be increased.

If mobility of an implant is detected at the follow-up appointment, the implant should be considered a failure. However, in the case of slight mobility, the following form of management can be considered: Deeper insertion under infiltration anesthetic will increase mechanical stabilization due to the unique design of the new type of implant. However, when insertion is made deeper, the chance of burial by soft tissue increases. This procedure should only be performed after the patient or parents of the patient have been notified. Use of a nickel-titanium coil spring is also recommended.

Fracture of the orthodontic implant

The causes of orthodontic implant fracture vary according to the fracture site (see Fig 3-35); elimination of the causes can prevent the problem. In most cases, fracture does not occur at orthodontic loading or at removal.

An orthodontic implant can be made of chromium-cobalt alloy, which increases the strength of the orthodontic implant so that the fracture rate is reduced.[16] However, the chromium-cobalt alloy demonstrated lower biocompatibility than the titanium alloy, and long-term stability is not guaranteed.[16,17]

Predrilling through cortical bone and use of proper surgical protocols can effectively prevent orthodontic implant fracture.

Injury of periodontal tissue

Orthodontic implants placed in interdental areas can cause direct or indirect injury to periodontal tissue (Figs 5-36 to 5-38). Root injury during implantation is rare but is often fatal to the tooth. The root damage itself may be reversible,[18,19] but the root can be cracked by an implant, which could give rise to irreversible damage of periodontal attachments.[6] Strict adherence to the suggested protocol for preventing root damage completely avoids these problems.

Infection and abscess

Once an abscess is found, an incision should be made and drainage should be performed; antibiotics should also be prescribed. At this time, if the patient does not feel any discomfort or pain, does not show any general signs indicating infection, and the neighboring periodontal tissues are sound, the orthodontic implant does not have to be removed (Figs 5-39 to 5-41). However, if the neighboring periodontal tissues are disrupted, the ortho-

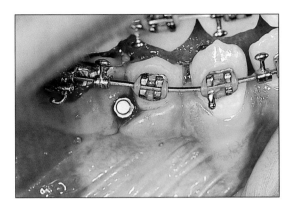

Fig 5-36a The orthodontic implant has come into contact with the tooth root after the teeth moved intrusively and distally.

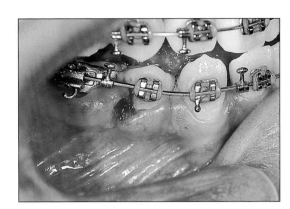

Fig 5-36b The implant has been removed. After the implant was removed, a normal probing depth was confirmed. Because anatomic structures, such as alveolar bone and tooth roots, are three-dimensional structures, the orthodontic implants rarely come into direct contact with the roots of the teeth during oblique insertion. Even if they do make contact, the damage may be resolved spontaneously.

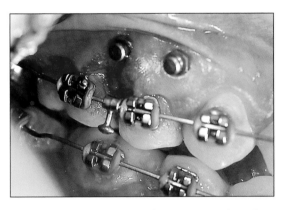

Fig 5-37 Oral hygiene has not been maintained, resulting in severe gingivitis.

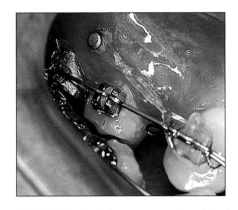

Fig 5-38 Elastic chains are apt to deposit food materials, and they hinder oral hygiene measures.

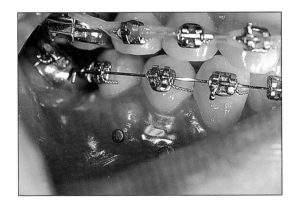

Fig 5-39 If an abscess is formed in the tissue surrounding the orthodontic implant, periodontal examinations should be performed with a periodontal probe. In this case, all adjacent teeth are sound, and the abscess is limited to the gingival tissue. Incision and drainage will be performed, and systemic antibiotics will be prescribed. The orthodontic implant will not be removed.

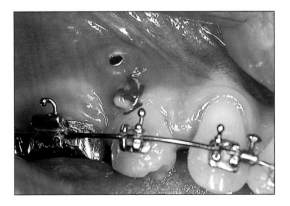

Fig 5-40 An abscess has formed and pus is being discharged through the adjacent tissue. Because the probing depth is within normal limits, the abscess will be resolved through incision and drainage and administration of systemic antibiotics. The orthodontic implant will not be removed.

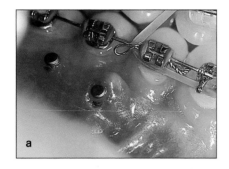

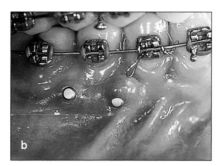

Fig 5-41a An abscess has formed and will be treated with incision and drainage and administration of systemic antibiotics.

Fig 5-41b The lesion has transformed to chronic inflammation. Because the patient has reported no pain, the orthodontic implant will not be removed.

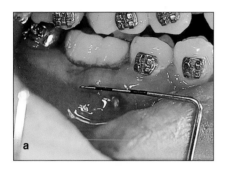

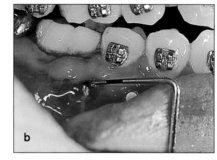

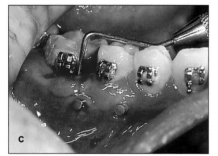

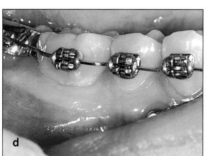

Figs 5-42a to 5-42d An abscess has formed and discharged purulent exudate in the area of the adjacent tooth. (a) During probing, the probe tip contacts the orthodontic implant because of the breakdown of the alveolar bone. (b) Destruction of the buccal bone at 5 mm from the implant. (c) The orthodontic implant will be removed and curettage will be performed. (d) At follow-up, the probing depth is within normal limits and the periodontal tissue shows normal conditions.

dontic implant should be removed immediately (Fig 5-42). In all cases, hygienic care of the surrounding tissue must be maintained.

Damage to anatomic structures

Anatomic structures can be injured by implants, so operators should be well acquainted with the anatomy of the insertion site (Fig 5-43).

Damage to adjacent soft tissue

Because of the physical irritation produced by the head of the implant, soft tissue such as the inner side of cheek may be damaged (Figs 5-44 to 5-46). In particular, the labial mucosa near the six anterior teeth, where many muscles are distributed, is apt to be damaged (Fig 5-47).

In some cases, aphthous ulcerations may arise from stress during the implantation procedure. Covering the head portion (Fig 5-48) and application of ointment are appropriate ways to heal the lesions; in most cases, the lesions heal spontaneously after 1 to 2 weeks.

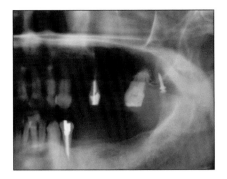

Fig 5-43a An implant was inserted on the maxillary tuberosity, but the panoramic radiograph has revealed that the implant is inside the sinus.

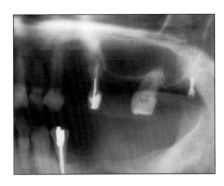

Fig 5-43b The implant has been removed and reinserted at a different position, and the patient has been instructed not to blow her nose. There are no objective or subjective symptoms, and no problems related to this issue have been found.

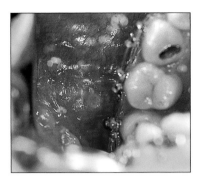

Fig 5-44 Ulcerations have resulted in the cheek area because of irritation from the head of an orthodontic implant. If the orthodontic implant is placed before the general orthodontic appliances, such as brackets, the patient should be informed of these potential side effects in advance.

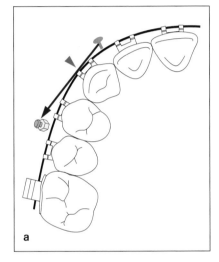

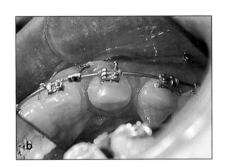

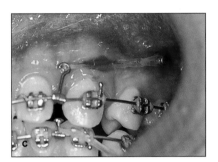

Figs 5-45a to 5-45c Because of the curvature of the alveolar bone surface, an elastic chain can injure the gingival tissue or alveolar bone. (*Arrowhead* indicates where the elastic chain is too close to the soft tissue.)

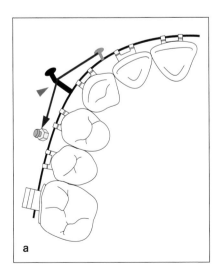

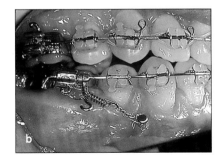

Figs 5-46a and 5-46b Crimped hooks such as a lever arm can prevent the type of impairment shown in Fig 5-45. (*Arrowhead* indicates where the lever arm holds the elastic chain away from the soft tissue.)

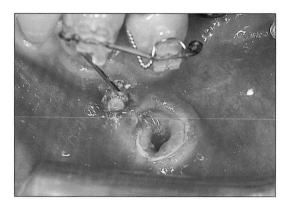

Fig 5-47 If exposure of the head portion is large and the muscular activity is high, the area of damage may be larger. In this case, the head of the implant can be covered with flowable resin to reduce discomfort. The orthodontic implant must be removed if the patient continues to complain of pain.

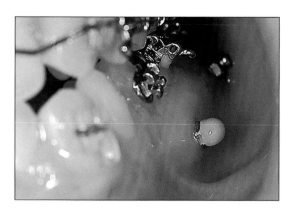

Fig 5-48 Covering the head portion with flowable resin reduces patient discomfort. If the flowable resin is to be removed, a high-speed engine must be used instead of a low-speed engine.

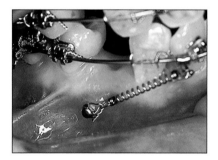

Fig 5-49 If the head is sufficiently exposed and oral hygiene is well maintained, even if the orthodontic implant is placed in the mucosal area, treatment may proceed without problems.

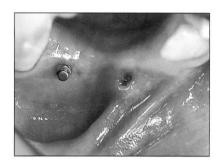

Fig 5-50 The edentulous ridge has been resorbed so that the vestibular height is reduced. If the vestibular height is shallow, the orthodontic implant is likely to be buried in gingival tissue.

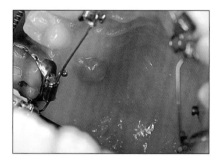

Fig 5-51 Problems associated with soft tissue seldom occur in the palatal interdental area because this area has a thick, keratinized gingiva. If problems arise after incision of the soft tissue, the head of the orthodontic implant should be exposed and treatment can be continued with a nickel-titanium coil spring. Soft tissue problems in the palatal interdental area rarely progress further.

Orthodontic implant covered with soft tissue

If the orthodontic implant is inserted too deeply for any reason, the head of the orthodontic implant may be buried (Figs 5-49 to 5-51). When the head is buried, inflammatory hypertrophy can arise because of poor oral hygiene and because the head of the orthodontic implant is covered. If the hypertrophy does not show any signs of infection, the patient will experience no pain. Therefore, after administration of minimal anesthetic, the operator makes an incision to expose the head of the implant and treatment should then be continued with a nickel-titanium coil spring, not elastic chains (Figs 5-52 and 5-53).

Pain during implantation

Incomplete anesthesia may allow the patient to experience too much pain. Even with adequate anesthesia, other remaining sensations can be mistaken for pain. With local anesthesia, the sense of pain should disappear, but the sense of touch usually does not. The anxiety of a patient may also decrease his or her pain threshold.

There is no definite evidence that pain from a procedure indicates contact between roots and implants. Adherence to the standard protocols for reducing root injuries during implantation can relieve orthodontists from anxiety regarding root injuries.

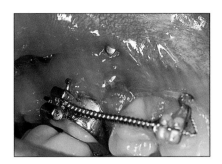

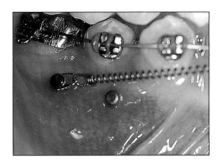

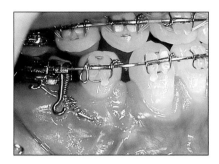

Fig 5-52a If exposure of the head of the implant is inadequate, an elastic chain is not suitable because oral hygiene becomes difficult.

Fig 5-52b If the implant head is poorly exposed, the nickel-titanium coil spring is better because it is more hygienic.

Fig 5-52c With the nickel-titanium coil spring, even if soft tissue covers the head of the orthodontic implant, treatment can continue without problems.

Figs 5-53a and 5-53b Orthodontic implants have been placed on the distal area of the maxillary canines to allow application of vertical forces to intrude the anterior teeth. Most patients complain of implants in this area, so exposure of the head portion in the area must be minimized and the orthodontic implant should be placed deeply. The soft tissue shows poor conditions.

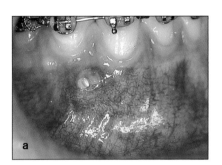

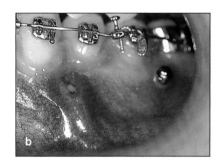

Figs 5-53c and 5-53d Because the orthodontic implants are placed in the mucosal area, treatment is continued with nickel-titanium coil springs.

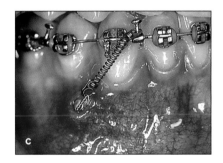

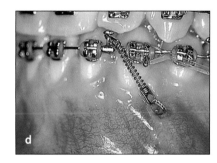

If the patient feels pain in the mandibular premolar areas, infiltration anesthetic is especially necessary on the corresponding areas of the lingual side; otherwise block anesthetic of the mandibular alveolar nerve is needed.

Pain during mastication

Pain during mastication indicates impairment of the periodontal membrane. The use of periapical radiographs at different horizontal angles is helpful for differential diagnosis, but this method is not always effective. In other words, visual proximity between the roots of the teeth and the orthodontic implant in periapical radiographs does not always indicate actual contact between the two structures.

Above all, adherence to a standardized procedure can give the clinician confidence that the root is not damaged. The patient should be informed that the situation is not exceptional and that even if the area is injured, the injury is reversible. The orthodontist should observe the healing state and may prescribe an analgesic. In most cases, impairment localized in the periodontal membrane and injuries limited to the root are reversible.

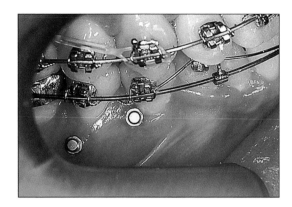

Fig 5-54 Orthodontic implants have been placed for distalization of the whole dentition. One of the orthodontic implants has been placed in an inappropriate area that impedes tooth movement, so the amount of distalization is limited.

Implantation in an inappropriate area

If the treatment plan involves the movement of adjacent teeth, it is very important that the orthodontic implant be placed in an appropriate area so that it does not impede tooth movement along the alveolar bone (Fig 5-54). Precise placement in a proper area is most important, and, according to the circumstances, placement in a site other than that originally planned may be considered.

SUMMARY

The use of orthodontic implants to facilitate orthodontic treatment is becoming universal. Surgical procedures for implantation of orthodontic mini-implants should be based on the following principles: *(1)* Aseptic principle; *(2)* atraumatic procedures; *(3)* thorough preoperative examination and precise implant positioning; *(4)* premedication for pain control; and *(5)* standardized surgical procedures. These standardized surgical procedures involve a five-stage approach: *(1)* Preoperative examination stage; *(2)* marking stage; *(3)* perforating stage; *(4)* guiding stage; and *(5)* finishing stage. Strict adherence to the recommended protocols, in particular the protocol for prevention of root injuries, will help to ensure the success of the orthodontic mini-implant.

REFERENCES

1. Brånemark PI, Zarb GA, Albrektsson T. Tissue-Integrated Prostheses: Osseointegration in Clinical Dentistry. Chicago: Quintessence, 1985:130–136.
2. Sharawy M, Misch CE, Weller N, Tehemar S. Heat generation during implant drilling: The significance of motor speed. J Oral Maxillofac Surg 2002;60:1160–1169.
3. Iyer S, Weiss C, Mehta A. Effects of drill speed on heat production and the rate and quality of bone formation in dental implant osteotomies. Part II: Relationship between drill speed and healing. Int J Prosthodont 1997;10:536–540.
4. Kerawala CJ, Martin IC, Allan W, Williams ED. The effects of operator technique and bur design on temperature during osseous preparation for osteosynthesis self-tapping screws. Oral Surg Oral Med Oral Pathol Oral Radiol Endod 1999;88:145–150.
5. Tehemar SH. Factors affecting heat generation during implant site preparation: A review of biologic observations and future considerations. Int J Oral Maxillofac Implants 1999;14:127–136.
6. Lee JS. Development of Orthodontic Mini-Implant Anchorage System. Pre-Conference: Basic Researches on Implant Orthodontics. The 4th Asian Implant Orthodontics Conference, Seoul, Korea, December 3–4, 2005.
7. Brunski JB, Puleo DA, Nanci A. Biomaterials and biomechanics of oral and maxillofacial implants: Current status and future developments. Int J Oral Maxillofac Implants 2000;15:15–46.
8. Sowden D, Schmitz JP. AO self-drilling and self-tapping screws in rat calvarial bone: An ultrastructural study of the implant interface. J Oral Maxillofac Surg 2002;60:294–299.
9. Heidemann W, Terheyden H, Gerlach KL. Analysis of the osseous/metal interface of drill free screws and self-tapping screws. J Craniomaxillofac Surg 2001;29:69–74.
10. Kim JW, Ahn SJ, Chang YI. Histomorphometric and mechanical analyses of the drill-free screw as orthodontic anchorage. Am J Orthod Dentofacial Orthop 2005;128:190–194.
11. Perry CR, Gilula LA. Basic principles and clinical uses of screws and bolts. Orthop Rev 1992;21:709–713.
12. Miyawaki S, Koyama I, Inoue M, Mishima K, Sugahara T, Takano-Yamamoto T. Factors associated with the stability of titanium screws placed in the posterior region for orthodontic anchorage. Am J Orthod Dentofacial Orthop 2003;124:373–378.
13. Cheng SJ, Tseng IY, Lee JJ, Kok SH. A prospective study of the risk factors associated with failure of mini-implants used for orthodontic anchorage. Int J Oral Maxillofac Implants 2004;29:100–106.
14. Ottoni JM, Oliveira ZF, Mansini R, Cabral AM. Correlation between placement torque and survival of single-tooth implants. Int J Oral Maxillofac Implants 2005;20:769–776.
15. Motoyoshi M, Hirabayashi M, Uemura M, Shimizu N. Recommended placement torque when tightening an orthodontic mini-implant. Clin Oral Implants Res 2006;17:109–114.
16. Simon SR. Orthopaedic Basic Science, ed 1. Chicago: American Academy of Orthopaedic Surgeons, 1994:467–470.
17. Brånemark PI, Zarb GA, Albrektsson T. Tissue-Integrated Prostheses: Osseointegration in Clinical Dentistry. Chicago: Quintessence, 1985:137–140.
18. Asscherickx K, Vannet BV, Wehrbein H, Sabzevar MM. Root repair after injury from mini-screw. Clin Oral Implants Res 2005;16:575–578.
19. Roberts WE, Helm FR, Marshall KJ, Gongloff RK. Rigid endosseous implants for orthodontic and orthopedic anchorage. Angle Orthod 1989;59:247–56.

MECHANICS AND LIMITATIONS 6

MECHANICS OF THE NEW TYPE OF ANCHORAGE

The orthodontic mini-implant has two major characteristics that affect the mechanics of this new anchorage system (Fig 6-1):

1. Similar to an ankylosed tooth (see Fig 6-1b) or a prosthodontic implant (see Fig 6-1c), the new type of anchorage does not move.[1] Because the orthodontic force is not applied from the dentition but from the orthodontic implant, undesirable movement in reaction to applied force can be avoided.
2. The anchorage unit is generally located in the apical area between the teeth (Fig 6-2). Intrusive mechanics can be applied more easily because of the positioning of the mini-implants.

Mechanics based on rigid orthodontic anchorage

Because the problems related to anchorage are reduced, the mechanics become simpler. Additionally, teeth can be moved more efficiently because force can be applied directly in the direction of the position indicated by the treatment objectives. Fundamentally, the force system with implants has consistent single forces, and the efficiency of the mechanics is improved.

Collective and three-dimensional movement

The entire dentition can be moved at one time because the problems related to anchorage are resolved. Moreover, the teeth can be simultaneously moved three-dimensionally for several treatment objectives.

Asymmetric movement

In conventional treatment, teeth were used as anchorage units, which made asymmetric movement of the teeth very difficult. However, the orthodontic implant provides rigid anchorage and simplifies control of asymmetric mechanics.

Mechanics based on the apical implant position

Conventional edgewise mechanics are mostly extrusive mechanics.[2] In general, during the movement of the tooth, it is likely that an extrusive force vector will be produced. However, the mechanics with the orthodontic mini-implant can be intrusive. Therefore, the intrusive movement thought to be difficult in conventional edgewise treatment can be easily achieved with mini-implants.

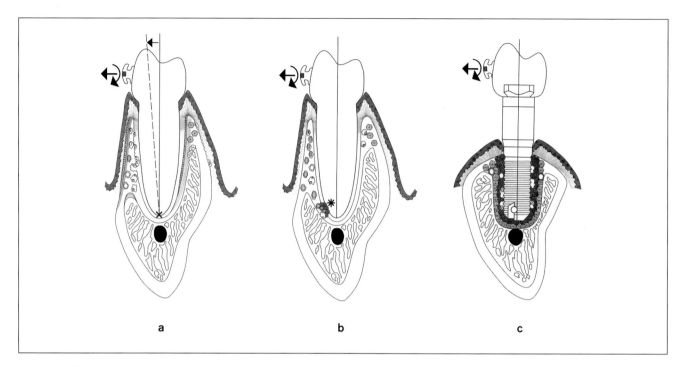

Fig 6-1 In all cases, applied energy should be delivered identically to the adjacent tissues. *(a)* If orthodontic force is applied to a normal tooth, a continuous periodontal ligament allows the tooth to move relative to the basal bone. *(b)* If that orthodontic force is applied to an ankylosed tooth, the tooth will not move. Although the area of ankylosis is typically small *(asterisk)*, the lack of a continuous periodontal ligament prevents tooth movement. *(c)* An endosseous implant maintains the intense bone-remodeling response at and near the interface. Because there is no continuous periodontal ligament separating the implant from the bone, the implant does not move and is a source of rigid orthodontic anchorage. However, if the mini-implant is separated from the bone by continuous fibrous tissue, orthodontic force can move the implant.[1] (From Roberts.[1] Reprinted with permission.)

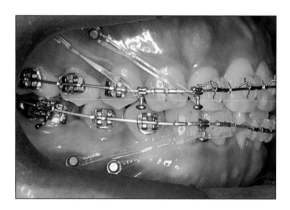

Fig 6-2 The orthodontic implant is generally placed in the apical area, a good position for the application of intrusive force.

LIMITATIONS OF TREATMENT

The new type of anchorage system has overcome the biomechanical limitations of conventional orthodontic mechanotherapy in terms of anchorage. However, this system does not resolve all of the problems related to orthodontic treatment.

Biomechanical limitations

Rotational tendency

For most treatment objectives, bodily movement is generally required, and force must be applied through the center of resistance. To apply force through the center of resistance, the point of force application should be con-

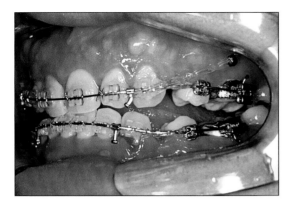

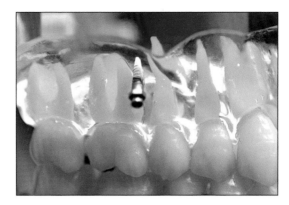

Fig 6-3 During en masse anterior retraction, canines have tipped distally, and vertical bowing has occurred as a consequence. An intrusive force vector and deflection of the wire have caused the maxillary molars to intrude. The orthodontic implant generally resolves only one-dimensional problems but does not resolve three-dimensional problems.

Fig 6-4 The orthodontic implant is generally placed between the teeth, which partially limits the mesiodistal movement of adjacent teeth.

trolled[3]; however, the possible locations of implant placement are limited. Forces away from the center of resistance produce rotation but do not produce translation.[3] Undesirable side effects may occur (Fig 6-3).

The implant itself can provide ideal orthodontic anchorage but cannot provide the ideal force system for tooth movement. Rigid anchorage is not the only factor in successful treatment; teeth should be controlled three-dimensionally with the assistance of rigid anchorage.

Implant positioning

The positioning of the orthodontic mini-implant is relatively unrestricted compared to that of other bone-supported anchorage systems. However, the implant cannot be positioned at every location in the mouth (Fig 6-4). The point of force application may be limited, and the line of action cannot be designed at random. To compensate for this weakness, indirect anchorage, attachments, or continuous arch mechanics can be used.

Interdental implants may restrict the mesiodistal movement of adjacent teeth. However, if proper protocols for surgical placement are followed, 3 mm of movement rarely causes problems.

Intrusive mechanics

The orthodontic implant placed in the interdental area is beneficial for retractive and intrusive mechanics but is un-

favorable for pushing and extrusive mechanics. Basically, mechanics with the orthodontic implant are intrusive, and the retractive mechanics are the intrinsic limitation.

An intrusive force vector from implants may cause side effects that have not occurred with conventional mechanics, and unwanted intrusion is a possibility (Figs 6-5 and 6-6).

Conventional extrusive mechanics, such as maxillomandibular elastics, are very useful in conjunction with intrusive mechanics from implants. These can provide synergistic effects to increase the efficiency of treatment.

Extrusive mechanics can be designed with implants. Indirect anchorage (Fig 6-7), push springs (Figs 6-8 and 6-9), and lever arm mechanics (Fig 6-10) can be used for extrusive mechanics.

Force threshold

It is likely that an orthodontic mini-implant can withstand approximately 200 to 400 mg of orthodontic force, depending on the bone conditions and the diameters of the mini-implants.[4-8] The interface between bone tissue and the orthodontic implant is weak to impact stress, so orthodontic application may be limited.[9] If two implants are splinted or extra implants are placed, more force can be used in treatment (Fig 6-11).

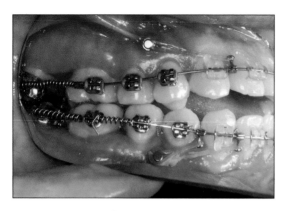

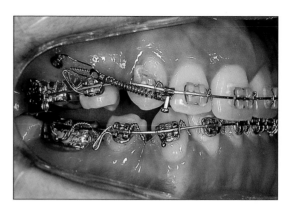

Fig 6-5a An intrusive force does not always have favorable results. In a patient who did not undergo orthodontic tooth extraction, the anterior occlusion has been opened by the retractive force generated by implants, which contains an intrusive force vector.

Fig 6-5b In a case involving extraction treatment, the first molar has been intruded by retractive force from implants.

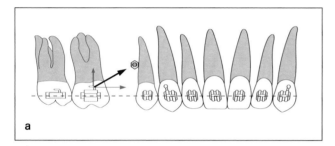

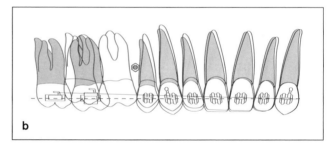

Figs 6-6a and 6-6b It would be extremely hazardous if the intrusive effects of orthodontic implants occurred on only one side. When **(a)** the posterior teeth are protracted unilaterally or in a unilateral extraction case, **(b)** occlusal plane canting can occur. This is very difficult to correct.

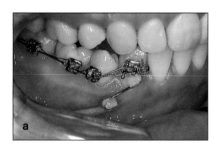

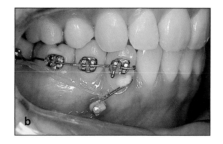

Figs 6-7a and 6-7b Orthodontic implant anchorage can be used as indirect anchorage to generate extrusive mechanics.

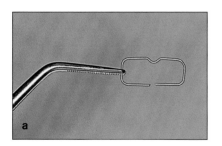

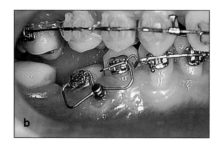

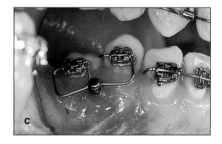

Figs 6-8a to 6-8c Orthodontic implant anchorage can be used for extrusive mechanics if a push spring is inserted between the teeth and the orthodontic implant. Maxillomandibular elastics were ineffectual because of the poor cooperation of the patient. Therefore, a spring for extrusion **(a)** has been made of 0.018-inch TMA wire and **(b)** inserted beneath the button of the orthodontic implant. **(c)** The first premolar has been extruded by the spring on the implant. The second premolar is ankylosed.

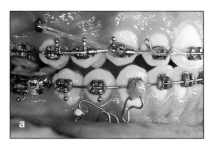

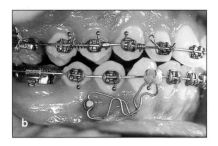

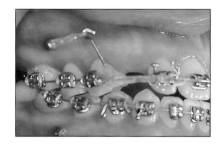

Figs 6-9a and 6-9b The mandibular canine is moved in the occlusal and mesial directions by the effect of a push spring made of 0.018-inch TMA wire connected to an implant.

Fig 6-10 The lever arm can be designed to have an extrusive force vector.

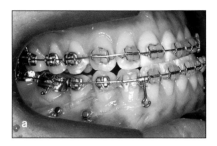

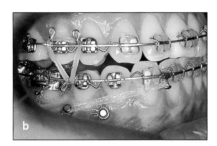

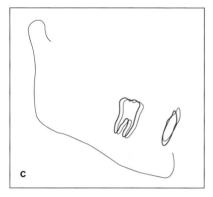

Figs 6-11a to 6-11c Two implants have been placed on each side to apply 700 g of force for distalization of the entire dentition.

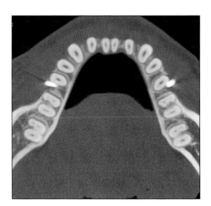

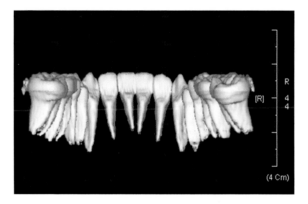

Fig 6-12a The retraction of mandibular incisors is limited within the lingual cortical bone. The mandibular incisors in this patient are out of the alveolar process; therefore, further retraction is impossible.

Fig 6-12b Fortunately, despite their location outside the alveolar process, the incisors exhibit no root resorption.

Biologic limitations

Movement within the alveolar trough
Tooth movement should take place within the alveolar trough, as in all mechanotherapy[10–13] (Fig 6-12).

Orthopedic effects
Much research has been conducted regarding orthopedic treatment using implants.[14–17] However, clinical guidelines for orthopedic treatment using mini-implants have not yet been established. Moreover, controversy remains concerning the amount of force needed to achieve an orthopedic effect.[18,19]

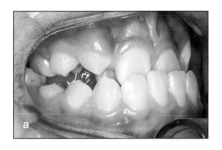

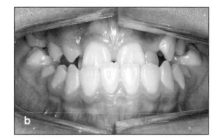

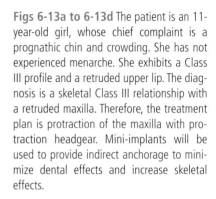

Figs 6-13a to 6-13d The patient is an 11-year-old girl, whose chief complaint is a prognathic chin and crowding. She has not experienced menarche. She exhibits a Class III profile and a retruded upper lip. The diagnosis is a skeletal Class III relationship with a retruded maxilla. Therefore, the treatment plan is protraction of the maxilla with protraction headgear. Mini-implants will be used to provide indirect anchorage to minimize dental effects and increase skeletal effects.

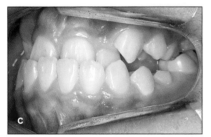

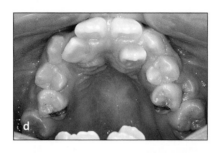

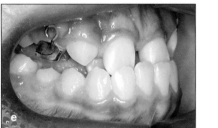

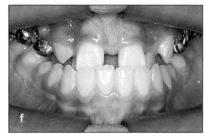

Figs 6-13e to 6-13h After rapid maxillary expansion is accomplished, the expansion area is splinted with mini-implants and resin composite. Then, maxillary protraction is performed using a facemask.

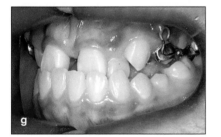

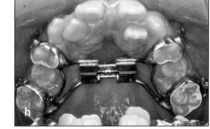

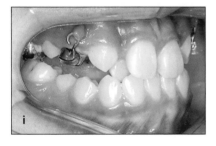

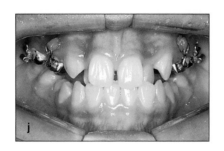

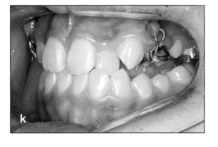

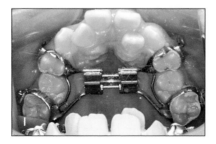

Figs 6-13i to 6-13l After 2 months of protraction, the anterior crossbite is corrected.

Figs 6-13m and 6-13n Although mini-implants have been used to minimize dental effects, the maxillary molars are extruded. Orthopedic effects are not significant compared to conventional facemask treatment. *(black)* Before retraction; *(purple)* after retraction.

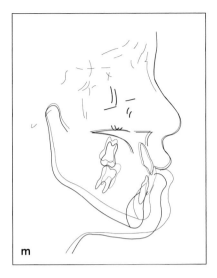

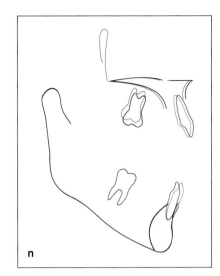

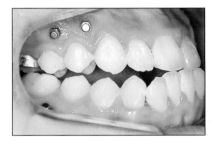

Fig 6-14a The postmenarche patient has an anterior edge-to-edge occlusion. Maxillary protraction with orthodontic implants was attempted. Four orthodontic implants have been placed to maximize the orthopedic effect and to minimize the dental side effects.

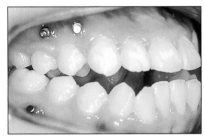

Fig 6-14b A labiolingual appliance was firmly connected to the orthodontic implants using resin, and protraction headgear was designed with 800 g of protraction force on each side. Appearance after 6 months of protraction.

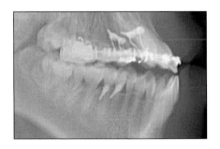

Fig 6-14c Cephalometric radiograph at the beginning of protraction.

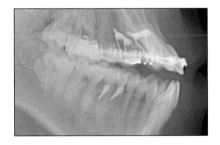

Fig 6-14d Cephalometric radiograph after 6 months of protraction. Because of the lack of orthopedic effect, the treatment has been discontinued and the labiolingual appliance removed. None of the orthodontic implants show any mobility.

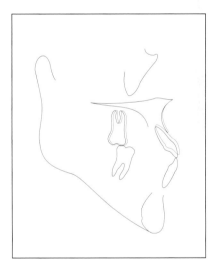

Fig 6-14e Superimposition before protraction *(black)*; after 6 months of protraction *(red)*. There has been little orthopedic effect on the body of the maxilla, despite good cooperation from the patient. Because orthodontic implants have been used as indirect anchorage, minor movement of the teeth has occurred.

Mini-implants are capable of applying orthopedic treatment in two ways. The first is direct application of orthopedic force to implants[17]; the second is splinting of teeth by indirect application to minimize tooth movement, a side effect of orthopedic treatment[4] (Figs 6-13 and 6-14). There are few established protocols regarding orthopedic treatment with mini-implants. More studies are required to clarify whether skeletal growth can be modified by

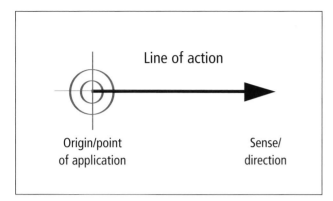

Fig 6-15 A force is a vector that has both magnitude and direction. Force vectors are characterized by their magnitude, line of action, point of application, and direction. By changing the point of application, the operator can control the line of action to obtain the type of movement that has been planned.

Table 6-1	Characteristics of the mechanics of force-driven and shape-driven appliances	
Characteristic	Force-driven appliance	Shape-driven appliance
Engagement into brackets	At least one point contact at one side	Insertion at both sides
Precise control	Possible	Impossible
Treatment efficiency	High	Low
Treatment simplicity	Low	High
Anchorage control	Favorable	Unfavorable
	Technique sensitive	Not technique sensitive
	Not fail-safe	Fail-safe

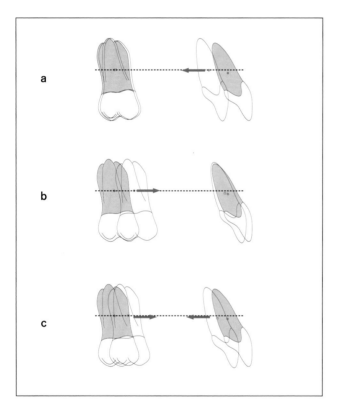

Fig 6-16 In tooth movement, there is an active unit and a reactive unit. The active unit is a part that is being moved for treatment objectives. The reactive unit is an anchor part used for moving the active part. Depending on the treatment objective, slight movement of the reactive unit may be permitted. *(a)* For example, in a patient with bialveolar protrusion, anterior teeth are the active unit and posterior teeth are the reactive unit. *(b)* In the patient with a balanced profile, posterior teeth are the active unit and anterior teeth are the reactive unit. *(c)* In the patient with moderate protrusion, anterior teeth are the active unit and reactive unit at the same time. *(red arrows)* Movement of the active unit.

treatment with orthodontic implants and how the orthopedic effects can be maximized. Studies for long-term stability are also required.

Complications

Root injuries during surgical placement of orthodontic implants are very rare but also quite critical.[8] The protocol for prevention of root injury avoids these problems.

In addition, the orthodontic implant can move teeth further. Therefore, there is an increase in the possibility of root resorption or periodontal problems related to orthodontic mechanotherapy.

CLASSIFICATION OF MECHANICS

Orthodontic mechanotherapy should be based on biologic and biomechanical principles[20,21] (Figs 6-15 and 6-16). Conventional mechanics can be classified into two groups[21–24] (Table 6-1 and Figs 6-17 to 6-20):

1. *Force-driven mechanics*, which have a statically determinate force system. With a statically determinate force system, the entire force system can be calculated by the use of the principles of statics or equilibrium.

Figs 6-17a and 6-17b In force-driven mechanics, the force is applied as a single force by one-point contact to the moving part, so that the entire force system can be precisely calculated at chairside using the principles of statics or equilibrium. *(blue arrow)* Active movement; *(red arrow)* reactive movement.

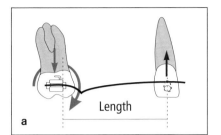

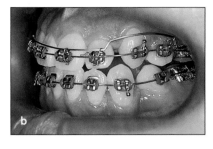

Figs 6-17c and 6-17d In shape-driven mechanics, the wire is fully engaged in the brackets both at the active and the reactive sides of the system. The forces and moments are developed at both sides and cannot be calculated directly because of interaction between force systems developed at the active or reactive unit. Because the precise force system cannot be known, precise control and adjustment are impossible. *(blue arrow)* Active movement; *(red arrow)* reactive movement.

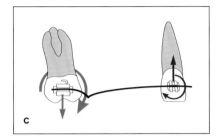

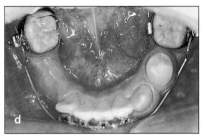

Fig 6-18a In a statically determinate force system, the force system is almost totally consistent, and the direction and amounts of forces and moments *(arrows)* are changed only slightly.

Fig 6-18b In addition to the fact that direct calculation of a full force system at chairside is impossible in a statically indeterminate force system, the fact that the force system changes continuously as teeth move may be highly problematic from the clinical point of view. The direction of the moments *(arrows)* may be changing, as are the amounts of forces and moments, which may either be beneficial to treatment or may reduce treatment efficiency.

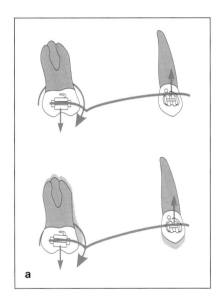

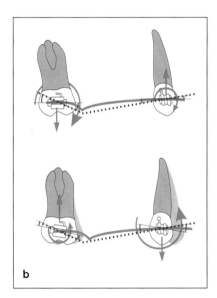

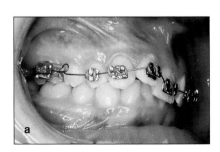

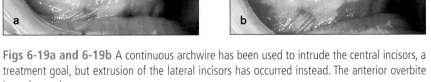

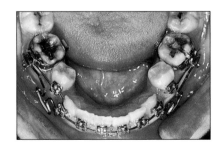

Figs 6-19a and 6-19b A continuous archwire has been used to intrude the central incisors, a treatment goal, but extrusion of the lateral incisors has occurred instead. The anterior overbite is unchanged.

Fig 6-20 In force-driven mechanics, unwanted effects occur if appliances are deformed by chewing or by other forces. Shape-driven mechanics are more reliable. The transpalatal arch was dislocated, but the patient did not come to the office for correction, and the posterior segments were severely rotated mesially as a result.

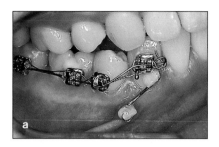
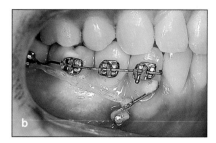

Figs 6-21a and 6-21b Shape-driven mechanics with indirect anchorage.

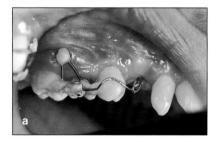
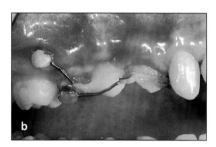

Figs 6-22a and 6-22b Force-driven mechanics with indirect anchorage.

2. *Shape-driven mechanics*, which have a statically indeterminate force system. With a statically indeterminate force system, the entire force system cannot be easily calculated because of interaction between the force systems developed at the active or reactive unit.

Shape-driven mechanics are disadvantageous with regard to biomechanics; the precise force system cannot be known. Therefore, precise control and adjustment are impossible. Moreover, the force system may change significantly as the teeth move; therefore, treatment efficiency may be reduced.[21,24] In general, sectional mechanics have a statically determinate force system and continuous arch mechanics have a statically indeterminate force system.

In shape-driven mechanics, delicate control is difficult to achieve, and the reactive force against the active force can be concentrated on adjacent teeth. In force-driven mechanics, monitoring and adjustment are complex and critical. Furthermore, depending on the force system, side effects can occur irrespective of the type of mechanics.

An extraoral appliance is useful if it is used full time and the applied force is precisely controlled. Because it has an unchanging force system and is a form of stationary anchorage, the extraoral appliance increases treatment efficiency. Basically, retractive forces and pushing forces from implants are similar to those derived from extraoral appliances. The point of applied force can be

controlled by changing the implant insertion site, to control the direction of action. Implants can also be used to compensate for the side effects of conventional mechanics. Moreover, with implants, mechanics that have advantages of both systems can be devised. Clinically, the mechanics designed with mini-implants can be classified into five groups:

1. Shape-driven mechanics with indirect anchorage (Fig 6-21): Because of the indirect anchorage achieved with implants, unwanted tooth movement can be minimized.
2. Force-driven mechanics with indirect anchorage (Fig 6-22): This type of mechanics is similar to shape-driven mechanics with indirect anchorage.
3. Force-driven mechanics with direct anchorage, type I (Figs 6-23 and 6-24): This type of mechanics consists of only single forces from implants. A single force causes uncontrolled tipping, but, if these single forces are combined, the type of tooth movement can be controlled.
4. Force-driven mechanics with direct anchorage, type II (Fig 6-25): These are single forces from implants to anchor teeth in a force system with this type of mechanics. However, there may be unfavorable movement of anchor teeth. This type of mechanics is rarely seen in clinical situations.

Figs 6-23a and 6-23b Force-driven mechanics with direct anchorage, type I: A single force causes uncontrolled tipping.

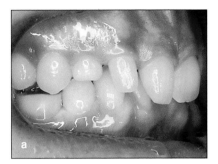
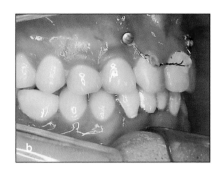

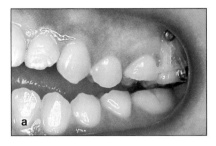
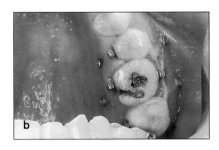
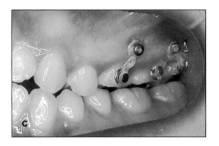

Figs 6-24a to 6-24c Force-driven mechanics with direct anchorage, type I: Translation can be obtained by combining single forces.

Fig 6-25 Force-driven mechanics with direct anchorage, type II: For a sectional arch, indirect anchorage is more appropriate.

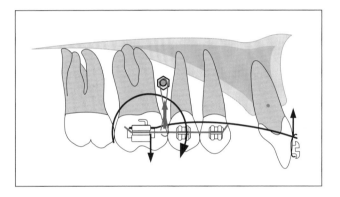

Figs 6-26a and 6-26b Combined mechanics. **(a)** Shape-driven mechanics were used on the labial side, and **(b)** force-driven mechanics were used on the lingual side.

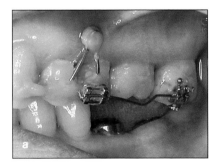
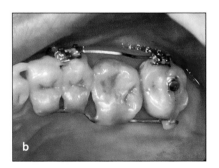

5. Combined mechanics with direct anchorage (Fig 6-26): This group of mechanics is similar to continuous arch mechanics with an extraoral appliance. To incorporate consistent single force into shape-driven mechanics, combined mechanics with direct anchorage can have the advantages of both systems. That is, a single force from implants increases treatment efficiency, and continuous arch mechanics can make treatment simple and fail-safe.

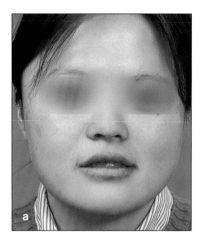

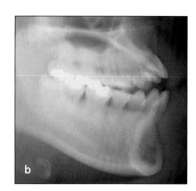

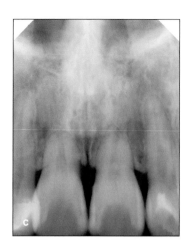

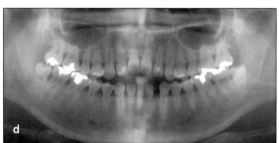

Figs 6-27a to 6-27d The patient is a 25-year-old woman, whose chief complaints are an anterior open bite and mandibular anterior spacing. Following consideration of facial esthetics, the decision was made to extrude the maxillary anterior teeth. Force-driven mechanics were chosen to control the force system precisely to minimize the risk of further root resorption.

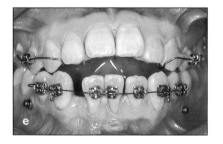

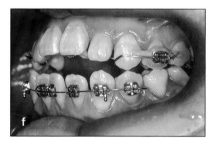

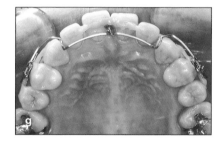

Figs 6-27e to 6-27g A cantilever extrusion spring made of 0.016 × 0.022-inch TMA wire was activated to apply 20 g of extrusion force. The spring is also tied to the button for single-point contact. Because the spring is made of TMA, it is possible to apply light continuous force.

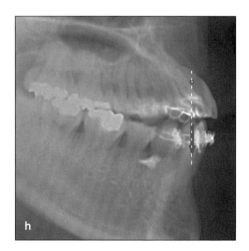

Fig 6-27h A cephalometric radiograph confirms the line of action.

SELECTION OF MECHANICS

The following factors should be considered during the selection of mechanics, although monitoring and adjustment are more important than the selection of mechanics.[20,21,24] Depending on the force system, side effects can occur irrespective of the type of mechanics used.

1. Treatment efficiency: The force-driven appliance is more efficient for moving teeth.
2. Force system control: Force-driven mechanics can precisely control the force system. For cases requiring precise control, force-driven mechanics should be selected (Fig 6-27).
3. Convenience: Generally, continuous arch mechanics are convenient for orthodontists and comfortable for patients.
4. Technique sensitivity: Force-driven mechanics require monitoring and precise adjustment, which require skill and experience.

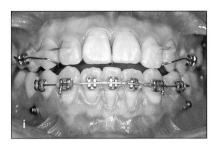
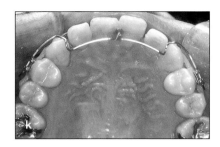
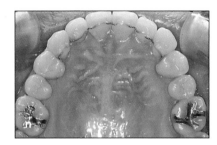

Figs 6-27i to 6-27k After extrusion of four anterior teeth, the central incisors are extruded further by the extrusion spring.

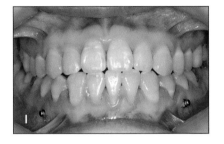
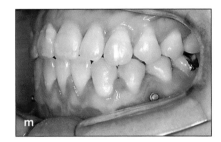
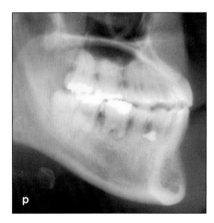

Figs 6-27l to 6-27p After treatment, the anterior vertical relationships are improved.

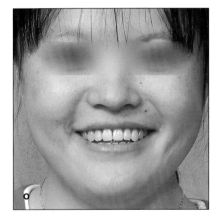

Figs 6-27q and 6-27r At the end of treatment, there is no evidence of further root resorption.

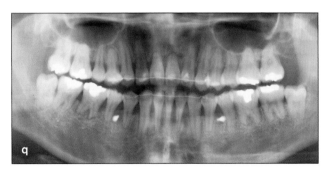
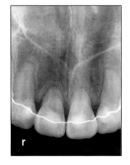

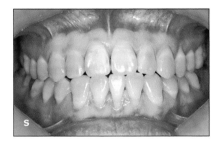
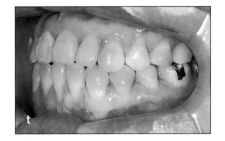
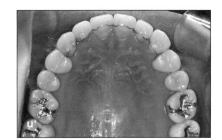

Figs 6-27s to 6-27u After 5 months of follow-up, the result is well maintained.

SIGNIFICANCE OF TREATMENT WITH ORTHODONTIC IMPLANTS

When a stable anchorage system is present, loss of anchorage is no longer a concern. This frees orthodontic mechanotherapy from the biomechanical limitations of anchorage. Thanks to orthodontic mini-implants, rigid anchorage can be easily acquired, even if no teeth remain. Treatment mechanics become simpler and less technique sensitive.

Efficiency

Based on the new type of anchorage, orthodontic treatment can be conducted more easily, and also more predictably, because treatment becomes independent of the cooperation of the patient. Furthermore, molar distalization becomes simpler even in adult patients, and it can be a very useful option for treatment of moderate crowding or camouflage treatment of anteroposterior skeletal discrepancies. Molar distalization can often eliminate the need for second premolar extraction. Therefore, the treatment period can be shortened as well.

Expanded range of orthodontic mechanotherapy

New mechanics based on rigid anchorage have expanded the range of orthodontic mechanotherapy[25] (Fig 6-28). The most drastic change is that it becomes possible to intrude posterior teeth bilaterally with mechanotherapy alone (see chapters 7 and 9). Intrusion of the posterior segment was previously considered clinically impossible because it is difficult to gain anchorage for intrusion. As molar intrusion becomes easier to obtain, vertical excess can be resolved nonsurgically. Through intrusion of the entire dentition or intrusion of the posterior teeth, mechanotherapy can indirectly change the position of the chin point, similar to surgical repositioning of the maxilla. In other words, nonsurgical mechanotherapy can change the relationship between the basal bones.

Orthodontic mini-implants have not changed the envelope of anterior tooth movement, but their use allows posterior teeth to be controlled vertically using only mechanotherapy.[26,27] The entire posterior segment, as well as the posterior teeth, can be intruded; this allows control of anterior facial height. It also becomes possible to distalize the entire posterior segment, so that the orthodontic extraction rate will be decreased. Several studies to expand the lateral movement envelope of the posterior teeth have been conducted, but no definite conclusion has been drawn regarding the lateral envelope.[28]

Stable anchorage

Obtaining orthodontic anchorage is particularly difficult in adult patients with severe periodontal disease. Removable appliances can be used to solve such problems, but they tend to be ineffective (Fig 6-29). The orthodontic mini-implant can provide sufficient orthodontic anchorage, regardless of the condition of the dentition (Fig 6-30).

Simplified treatment

In general, for adjunctive orthodontic treatment, movement of only one or two teeth is required; movement of the other teeth is undesirable. For this situation, delicate and precise anchorage control is indispensable (Fig 6-31). If orthodontic implants are used as anchorage, the treatment can be simplified and the expertise of the orthodontists has little influence on anchorage control (Fig 6-32).

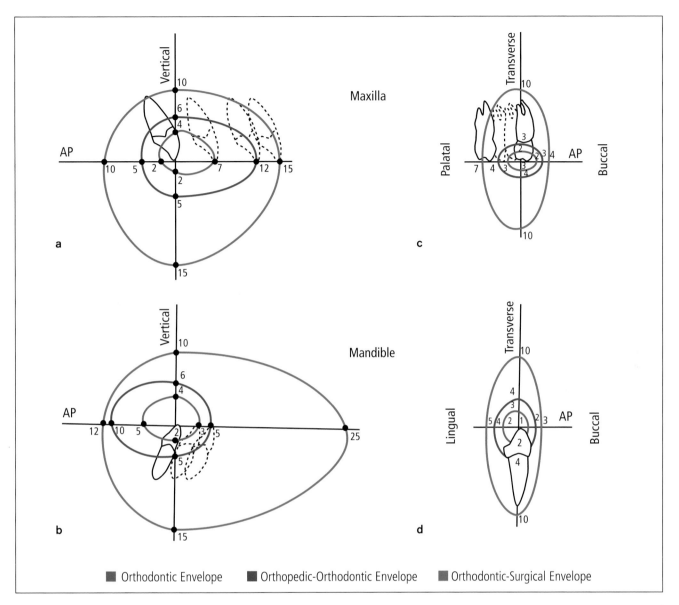

■ Orthodontic Envelope ■ Orthopedic-Orthodontic Envelope ■ Orthodontic-Surgical Envelope

Fig 6-28 As described by Graber et al,[25] the *envelopes of discrepancy* for the maxilla and mandible in three planes of space. The ideal position of the maxillary and mandibular incisors in the anteroposterior (AP) and vertical planes is shown in the center of the incisor diagrams *(a and b)*. The millimeters of change required to retract a protruding incisor, move forward a posteriorly positioned incisor, or extrude/intrude an incorrectly vertically positioned incisor are shown along the horizontal and vertical axes, respectively. The limits of orthodontic tooth movement alone are represented by the inner envelope; possible changes in the incisor position from combined orthopedic and orthodontic treatment in growing individuals are shown by the middle envelope; and the limits of change with combined orthodontic and surgical treatment are shown by the outer envelope.

The inner envelope for the maxilla suggests that maxillary incisors can be brought back a maximum of 7 mm by orthodontic tooth movement alone to correct protrusion but can be moved forward only 2 mm. The limit for retraction is established by the lingual cortical plate and is observed in the short term; the limit for forward movement is established by the lip and is observed in long-term stability or relapse. Maxillary incisors can be extruded 4 mm and depressed 2 mm, with the limits being observed in long-term stability rather than on initial tooth movement.

The envelopes of discrepancy for the transverse dimension in the premolar and canine areas *(c and d)* are much smaller than those for incisors in the AP plane. The transverse dimension can be crucial to long-term stability, periodontal health, and frontal dentofacial esthetics.

The orthodontic and surgical envelopes can be viewed separately for the maxilla and mandible, but the growth modification envelope is the same for both: 5 mm of growth modification in the AP plane to correct Class II malocclusion is the maximum that should be anticipated, whether occlusion is achieved by acceleration of mandibular growth or restriction of maxillary growth. The outer envelope suggests that 10 mm is the limit for surgical maxillary advancement or downward movement, although the maxilla can be retracted or moved up as much as 15 mm; the mandible can be surgically set back 25 mm but can be advanced only 12 mm.

These numbers are merely guidelines and underestimate or overestimate the possibilities for any given patient; however, they help place the potential of the three major treatment modalities in perspective. (From Graber et al.[25] Reprinted with permission.)

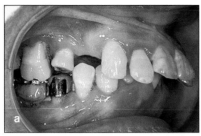

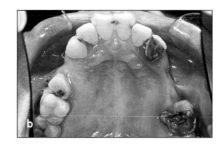

Figs 6-29a and 6-29b The vertical dimension is collapsed with posterior bite collapse, and the anterior teeth protrude in sequence. Because the periodontal conditions are not healthy and there are few teeth, anchorage cannot be secured from the teeth. Therefore, tissue-borne anchorage will be used.

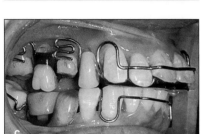

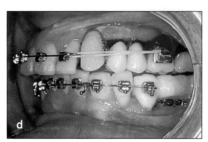

Figs 6-29c and 6-29d A removable appliance is used as anchorage so that the maxillary posterior teeth are extruded to restore the posterior bite. A removable appliance is also used as anchorage to retract the anterior teeth.

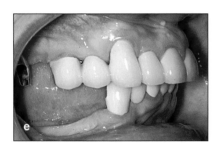

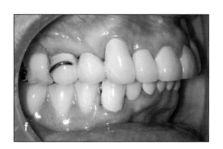

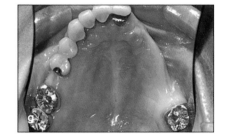

Figs 6-29e to 6-29g Following orthodontic treatment, prosthodontic treatment is completed.

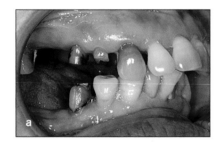

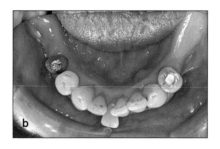

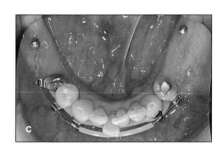

Figs 6-30a and 6-30b The situation is almost the same as that shown in Fig 6-29. Prepros-thetic orthodontic treatment is necessary; however, it is difficult to obtain saggital anchorage from the dentition alone.

Fig 6-30c The orthodontic implants are placed in the edentulous areas and used as anchorage for distalization of the teeth.

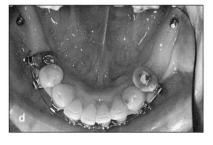

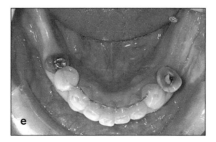

Figs 6-30d and 6-30e After space is gained by distalization of the premolars, the anterior teeth are aligned.

Figs 6-30f and 6-30g After the orthodontic treatment is completed, missing teeth are restored with a removable partial denture.

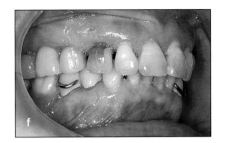

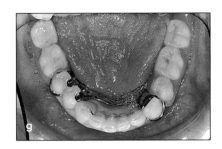

Figs 6-31a and 6-31b Because the first and second molars are missing, the third molar is important to prosthodontic treatment. To allow restoration of missing teeth with a fixed partial denture, the treatment plan is to protract the third molar to the second molar position and maintain the other teeth in their current positions.

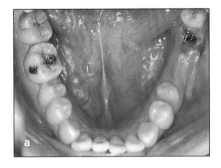

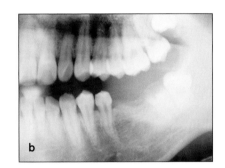

Figs 6-31c and 6-31d To reinforce anchorage, the following techniques are used: crossarch splinting from canine to canine by 0.016 × 0.022-inch SS wire, splinting from canine to second premolar by 0.019 × 0.025-inch SS wire, the Burstone T-loop to control the moment-to-force ratio, and minimal protraction force. The A-type T-loop is used first to control the root position of the third molar. The C-type T-loop is then used to control the anterior anchorage unit.

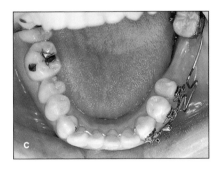

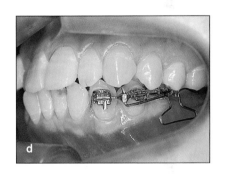

Figs 6-31e and 6-31f Without undesirable movement of the other teeth, only the third molar has been protracted by various efforts, including anchorage control, monitoring, and adjustment.

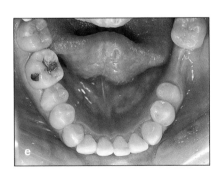

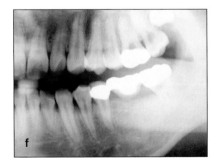

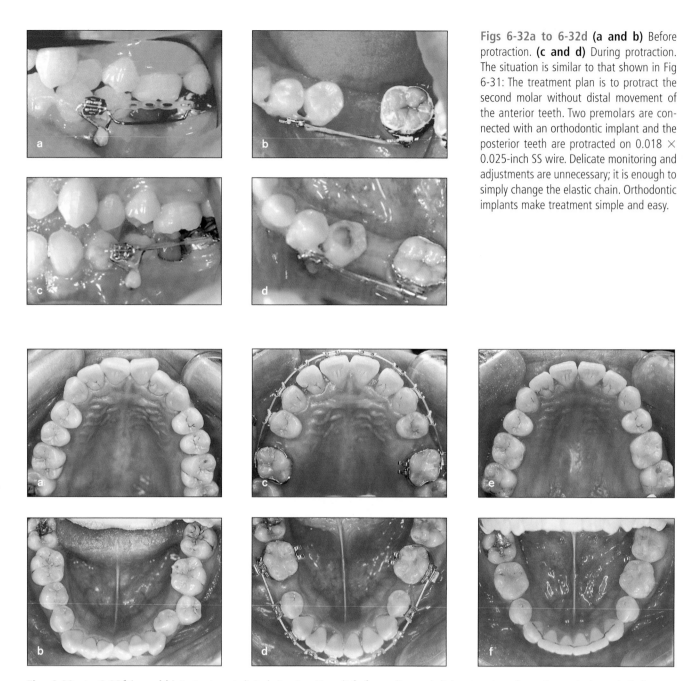

Figs 6-32a to 6-32d (a and b) Before protraction. (c and d) During protraction. The situation is similar to that shown in Fig 6-31: The treatment plan is to protract the second molar without distal movement of the anterior teeth. Two premolars are connected with an orthodontic implant and the posterior teeth are protracted on 0.018 × 0.025-inch SS wire. Delicate monitoring and adjustments are unnecessary; it is enough to simply change the elastic chain. Orthodontic implants make treatment simple and easy.

Figs 6-33a to 6-33f (a and b) Pretreatment clinical situation. For relief of crowding and slight retraction of anterior teeth, (c and d) the second premolars are extracted and sliding mechanics are used to close the extraction space. It took approximately 19 months to complete treatment (e and f).

Space gaining through distalization of posterior teeth

In adult patients, extraction of the second premolars is useful when a moderate space of about 6 mm is needed or excessive retraction of anterior teeth has to be avoided (Fig 6-33). Sometimes, however, relapse or periodontal problems occur after second premolar extraction, partic-ularly in the mandible. Moreover, in the case of second premolar extraction, more than half of the space obtained is lost by protraction of the posterior teeth. However, when an orthodontic implant is used as anchorage, the posterior teeth can be distalized predictably regardless of the cooperation of the patient. Therefore, moderate crowding can be resolved through distalization of the posterior teeth (Fig 6-34).

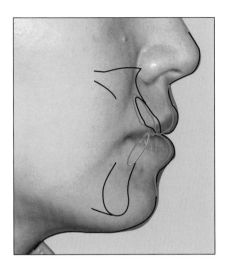

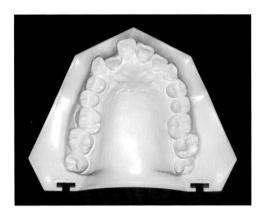

Fig 6-34a The treatment plan is to retract the upper and lower lips by 2 mm. *(black)* Pretreatment situation; *(green)* treatment objective.

Fig 6-34b To accomplish the planned retraction, the anteroposterior position of the mandibular incisor should be maintained, and the maxillary incisors should be retracted.

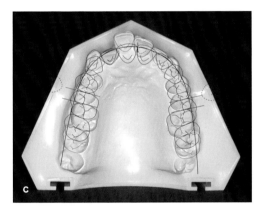

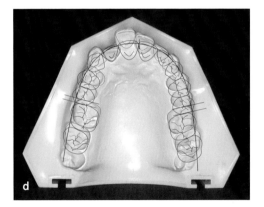

Figs 6-34c and 6-34d According to the visual treatment objective, a space of approximately 5 mm is needed in the maxillary area. **(c)** If the second premolar is to be extracted, an extraction space of 11 mm should be obtained. **(d)** However, if mini-implants are used as anchorage, a space of 5 mm can be obtained by distalization of the posterior teeth without extraction.

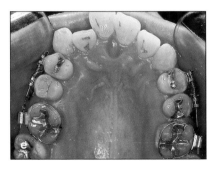

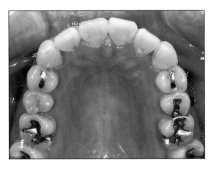

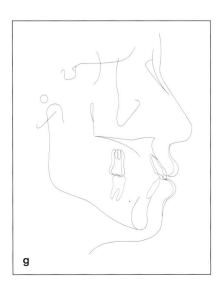

Figs 6-34e to 6-34g Through **(e)** distalization, the required space has been gained and the treatment is **(f)** finished exactly as planned according to the visual treatment objective. It took about 13 months to complete the treatment. With mini-implants, precise treatment can be performed and the duration of treatment can be shortened. **(g)** Superimposition at beginning of treatment *(black)*; at completion of treatment *(red)*.

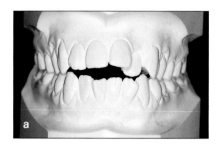

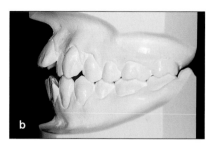

Figs 6-35a and 6-35b The patient exhibits anterior open bite, long face, and lip protrusion. The first treatment option was surgical correction of her long face. However, the patient desired orthodontic camouflage treatment. At that time, orthodontic implants were not available, so the treatment plan consisted of extraction of the four premolars and extrusion of the anterior teeth.

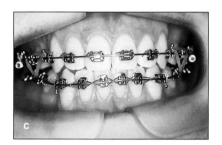

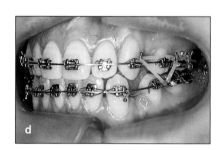

Figs 6-35c and 6-35d At that time, when the occlusal plane of the anterior teeth and that of the posterior teeth were different, an anterior extrusion was achieved more easily by leveling with continuous arch and intermaxillary elastics.

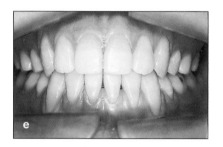

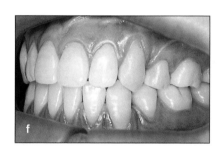

Figs 6-35e to 6-35i Because of the resulting extrusion of the anterior teeth, the smile line has worsened and the facial profile has not improved esthetically. **(e and f)** Post-treatment frontal and lateral views. Facial views **(g)** before and **(h)** after treatment. **(i)** Superimposition before treatment *(black)*; at completion of treatment *(red)*.

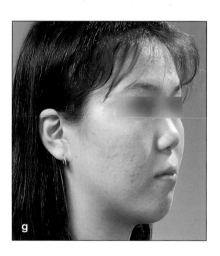

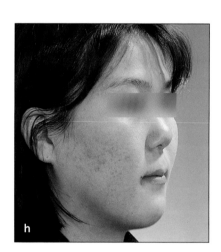

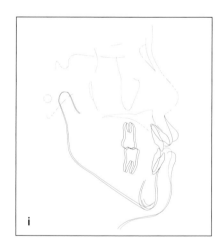

Nonsurgical correction of vertical excess

In conventional mechanotherapy, intrusion of the posterior teeth is regarded as impossible because of the biomechanical limitations of anchorage. If orthognathic surgery is not performed, an open bite should be treated by extrusion of the anterior teeth, which is referred to as *camouflage treatment* (Fig 6-35). When the orthodontic implant is used as anchorage, strong intrusive mechanics become incorporated into modern mechanotherapy, so that posterior intrusion can be performed in a predictable manner (Fig 6-36).

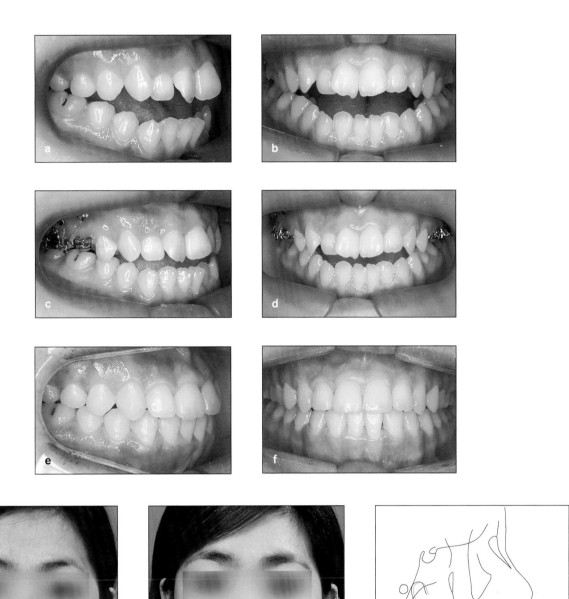

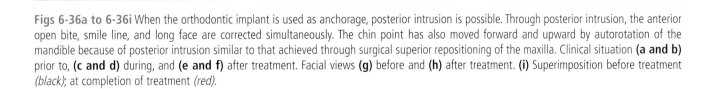

Figs 6-36a to 6-36i When the orthodontic implant is used as anchorage, posterior intrusion is possible. Through posterior intrusion, the anterior open bite, smile line, and long face are corrected simultaneously. The chin point has also moved forward and upward by autorotation of the mandible because of posterior intrusion similar to that achieved through surgical superior repositioning of the maxilla. Clinical situation **(a and b)** prior to, **(c and d)** during, and **(e and f)** after treatment. Facial views **(g)** before and **(h)** after treatment. **(i)** Superimposition before treatment *(black)*; at completion of treatment *(red)*.

CASE REPORTS

Particularly in treatment based on conventional treatment concepts, the orthodontic mini-implant anchorage system makes treatment simple and efficient.

Nonextraction treatment

The most prominent characteristic related to treatment based on conventional treatment concepts is molar distalization. The orthodontic mini-implant allows molar distalization to progress predictably. Reliable and predictable molar distalization could be very useful in the following cases:

1. Gaining moderate space without extraction of second premolars (Case 6-1)
2. Camouflage treatment of asymmetry, Class II, and Class III problems (Case 6-2)
3. Treatment of relapse (Case 6-3)

Case 6-1

A 20-year-old woman had a chief complaint of crowding in the maxillary and mandibular arches (Figs 6-37a to 6-37d). Her face exhibited normal vertical and anteroposterior relationships. An Angle Class I molar relationship, a normal overjet and overbite, and moderate crowding were observed. The treatment objectives were relief of crowding in the maxillary and mandibular dentitions and maintenance of the soft tissue profile. An increase of approximately 2.0 mm of space per quadrant was required to achieve the treatment objectives. Therefore, it was decided that the maxillary and mandibular molars would be distalized with mini-implants.

Initially, the mandibular third molars were extracted. ORLUS mini-implants (Ortholution) were then placed between the second premolar and first molar about 1.0 mm distal to an off-center position between the teeth (Figs 6-37e and 6-37f). ORLUS mini-implants of 1.8 mm in diameter and 7.0 mm in length were used for the maxilla,

while ORLUS mini-implants of 1.6 mm in diameter and 7.0 mm in length were used for the mandible.

The 0.022-inch slot preadjusted appliances were placed, and 0.018 × 0.025-inch Bioforce nickel-titanium (NiTi) wires (GAC) were engaged with the bypass of the anterior teeth. Leveling, alignment, and distalization of the second molar were performed on the initial wire. Ni-Ti open coil springs were used to distalize the second molar, and posterior retractive forces from the implants were applied to the first premolars and crimpable hooks on the wires.

After 6 weeks of treatment, 0.017 × 0.025-inch titanium-molybdenum alloy (TMA) wires (Ormco) were engaged and NiTi open coil springs were added between the second premolar and first molar to move the first molar distally. Posterior retractive forces from implants were applied to the first premolars and crimpable hooks on the wires, and a constriction curve and toe-in bend were formed in the main wire to control arch form.

After 4 months of treatment, space for alignment was secured by molar distalization, and brackets were bonded to the anterior teeth (Figs 6-37g and 6-37h). In the maxillary arch, 0.018 × 0.025-inch Bioforce NiTi wires were engaged for leveling of the canines, and NiTi open coil springs were used to maintain the anteroposterior position of the central incisor. In the mandibular arch, a 0.014-inch NiTi wire was overlaid on a 0.016 × 0.022-inch TMA wire for alignment. Posterior retractive forces from the implants were applied continuously.

After 8 months of treatment, brackets were bonded to the maxillary lateral incisors and a 0.016 × 0.022-inch Bioforce wire was placed for leveling and alignment (Figs 6-37i to 6-37l). The treatment proceeded predictably because the molars were moved to the position planned in the treatment objectives.

At 14 months, active treatment was completed to the position that had been planned (Figs 6-37m to 6-37t). Much time was spent controlling the axis of the distally tipped mandibular left canine. The root of the second premolar on the left side of the mandible did not show a significant change. A fixed retainer from first premolar to first premolar was used in the maxilla and mandible. A circumferential retainer in the maxillary arch was also worn at night.

Case 6-1   Gaining moderate space without extraction of second premolars.

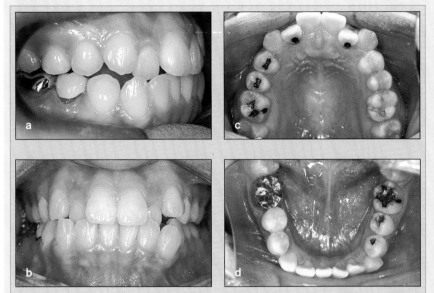

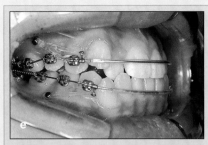

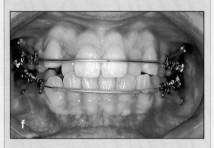

Figs 6-37a to 6-37d Clinical situation prior to treatment.

Figs 6-37e and 6-37f Beginning of treatment.

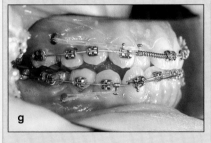

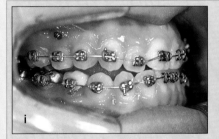

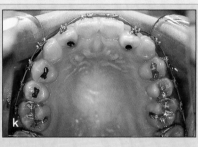

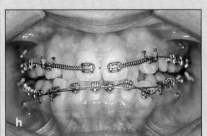

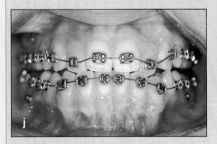

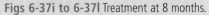

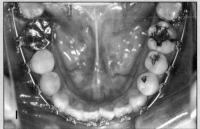

Figs 6-37g and 6-37h Treatment at 4 months.

Figs 6-37i to 6-37l Treatment at 8 months.

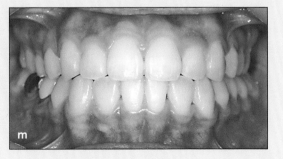

Fig 6-37m Result at the completion of active treatment.

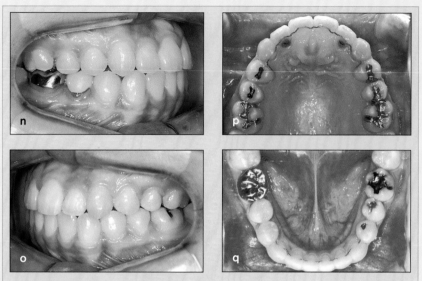

Figs 6-37n to 6-37q Lateral and occlusal views at the completion of active treatment.

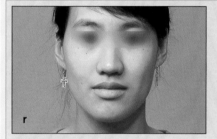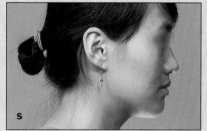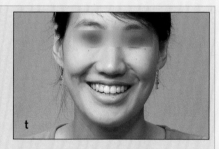

Figs 6-37r to 6-37t Facial views at the completion of active treatment.

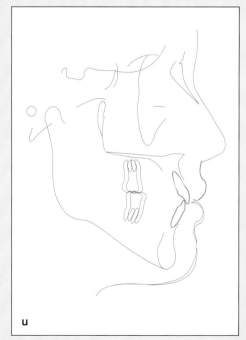

Fig 6-37u Superimposition before treatment *(black)*; at the completion of treatment *(red)*.

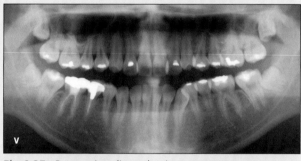

Fig 6-37v Panoramic radiograph prior to treatment.

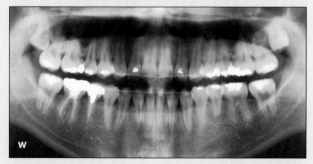

Fig 6-37w Panoramic radiograph at the completion of active treatment.

Case 6-2

The patient was a 22-year-old man whose chief complaints were an anterior crossbite and prominent chin (Figs 6-38a to 6-38d). He had a Class III profile and a short face (see Figs 6-38s and 6-38t). His incisors could be placed edge-to-edge in centric relation, but a significant anterior slide was noted from centric relation to maximum intercuspation. There were no signs or symptoms of temporomandibular disorders. The treatment objectives consisted of improvement of facial esthetics and establishment of a normal anterior occlusion. The first treatment option was surgical correction for a long mandibular body, but the patient opted for nonsurgical correction. Therefore, the decision was made to distalize the mandibular dentition by approximately 3.0 mm per side through the use of mini-implants.

ORLUS mini-implants, 1.8 mm in diameter and 7.0 mm in length, were placed in the mandible for distalization (Figs 6-38e and 6-38f). The 0.022-inch slot preadjusted appliances were bonded, and a 0.0175-inch twist-flex wire with an advancing U loop was placed to flare out the anterior teeth. In the mandible, a 0.018 × 0.025-inch Bioforce NiTi wire was placed for leveling, alignment, and distalization; posterior retractive forces from implants were applied to the canines and crimpable hooks on the wires. On the right side, approximately 500 g of force was applied; on the left side, approximately 300 g of force was applied, because there was space distal to the canine. After leveling, the mandibular main wires were changed to plain 0.017 × 0.025-inch TMA wires. After 4 weeks, a reverse curve and constriction bend were added to the 0.017 × 0.025-inch TMA wire.

After 6 months of treatment, the anterior crossbite was corrected (Figs 6-38g and 6-38h). Cephalometric examination revealed distal movement of the entire mandibular dentition (see Fig 6-38x). However, clinical examination showed insufficient exposure of the maxillary anterior teeth and excessive exposure of the mandibular anterior teeth. An ORLUS mini-implant, 1.8 mm in diameter and 8.0 mm in length, was placed between the maxillary right second premolar and first molar. Posterior retractive forces from the implants were applied to the maxillary right side and mandibular left side to correct midline discrepancies.

Following 7 months of treatment, a 0.016 × 0.022-inch TMA L loop was placed in the mandibular arch for intrusion of the anterior teeth (Figs 6-38i and 6-38j). For anchorage control, intrusive forces from the implants were applied to premolar areas.

After 12 months of treatment, a sectional wire was placed from first premolar to first premolar in the maxillary arch to aid in extrusion of the anterior teeth (Figs 6-38k and 6-38l). Box elastics were used to extrude the maxillary anterior teeth, while a removable posterior bite block was used to disocclude the anterior teeth. Intrusive forces from the implants were applied to the mandibular dentition.

Seventeen months after the start of treatment, appliances were removed because of decreasing interest by the patient, although further extrusion of the maxillary anterior teeth and an increase in the overall vertical dimensions were planned (Fig 6-38m). Fixed retainers were used to provide lifetime retention. Additionally, a circumferential retainer in the maxillary arch was worn at night.

At a follow-up examination 6 months after the end of treatment, the results were well maintained (Figs 6-38n to 6-38r).

Case 6-2   Camouflage treatment of Class III problems.

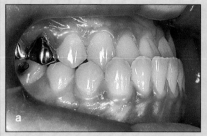

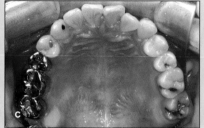

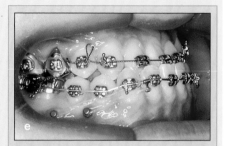

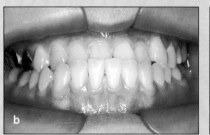

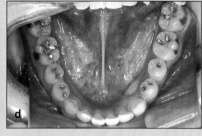

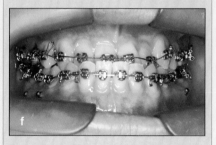

Figs 6-38a to 6-38d Clinical situation prior to treatment.

Figs 6-38e and 6-38f First appliance.

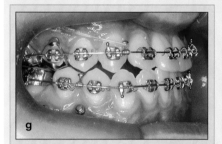

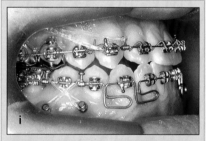

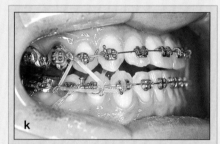

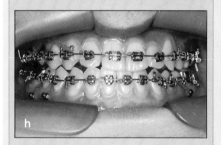

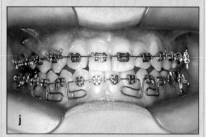

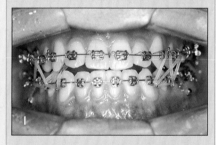

Figs 6-38g and 6-38h Treatment at 6 months.

Figs 6-38i and 6-38j Treatment at 7 months.

Figs 6-38k and 6-38l Treatment at 12 months.

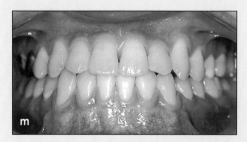

Fig 6-38m Result at the completion of active treatment.

Case 6-2   *(cont)*

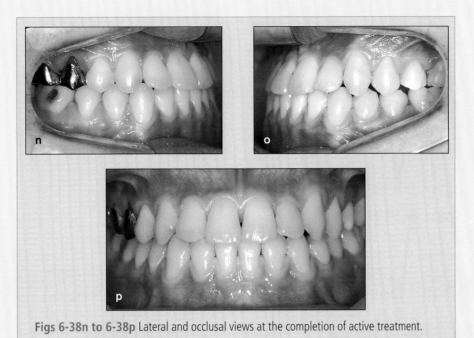

Figs 6-38n to 6-38p Lateral and occlusal views at the completion of active treatment.

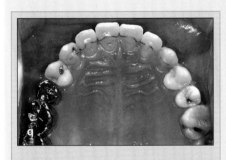
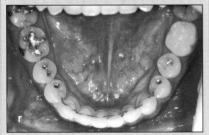

Figs 6-38q and 6-38r Occlusal views at 6-month follow-up.

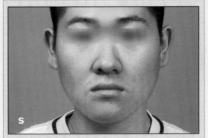
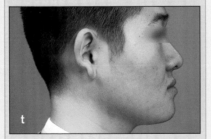

Figs 6-38s and 6-38t Facial views prior to treatment.

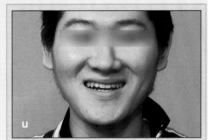
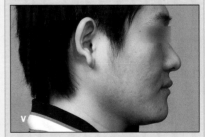

Figs 6-38u and 6-38v Facial views at the completion of active treatment.

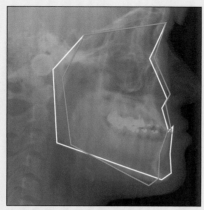

Fig 6-38w Cephalometric analysis prior to treatment. *(white)* Patient; *(green)* normal template.

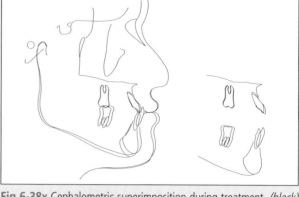

Fig 6-38x Cephalometric superimposition during treatment. *(black)* Prior to treatment; *(red)* after 6 months of treatment.

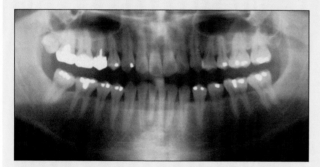

Fig 6-38y Panoramic radiograph prior to treatment.

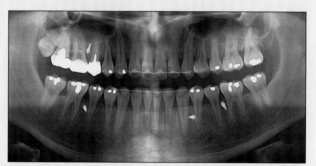

Fig 6-38z Panoramic radiograph at the completion of active treatment.

Case 6-3

The patient was a 23-year-old woman whose chief complaint was that her dental midlines deviated and were likely to worsen (Figs 6-39a to 6-39d). She showed a slightly asymmetric face, and the mandibular dental midline deviated to the left (see Figs 6-39n to 6-39p). She exhibited a Class III molar relationship and bruxism, but there were no significant signs or symptoms of temporomandibular disorders. The treatment objectives were to improve facial esthetics and establish normal anterior occlusion. The patient desired nonsurgical correction. Therefore, it was decided that the mandibular dentition would be distalized through the use of mini-implants.

Initially, two ORLUS mini-implants of 1.6 mm in diameter and 7.0 mm in length were placed on the right side, and one ORLUS mini-implant of the same diameter and length was placed on the left for asymmetric distalization (Figs 6-39e and 6-39f). The 0.022-inch slot preadjusted

appliances were placed in the mandibular arch, and 0.018 × 0.025-inch Bioforce NiTi wire was engaged as an initial wire. Then, 200 g of distalizing force was applied to each implant, resulting in 400 g of force on the right side and 200 g on the left side for midline correction. Open coil springs were also inserted to distalize the second molars.

After 4 months of treatment, molar relationships and midline discrepancies had been improved by asymmetric molar distalization (Figs 6-39g and 6-39h). A 0.017 × 0.025-inch TMA wire was placed to control the arch form and the axes of molars. The 0.022-inch slot preadjusted appliances were then placed in the maxillary arch, and treatment continued. Extrusion of the maxillary incisors was planned to improve the smile esthetics.

After 16 months of treatment, the planned position was achieved and treatment completed (Figs 6-39i to 6-39m).

Case 6-3 Distalization of the mandibular dentition to establish normal anterior occlusion and improved facial esthetics.

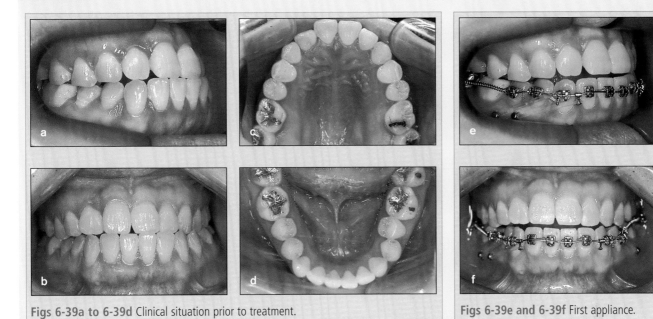

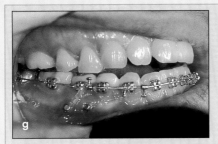

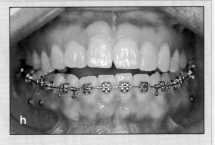

Figs 6-39a to 6-39d Clinical situation prior to treatment.

Figs 6-39e and 6-39f First appliance.

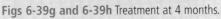

Figs 6-39g and 6-39h Treatment at 4 months.

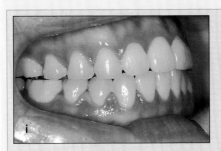

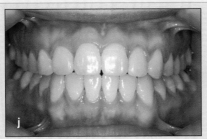

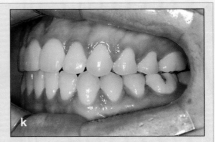

Figs 6-39i to 6-39k Result at the completion of active treatment.

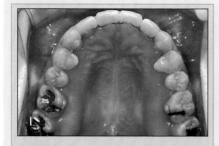

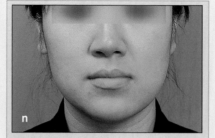

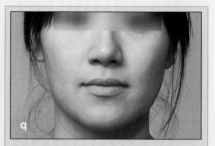

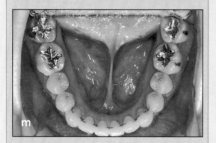

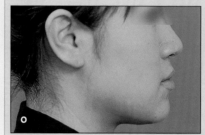

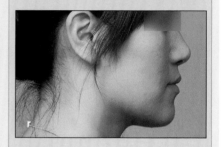

Figs 6-39l and 6-39m Occlusal views at the completion of active treatment.

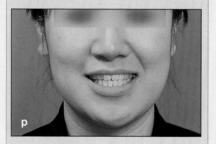

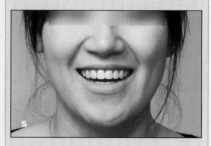

Figs 6-39n to 6-39p Facial views prior to treatment.

Figs 6-39q to 6-39s Facial views at the completion of active treatment.

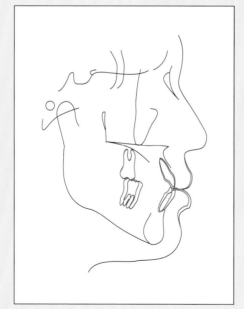

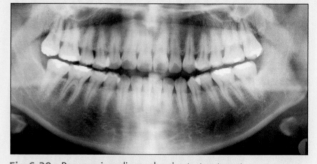

Fig 6-39u Panoramic radiograph prior to treatment.

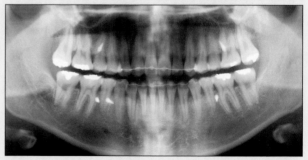

Fig 6-39t Cephalometric superimposition at the completion of active treatment. *(black)* Prior to treatment; *(red)* at the completion of active treatment.

Fig 6-39v Panoramic radiograph at the completion of active treatment.

Extraction treatment

The problems in conventional extraction treatment are that maxillary molars easily move mesially while mandibular molars are difficult to move mesially. Orthodontic implants can solve these problems without difficulty (Case 6-4). Furthermore, orthodontic implants make it easy to retract anterior teeth maximally (Case 6-5).

Case 6-4

A 16-year-old girl had chief complaints of maxillary spacing and rotation (Figs 6-40a to 6-40d). Beginning at the age of 11 years, she had undergone orthodontic treatment for about 2.5 years at another clinic; this treatment involved the use of removable appliances after the extraction of four premolars. She had a nail- and lip-biting habit, and the roots of the maxillary central incisors were short. The mandibular extraction site had become narrowed, because much time had passed since extraction. She also had slightly protruded lips. The treatment plan was to retract the maxillary lip by 1.5 mm; therefore, the decision was made to distalize the maxillary molars and protract the mandibular molars using 0.022-inch slot preadjusted appliances and mini-implants.

After 1 month of treatment, 0.018×0.025-inch Bioforce NiTi wires were placed (Figs 6-40e and 6-40f). In the maxillary arch, distalizing forces were applied to hooks on the wire; protractive forces were applied to the mandibular molars. Two ORLUS mini-implants of 1.8 mm in diameter and 7.0 mm in length were placed in the maxillary arch, while two ORLUS mini-implants of 1.6 mm in diameter and 7.0 mm in length were placed in the mandibular arch.

Six months after the start of treatment, 0.017×0.025-inch TMA wires were placed in the maxillary and mandibular arches to control the arch forms and occlusal plane (Figs 6-40g and 6-40h). An anterior crossbite developed because the mandibular dentition moved anteriorly as a result of protractive forces to the first molars. Therefore, posterior bites were raised using resin for core buildup, and mandibular protractive forces from the mini-implants were discontinued.

After 12 months of treatment, 0.016×0.022-inch SS wires were placed in the maxillary and mandibular arches to control the arch forms and occlusal plane (Figs 6-40i and 6-40j). Class II maxillomandibular box elastics were also used for occlusal seating (Figs 6-40k to 6-40o).

After 16 months of treatment, the planned position was achieved and treatment completed.

Case 6-4 Distalization of maxillary molars and protraction of mandibular molars for retraction of the upper lip.

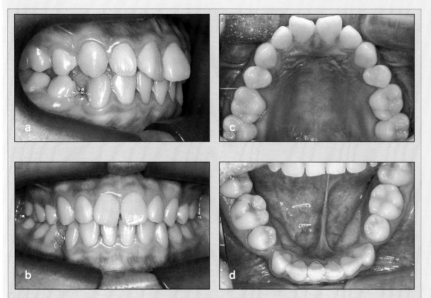

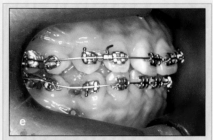

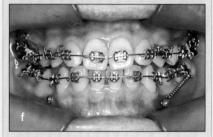

Figs 6-40a to 6-40d Clinical situation prior to treatment.

Figs 6-40e and 6-40f Treatment at 1 month.

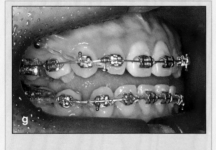

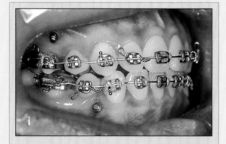

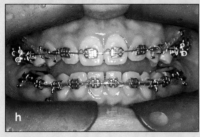

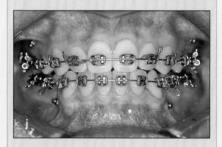

Figs 6-40g and 6-40h Treatment at 6 months.

Figs 6-40i and 6-40j Treatment at 12 months.

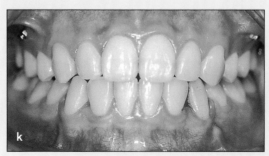

Fig 6-40k Result at the completion of active treatment.

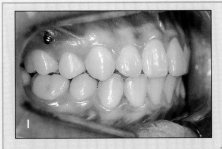

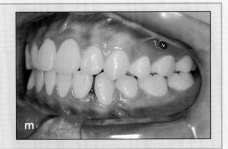

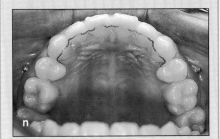

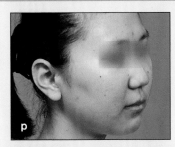

Fig 6-40p Facial view prior to treatment.

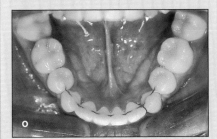

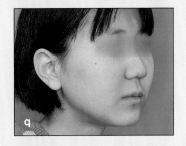

Fig 6-40q Facial view at the completion of active treatment.

Figs 6-40l to 6-40o Lateral and occlusal views at the completion of active treatment.

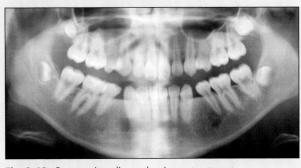

Fig 6-40s Panoramic radiograph prior to treatment.

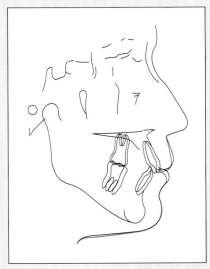

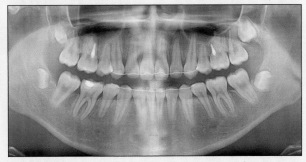

Fig 6-40r Cephalometric superimposition at the completion of active treatment. *(black)* Prior to treatment; *(red)* at the completion of active treatment.

Fig 6-40t Panoramic radiograph at the completion of active treatment.

Case 6-5

The patient was a 24-year-old woman whose chief complaints consisted of lip protrusion and an anterior open bite (Figs 6-41a to 6-41d). She showed protruded incisors and lips as well as lip incompetency. An Angle Class I molar relationship and a normal anteroposterior skeletal relationship were observed. The treatment objective was the improvement of facial esthetics, and extraction of the four first premolars was decided on for anterior retraction.

After 12 months of treatment, a 0.019 × 0.025-inch SS wire was engaged in the maxillary arch, while a 0.017 × 0.025-inch SS wire was engaged in the mandibular arch (Figs 6-41e and 6-41f). Extraction spaces were closed using sliding mechanics. In the maxillary arch, anchorage was reinforced by indirect anchorage using a midpalatal implant. For midline correction in the mandibular arch, anchorage was reinforced by direct anchorage using an interdental implant on the right side.

After 18 months of treatment, the extraction spaces were almost closed (Figs 6-41g and 6-41h). Interdental stripping was performed to improve the esthetics of the anterior interdental areas by reducing the contact points.

Treatment was completed after 22 months (Figs 6-41i to 6-41m).

| Case 6-5 | Extraction of four first premolars for anterior retraction to improve facial esthetics. (Courtesy of Dr BS Yoon, Seoul, Korea.) |

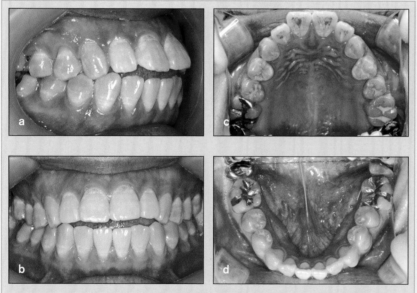

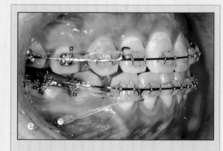

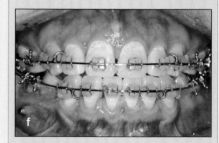

Figs 6-41a to 6-41d Clinical situation prior to treatment.

Figs 6-41e and 6-41f Treatment at 12 months.

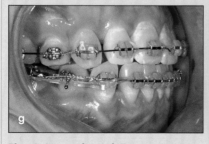

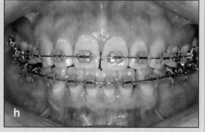

Figs 6-41g and 6-41h Treatment at 18 months.

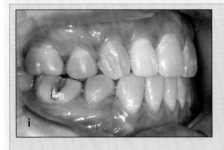
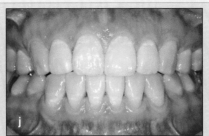
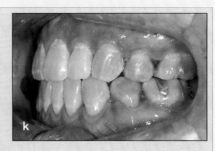

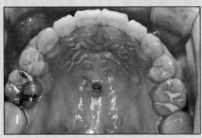

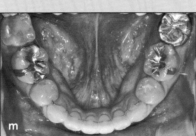

Figs 6-41i to 6-41m Result at the completion of active treatment.

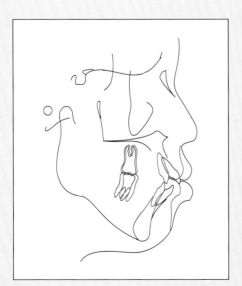

Fig 6-41n Cephalometric superimposition at the completion of active treatment. *(black)* Prior to treatment; *(red)* at the completion of active treatment.

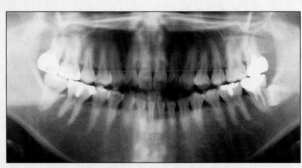

Fig 6-41o Panoramic radiograph prior to treatment.

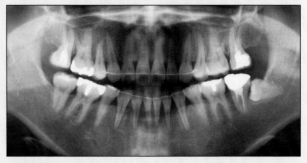

Fig 6-41p Panoramic radiograph at the completion of active treatment.

SUMMARY

The rigid anchorage and apical positioning of orthodontic mini-implants have two implications for orthodontic mechanics:

1. Because the orthodontic force is not applied from the anchorage of the dentition but from the orthodontic implant, undesirable movement in reaction to applied force can be avoided.
2. Because of the positioning of the implants, intrusive mechanics can be applied more easily. These factors simplify treatment and expand the range of treatment possibilities. However, treatment with orthodontic mini-implants does have biomechanical and biologic limitations, which should be considered during the treatment of each patient.

Conventional mechanics can be classified into two groups: shape-driven mechanics and force-driven mechanics, each of which has advantages and disadvantages. With mini-implants, mechanics that have advantages of both systems can be devised. Thus, mini-implants make treatment simpler and more efficient.

REFERENCES

1. Roberts WE. Bone dynamics of osseointegration, ankylosis, and tooth movement. J Indiana Dent Assoc 1999;78:24–32.
2. Melsen B. Current Controversies in Orthodontics. Chicago: Quintessence, 1991:155.
3. Smith RJ, Burstone CJ. Mechanics of tooth movement. Am J Orthod 1984;85:294–307.
4. Buchter A, Wiechmann D, Koerdt S, Wiesmann HP, Piffko J, Meyer U. Load-related implant reaction of mini-implants used for orthodontic anchorage. Clin Oral Implants Res 2005;16:473–479.
5. Akin-Nergiz N, Nergiz I, Schulz A, Arpak N, Niedermeier W. Reactions of peri-implant tissues to continuous loading of osseointegrated implants. Am J Orthod Dentofacial Orthop 1998;114:292–298.
6. Wehrbein H, Merz BR, Hammerle CH, Lang NP. Bone-to-implant contact of orthodontic implants in humans subjected to horizontal loading. Clin Oral Implants Res 1998;9:348–353.
7. De Pauw GA, Dermaut L, De Bruyn H, Johansson C. Stability of implants as anchorage for orthopedic traction. Angle Orthod 1999;69:401–407.
8. Lee JS. Development of Orthodontic Mini-Implant Anchorage System. Pre-Conference: Basic Researches on Implant Orthodontics. The 4th Asian Implant Orthodontics Conference, Seoul, Korea, December 3–4, 2005.
9. Gapski R, Wang HL, Mascarenhas P, Lang NP. Critical review of immediate implant loading. Clin Oral Implants Res 2003;14:515–527.
10. Wennstrom JL. Mucogingival considerations in orthodontic treatment. Semin Orthod 1996;2:46–54.
11. Steiner GG, Pearson JK, Ainamo J. Changes of the marginal periodontium as a result of labial tooth movement in monkeys. J Periodontol 1981;52:314–320.
12. Engelking G, Zachrisson BU. Effects of incisor repositioning on monkey periodontium after expansion through the cortical plate. Am J Orthod 1982;82:23–32.
13. Handelman CS. The anterior alveolus: Its importance in limiting orthodontic treatment and its influence on the occurrence of iatrogenic sequelae. Angle Orthod 1996;66:95–109.
14. Hong H, Ngan P, Han G, Qi LG, Wei SH. Use of onplants as stable anchorage for facemask treatment: A case report. Angle Orthod 2005;75:453–460.
15. Parr JA, Garetto LP, Wohlford ME, Arbuckle GR, Roberts WE. Sutural expansion using rigidly integrated endosseous implants: An experimental study in rabbits. Angle Orthod 1997;67:283–290.
16. De Pauw GA, Dermaut L, De Bruyn H, Johansson C. Stability of implants as anchorage for orthopedic traction. Angle Orthod 1999;69:401–407.
17. Kircelli BH, Pektas ZO, Uckan S. Orthopedic protraction with skeletal anchorage in a patient with maxillary hypoplasia and hypodontia. Angle Orthod 2006;76:156–163.
18. Aelbers CM, Dermaut LR. Orthopedics in orthodontics: Part I, Fiction or reality—A review of the literature. Am J Orthod Dentofacial Orthop 1996;110:513–519.
19. Dermaut LR, Aelbers CM. Orthopedics in orthodontics: Fiction or reality. A review of the literature—Part II. Am J Orthod Dentofacial Orthop 1996;110:667–671.
20. Hösl E, Baldauf A. Mechanical and Biological Basics in Orthodontic Therapy. Heidelberg: Hüthig, 1991:1–6.
21. Melsen B. Current Controversies in Orthodontics. Chicago: Quintessence, 1991:131–146.
22. Burstone CJ, Koenig HA. Force systems from an ideal arch. Am J Orthod 1974;65:270–289.
23. Burstone CJ, Koenig HA. Creative wire bending—The force system from step and V bends. Am J Orthod Dentofacial Orthop 1988;93:59–67.
24. Weiland FJ, Bantleon HP, Droschl H. Evaluation of continuous arch and segmented arch leveling techniques in adult patients—A clinical study. Am J Orthod Dentofacial Orthop 1996;110:647–652.
25. Graber TM, Vanarsdall RL, Vig KWL. Orthodontics: Current Principles and Techniques. St Louis: Mosby, 2005:973.
26. Lee JS, Kim DH, Park YC, Kyung SH, Kim TK. The efficient use of midpalatal miniscrew implants. Angle Orthod 2004;74:711–714.
27. Sugawara J, Baik UB, Umemori M, et al. Treatment and posttreatment dentoalveolar changes following intrusion of mandibular molars with application of a skeletal anchorage system (SAS) for open bite correction. Int J Adult Orthodon Orthognath Surg 2002;17:243–253.
28. Park JY, Lee KJ. Treatment effects of miniscrew assisted rapid palatal expansion in young adults [Master thesis]. Seoul: Yonsei University, 2006.

TREATMENT BASED ON A NEW PARADIGM

A *paradigm* can be thought of as a set of shared beliefs and assumptions that represents the conceptual foundation for an area of a science or clinical practice.[1,2] As the anchorage system with orthodontic implants has been introduced, a new technique has also been developed. As a consequence, the range of orthodontic mechanotherapy has been expanded. Based on the accumulated clinical evidence, a new paradigm for orthodontics can be established. Again, the modified paradigm creates new treatment principles and techniques and requires additional modalities for diagnosis. Traditionally, the paradigm for orthodontic mechanotherapy has been restricted by the biomechanical limitations of anchorage control, but this may now be changed, with the orthodontic implant anchorage system serving as momentum.

E.H. ANGLE PARADIGM VERSUS SOFT TISSUE TREATMENT PARADIGM

During the 20th century, the Edward H. Angle paradigm, which emphasized a static relationship and occlusion, was dominant.[1,2] The main concept of the E. H. Angle paradigm was expanded, and, until recently, the basic concept—that the dentition and facial skeleton determine treatment goals—remained intact.[1,2]

Proffit[2] suggested the biologically driven "soft tissue paradigm" as an alternative to the E. H. Angle paradigm (Table 7-1) and also suggested that the following additional factors should be considered during treatment[2,3]:

1. Norms instead of ideals
2. Pressure exerted on the teeth by the lips, cheeks, and tongue
3. Limitations of periodontal attachment
4. Neuromuscular influences on mandibular position
5. Contours of the soft tissue facial mask
6. Lip-tooth relationships and anterior tooth display during facial animation

Clinically, ideal occlusion is difficult to achieve because of biologic and biomechanical limitations (Fig 7-1). However, orthodontic mini-implants have made the approaches to treatment goals more straightforward. Orthodontic mini-implants make the process of "gross" anchorage control simple, easy, and less technique independent. Moreover, molar intrusion and molar distalization become possible through the use of orthodontic mini-implants, and the range of mechanotherapy has been expanded. Even without orthognathic surgery, vertical excess and retruded chins may be corrected based on soft tissue paradigm considerations. Orthodontic mini-implants will accelerate the paradigm shift to include assessment of the soft tissue paradigm.

Table 7-1   E. H. Angle paradigm versus the soft tissue paradigm[2]

Parameter	E.H. Angle paradigm	Soft tissue paradigm
Primary treatment goal	Ideal dental occlusion	Normal soft tissue proportions and adaptation
Secondary treatment goal	Ideal jaw relationships	Functional occlusion
Hard/soft tissue relationships	Ideal hard tissue proportions produce ideal soft tissues	Ideal soft tissue proportions define ideal hard tissue relationships
Diagnostic emphasis	Dental casts, cephalometric radiographs	Clinical examination of soft tissues
Treatment approach	Obtain ideal dental and skeletal relationships and the soft tissues will be acceptable	Plan ideal soft tissue relationships, then place the teeth and jaws accordingly
Function of emphasis	Temporomandibular joint in relation to dental occlusion	Soft tissue movement in relation to dental display
Stability of result	Related primarily to dental occlusion	Related primarily to soft tissue pressures/equilibrium effects

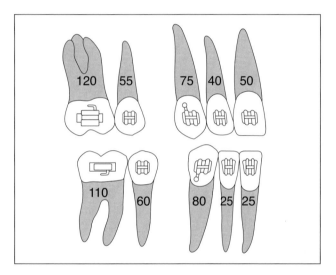

Fig 7-1a Biologic limitation. There are differences between the surface area of the maxillary teeth and that of the mandibular teeth. Numbers indicate surface area in mm[2]. (From Ricketts.[4] Modified with permission.)

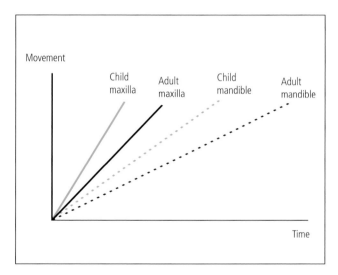

Fig 7-1b Rates of tooth movement differ because of a difference in bone turnover rates. (From Graber et al.[5] Modified with permission.)

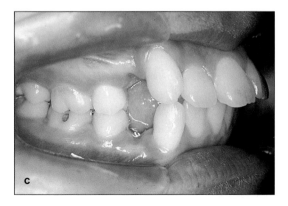

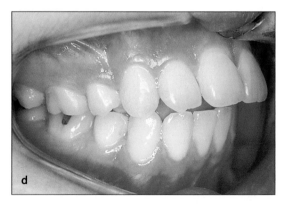

Figs 7-1c and 7-1d Because of the biologic limitations, Class II maxillomandibular relationships are difficult to correct. **(c)** Premolar extraction. **(d)** The Class II molar relationship was not improved after treatment.

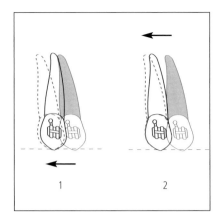

Fig 7-2a The classic strategy for anchorage control is (1) tipping and (2) uprighting. That is, if tooth movement *(arrows)* is divided into stages, anchorage is easily preserved.

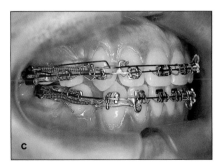

Fig 7-2b A typical example of the tipping and uprighting strategy is the tip edge bracket system. In this system, the crown is moved first.

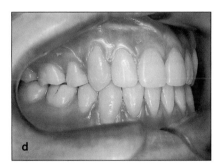

Fig 7-2c After the crown is moved, the root is moved with a root spring.

Fig 7-3 Classically, **(a)** orthodontic treatment that involves extractions progresses through three stages: **(b)** leveling and alignment, **(c)** space closure, and **(d)** finishing. These stages are divided for clinical convenience and are not directly related to treatment objectives.

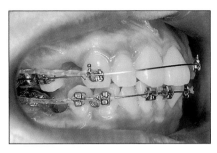

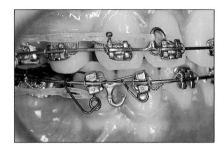

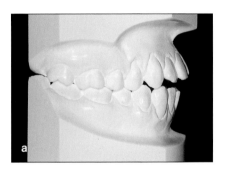

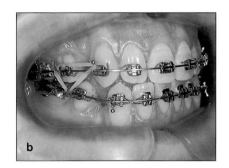

MECHANICS-CENTERED TREATMENT VERSUS OBJECTIVE-CENTERED TREATMENT

Orthodontic treatment during the 20th century, from treatment planning to treatment progress, has been restricted by the biomechanical limitations of the law of action and reaction (Fig 7-2). The biomechanical limitations nearly outnumber the biologic limitations. For example, in treatment planning, the visual treatment objective (VTO) should be within the clinical limits of the tooth movement, which makes it clinically possible to secure anchorage from the dentition. Biomechanical limitations should be considered during the planning of the treatment objectives. Molar intrusion has been regarded as clinically impossible because it is difficult to secure enough anchorage from the dentition. Furthermore, extraction treatment usually is achieved in three stages[6]: leveling, space closure, and finishing and management of anchorage problems, which are independent of the treatment objectives (Fig 7-3).

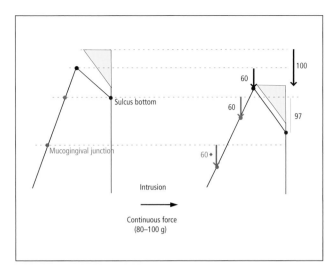

Fig 7-4 Local changes caused by intrusion, according to experiments in monkeys.[19]

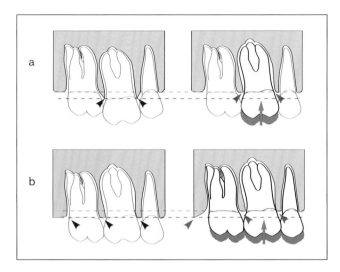

Fig 7-5 There is a difference between *(a)* intrusion of a single posterior tooth and *(b)* intrusion of posterior teeth that remodels all interseptal alveolar bone. *(blue arrowheads)* Initial alveolar crest level; *(red arrowheads)* postintrusion bone level.

The availability of a stable anchorage system suggests that loss of anchorage is no longer a concern. Based on the orthodontic implant type of anchorage, a new objective treatment technique is now possible. This may free orthodontists from the idea of anchorage loss.[5,7–9] That is, treatment is not focused on mechanics-centered thinking to preserve anchorage, but treatment objective–centered thinking in terms of clinical treatment technique. Objective-centered thinking makes it possible to take an approach to objective-centered mechanics.

Moreover, the precise three-dimensional control provided by orthodontic implants allows orthodontic treatment to achieve more esthetic results. For example, only mechanotherapy can comprehensively change the smile line.

NEW TREATMENT PARADIGM BASED ON THE ORTHODONTIC IMPLANT TYPE OF ANCHORAGE

Treatment based on a new treatment paradigm emphasizes the following:

1. Soft tissue paradigm[1,2]
2. Treatment objective–centered approach
3. Not only the occlusion, but also the face

4. Not only the facial profile, but also the frontal view
5. Not only the anteroposterior relationships, but also the vertical and transverse relationships
6. Not only the static relationships, but also the dynamic relationships
7. Not only the facial appearance of the present, but also the facial appearance with aging

MOLAR INTRUSION WITH FIXED MECHANOTHERAPY

Rationale

One of the most outstanding characteristics of orthodontic treatment with implants is the ability to achieve intrusion of molars.[10–18] Molar intrusion is needed for the following purposes:

1. Intrusion of teeth that have overerupted as a result of missing opposing teeth
2. Improvement of angular crest bone level with extruded teeth
3. Nonsurgical correction of anterior open bite in patients with skeletal open bite tendency
4. Nonsurgical correction of excess anterior facial height
5. Improvement of the smile line

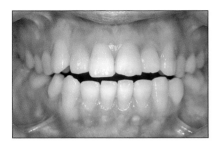

Fig 7-6a Intraoral view prior to molar intrusion.

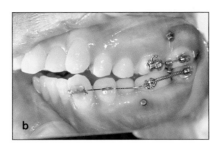

Figs 7-6b and 7-6c Single forces from buccal implants and palatal implants are used to intrude the molars.

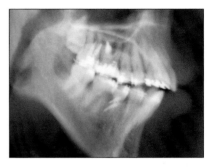

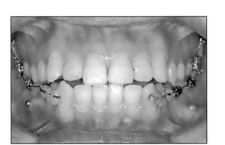

Fig 7-6d Changes after 2 months of treatment.

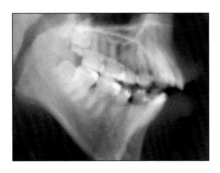

Fig 7-6e Cephalometric radiograph prior to treatment.

Fig 7-6f Cephalometric radiograph after 2 months of treatment.

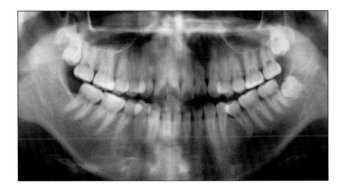

Fig 7-6g Panoramic radiograph prior to treatment.

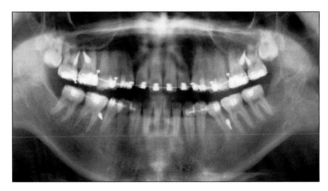

Fig 7-6h Panoramic radiograph after 2 months of treatment. When the third molar is erupting, there is no angular bony change. Note the change of the distal side of the maxillary second molar.

Effects

Local effects

As teeth move during molar intrusion, the alveolar bone level also remodels[10,19,20] (Fig 7-4), and there are no changes in healthy tissues in clinical crown length, significant root length, or crown-root ratio, measured from crown tip to crestal bone and from crestal bone to root tip[10,21] (Figs 7-5 to 7-7).

Alveolar bone may be angulated yet parallel to the cementoenamel junctions of the teeth and will appear as an angular crest (see Fig 7-5). The alveolar bone level may be remodeled after treatment, but periodontal pockets form easily in the absence of proper inflammatory periodontal control, because supragingival plaque may

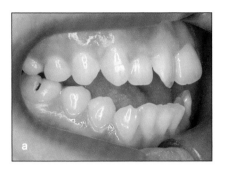
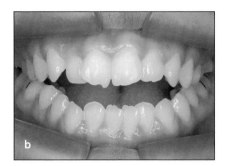

Figs 7-7a and 7-7b Intraoral views prior to treatment. Anterior open bite and vertical excess are to be corrected by molar intrusion.

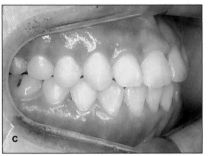
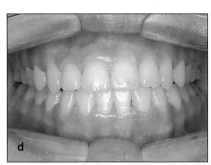

Figs 7-7c and 7-7d Intraoral views at the completion of active treatment (28th month). Note the periodontal changes of the most posterior tooth.

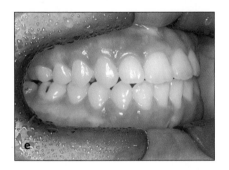
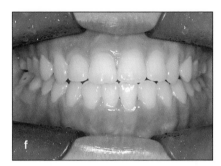

Figs 7-7e and 7-7f Intraoral views 12 months after completion of active treatment. At this time, the maintenance is acceptable. A tongue crib has not been used, and the mandibular incisors have flared out slightly.

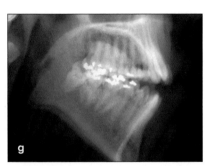
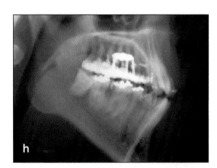

Fig 7-7g Cephalometric radiograph prior to treatment.

Fig 7-7h Cephalometric radiograph after 12 months of treatment. Note the relationship between the roots of the second molar and the maxillary sinus.

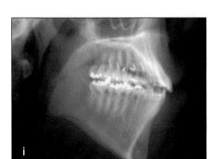
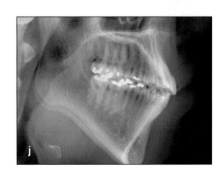

Fig 7-7i Cephalometric radiograph at the completion of active treatment (28th month).

Fig 7-7j Cephalometric radiograph 12 months after completion of active treatment.

Fig 7-7k Cephalometric superimposition of changes after treatment. *(black)* Prior to treatment; *(red)* completion of active treatment.

Fig 7-7l Cephalometric superimposition of changes during retention. *(red)* Completion of active treatment; *(green)* at 12-month follow-up.

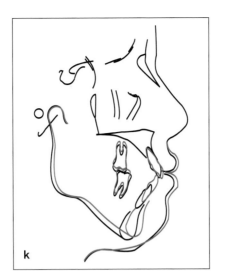

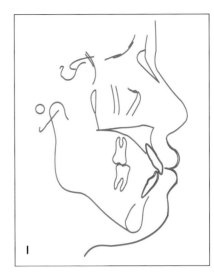

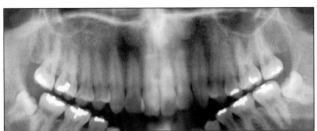

Fig 7-7m Panoramic radiograph prior to treatment.

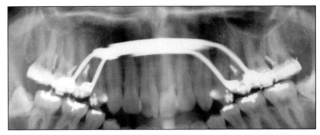

Fig 7-7n Panoramic radiograph after 4 months of treatment.

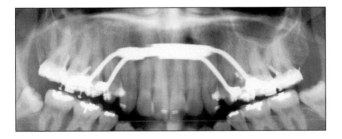

Fig 7-7o Panoramic radiograph after 7 months of treatment.

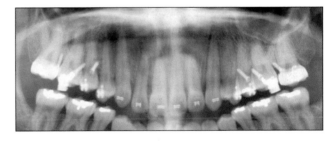

Fig 7-7p Panoramic radiograph after 12 months of treatment.

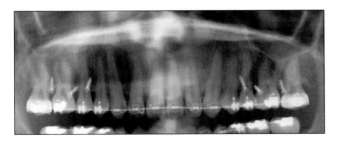

Fig 7-7q Panoramic radiograph after 24 months of treatment.

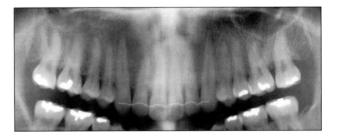

Fig 7-7r Panoramic radiograph at the completion of active treatment (28th month).

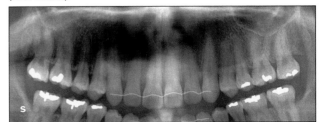

Fig 7-7s Panoramic radiograph 12 months after completion of active treatment.

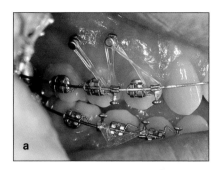

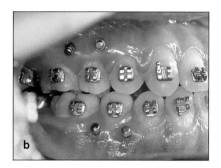

Figs 7-8a and 7-8b Local changes caused by intrusion of posterior teeth. As molars are intruded, probing depths may increase and the alveolar bone level may become inclined because the alveolar bone moves as a tooth moves. Recovery will occur following treatment if proper oral hygiene control is maintained. However, in adult patients, the width of attached gingiva diminishes without a change in the mucogingival junction.

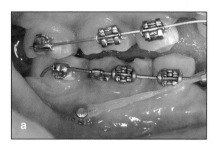

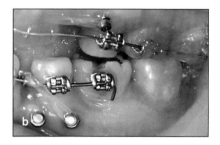

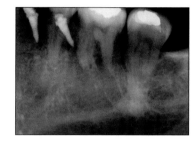

Figs 7-9a and 7-9b The intrusion of the entire dentition was planned, but the left second molar was excluded from the appliance because of the lack of attached gingiva and alveolar bone resorption. As the right second molar intruded, occlusal reduction was performed on the left second molar.

Fig 7-9c Note the alveolar bone level on the distal side of the mandibular left second molar.

create an environment conducive to subgingival plaque with the progression of intrusion. Therefore, appropriate periodontal care, including adequate subgingival plaque control, is necessary. If plaque is controlled, there will be less chance of detrimental influences on the periodontal attachment apparatus.[22]

In animal experiments, it has been reported that molar intrusion does not result in negative effects on the adjacent structures, such as the maxillary sinus or the mandibular canal.[23,24]

Molar intrusion is likely to decrease the width of the attached gingiva since the mucogingival junction is unchanged[25,26] (Fig 7-8). This might cause periodontal problems, particularly in the mandibular second molar area where there is less attached gingiva, and it may increase morbidity where furcation involvement is possible. Therefore, the width of the attached gingiva is a major limiting factor in molar intrusion (Figs 7-9 and 7-10).

General effects

In nongrowing patients, intrusion of the maxillary dentition and intrusion of the maxillary posterior teeth have similar effects, and the patients undergo similar physiologic changes to those experienced after maxillary superior repositioning via total or segmental maxillary osteotomy[27–30] (Fig 7-11). With surgical superior repositioning of the maxilla, or at least the posterior part of the maxilla, the mandible rotates around the horizontal condylar axis to align itself, so that the chin moves upward and forward.[27–30] Similar effects on the mandible can be obtained with orthodontic posterior intrusion.

Interocclusal rest space is maintained after surgery and posterior intrusion by the function of proprioceptors in the periodontal ligaments.[28–31] Occlusal force increases after maxillary surgery,[32,33] but a change in occlusal force after orthodontic molar intrusion has not been reported.

Short term, the effects of posterior intrusion in growing patients are the same as those in nongrowing patients. The long-term effects of posterior intrusion on remaining growth still must be evaluated, because they have not yet been established.

Surgical superior repositioning of the maxilla and consequent mandibular autorotations seem to have little detrimental effect on the temporomandibular joints and masticatory muscles.[34] Soft tissues are relaxed, and resting lip pressure decreases as the mandible rotated forward following superior repositioning of the maxilla.[35]

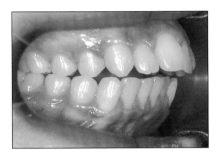

Fig 7-10a Intraoral view prior to treatment.

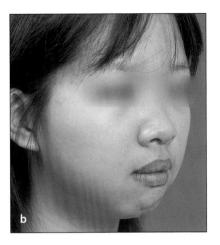

Figs 7-10b and 7-10c Facial views prior to treatment.

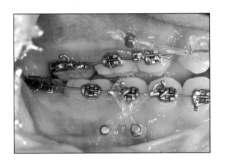

Fig 7-10d Intraoral view at 16 months of treatment. As the posterior teeth have been intruded, the width of attached gingiva has been reduced. Considering the width of attached gingiva, further intrusion of maxillary molars seems undesirable.

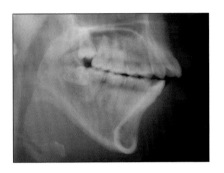

Fig 7-10e Cephalometric radiograph prior to treatment.

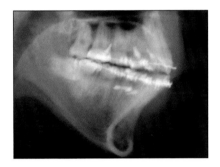

Fig 7-10f Cephalometric radiograph at 16 months of treatment.

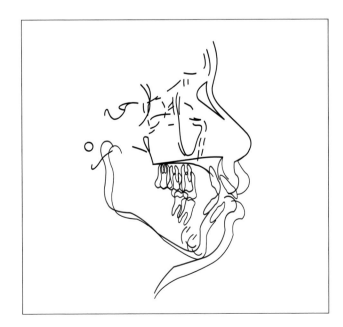

Fig 7-10g Cephalometric superimposition. (black) Prior to treatment; (blue) at 16 months of treatment.

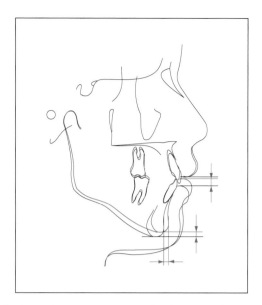

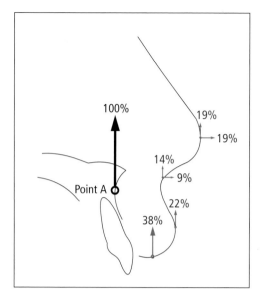

Fig 7-11a Following molar intrusion, it seems that there is no change in upper lip length or in the nose. As the mandible rotates upward and forward, soft tissue movements of the upper lip and nose parallel the adjacent hard tissue movements almost exactly. With nonsurgical correction, anterior facial height is reduced; neck length is increased; interlabial space is reduced; and interocclusal rest space is maintained. *(black)* Prior to treatment; *(red)* at completion of active treatment. (Modified from Lee et al.[27] Reprinted with permission.)

Fig 7-11b Following superior repositioning of the maxilla by Le Fort I osteotomy, the upper lip moved superiorly one third the distance that point A moved, but there was considerable variability. With surgical correction, in addition to changes in the mandibular position, the nose and the upper lip are changed. (Modified from Lee et al.[27] Reprinted with permission.)

Stability

It has been no more than a decade since the intrusion of the bilateral posterior segment was introduced, but the lack of long-term data and research regarding physiologic change remains. The stability of molar intrusion by mechanotherapy should be evaluated in terms of the potential for relapse of tooth movement, return of open bite, and change in facial height.

Tooth movement

Intrusion of the posterior teeth has relapse potential that is within an acceptable range compared to other types of orthodontic movement without surgery.

Orthodontic intrusion might possess several disadvantages compared to other types of tooth movement.[10] First, while the other types of tooth movement are accompanied by new bone formation that appears to reduce relapse, intrusion does not induce new bone formation but allows for remodeling during tooth movement. Second, periodontal fibers, which are generally thought to resist occlusal forces, can also strongly resist intrusive forces. Third, apical periodontal tissues are reorganized more slowly than are periodontal tissues in other sites.

However, intrusion possesses several advantages over extrusion.[36] First, with molar intrusion, overcorrection is possible and occlusal force may be helpful in the maintenance of the orthodontic result. Second, with intrusion, less stress is placed on supra-alveolar gingival tissue, which could lessen the tendency for relapse. With extrusion, on the contrary, supra-alveolar gingival tissue becomes stretched, resulting in a tendency to relapse. However, it is essential to provide sufficient time for reorganization of periodontal tissue to obtain stability after molar intrusion, just as it is after any type of tooth movement.

Anterior open bite correction

Following orthodontic correction of open bite patterns, relapse is common.[37–42] Even after surgical correction, relapse is very common in anterior open bite patients.[43–45] That is to say, there is no evidence suggesting that surgical correction is more stable than orthodontic correction by posterior intrusion. Rather, the fact that the soft tissue has sufficient time to adapt gradually is advantageous because orthodontic correction spans a long period of time.

After the improvement of the form, function may not be improved. For instance, tongue-thrusting habits can re-

Figs 7-12a and 7-12b The first and second molars were overcorrected in the finishing stage, and the result has been well maintained. Overcorrection of the molars is preferable to reduce the risk of relapse. Sugawara[10] recommended overcorrection during the end stage of treatment with the prediction of 25% relapse.

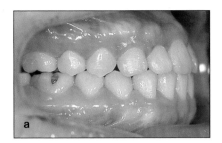

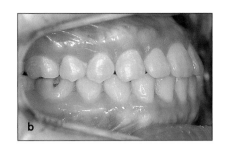

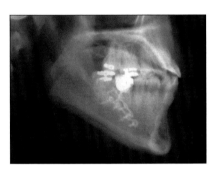

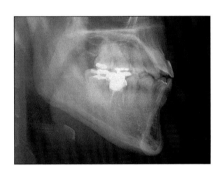

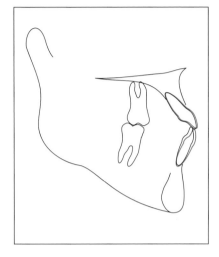

Fig 7-13a Cephalometric radiograph taken after completion of treatment.

Fig 7-13b Cephalometric radiograph at the 18-month follow-up. Relapse of the open bite is observed.

Fig 7-13c The cephalometric superimposition reveals that the relapse resulted from the labial tipping of the anterior teeth, which was probably caused by tongue thrusting during swallowing. The mandibular incisors have flared labially despite the lingual fixed retainer. *(black)* Immediately postsurgery; *(red)* at 18 months postsurgery.

main, which may cause a relapse of anterior open bite.[36,43,46,47] To ensure stability, tongue-thrusting habits should be controlled after correction of anterior open bite.[47,48] This is done with a retention appliance.

Reduction of anterior facial height

There have been many studies concerning the change in anterior facial height caused by autorotation of the mandible after surgical superior repositioning of the maxilla.[43–45,49,50] Surgical superior repositioning of the maxilla has been concluded to be one of the most stable types of treatment, because it relaxes the soft tissue and induces physiologic adaptations.[43,49,50]

Orthodontic correction of vertical excess may be more advantageous than surgical correction in terms of the stability of the reduced vertical dimension. Orthodontic correction takes place over a relatively long period of time, and adjacent tissues have a longer period to adapt in correction. Moreover, mandibular posterior alveolar excess is very difficult to correct surgically, but it can be corrected more easily by mechanotherapy.

Maintenance of molar intrusion

An adequate amount of time is required for the reorganization of periodontal tissue, so it is recommended that molar intrusion be performed as early as possible. This protocol then allows for the use of the other active treatment time as an additional retention period. Overcorrection in the second molar area is also a useful way to reduce potential relapse (Fig 7-12). Posterior bite blocks, which use occlusal force to achieve stability, do not appear to be very effective.

In the case of an open bite, functional correction should be accompanied by control of tongue-thrusting behaviors[43,47,48] (Fig 7-13). A retainer should have a

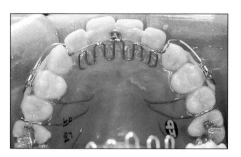

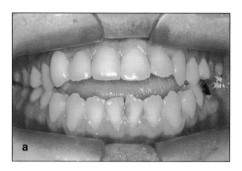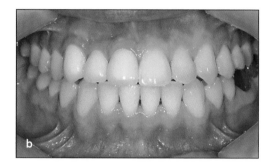

Fig 7-14 A tongue crib is necessary to control tongue-thrusting habits and tongue posture for maintenance of open bite after treatment. It is recommended that the tongue crib be incorporated in maxillary appliances to guide the tongue into proper position.

Figs 7-15a and 7-15b (a) Anterior open bite prior to treatment. **(b)** Frontal view after 12 months of follow-up. The anterior open bite has been corrected by orthodontic mechanotherapy, and the result is well maintained. For retention, the patient has been instructed in proper tongue posture and swallowing, and a circumferential retainer with a tongue crib is used at night to prevent unconscious tongue thrusting. A lingual fixed retainer extending from premolar to premolar has been placed.

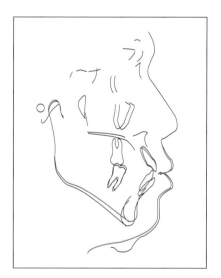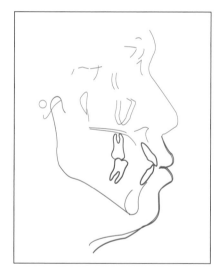

Fig 7-15c Cephalometric superimposition. *(black)* Prior to treatment; *(red)* at the end of active treatment.

Fig 7-15d Cephalometric superimposition. *(red)* At the end of active treatment; *(green)* at 12-month follow-up.

tongue crib to maintain position of the tongue in the appropriate position and prevent tongue thrusting during swallowing (Fig 7-14). It is recommended that the tongue crib be used for no less than 1 year. The tongue crib should be used together with a fixed (bonded) retainer that extends from premolar to premolar (Fig 7-15). It is also essential that a fixed retainer be used after intrusion of only one or two teeth.

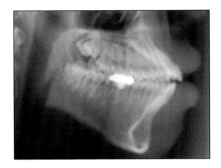

Fig 7-16a Cephalometric radiograph prior to treatment.

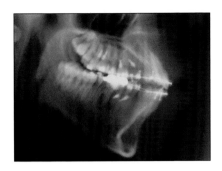

Fig 7-16b Cephalometric radiograph after 4 months of treatment. The maxillary teeth have been intruded successfully with the use of mini-implants, but the anterior facial height has been maintained because of extrusion of the mandibular posterior teeth. No particular extrusive mechanics were used in the mandibular arch.

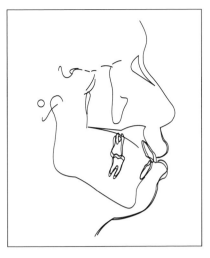

Fig 7-16c Cephalometric superimposition. *(black)* Prior to treatment; *(blue)* at 4 months of treatment.

Fig 7-17 Examination with a periodontal probe is absolutely necessary during molar intrusion. With inspection, there seemed to be no problem in the second molar area, but the probing depth was 5 mm in the distopalatal area and there was bleeding on probing. On the attached gingiva, redness and swelling were not visible in spite of inflammation because of the thick keratinized gingiva. A flap operation with crown lengthening is planned to control periodontitis during orthodontic treatment.

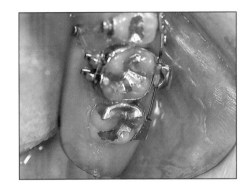

Risk factors and their solutions

Physiologic aspects

The change in vertical dimension resulting from mandibular autorotation is not just a morphologic change but a physiologic change as well.[10,28,29,35] That is, the vertical dimension tends to be maintained, so maxillary intrusion may cause physiologic mandibular extrusion (Fig 7-16). Therefore, in cases of maxillary intrusion, the mandibular vertical position should be controlled with mandibular intrusive force.[10]

Periodontal risks

Much research has been carried out to investigate the risks of anterior intrusion and their management.[21,51] As teeth intrude, supragingival plaque may be conducive to formation of subgingival plaque, so periodontitis may easily occur. This should be managed by periodic professional plaque control and an oral hygiene maintenance program. Most of all, special attention should be given to the distal surface of the most posterior molar.

If possible, bonding should be used instead of banding to the molar, and use of a minibracket or minitube is better for periodontal maintenance. Additionally, even when a band is used, the band margin should be situated sufficiently supragingivally to avoid infringement on the biologic width. It is recommended that stronger band cements, such as light-cured glass-ionomer cement, be used to prevent banding failure. Before treatment, the importance of periodontal inflammatory control should be sufficiently conveyed to the patient; the possibility of the need for periodontal surgery after treatment or during the treatment should also be stressed (Fig 7-17).

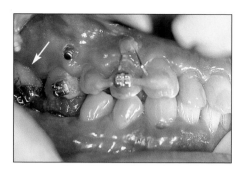

Fig 7-18 The second molar has been intruded, but buccal recession has occurred on the lingual aspect of the second molar *(arrow)*. This probably resulted from buccal deviation of the second molar caused by buccal intrusive force. The patient's heavy smoking habit may have contributed to the problem.

Root resorption

Although there have been few studies reporting the incidence of root resorption of posterior teeth after molar intrusion, it is presumed that the risk of root resorption is less than that of the anterior teeth.[10,21] In anterior intrusion, the stress is concentrated on the root apex; in posterior intrusion, however, the stress is noted first in the furcation area.[52] More research is needed to investigate the risk factors for molar root resorption, such as dilaceration of the root. Systematic risk management assessments for prevention are also required, including pre-orthodontic examination of short root length and periodic examinations with panoramic radiography to assess response to treatment.

Recession and dehiscence

Tooth movement beyond the alveolar trough causes recession and dehiscence. Maxillary buccal alveolar bone tends to be thin, and buccal intrusive force can easily tip teeth buccally (Fig 7-18). Therefore, there is a high risk of facial dehiscence in the maxillary molar areas, particularly for periodontally compromised patients.

Optimal orthodontic force for molar intrusion

Controversy remains regarding the mechanism of orthodontic tooth movements and the amount of optimal force.[53] Some explain tooth movements using the pressure-tension theory,[54] and others explain it through the Frost mechanostat theory.[55] According to the pressure-tension theory, the intrusive force for molar intrusion can be estimated from orthodontic force per unit of surface area[54]; according to the Frost theory, however, the intrusive force cannot be estimated in this manner.[55] As Sugawara[10,12] noted, the periodontal ligament of the molar is capable of resisting occlusal force, so it is more difficult to determine the optimal force for molar intrusion.

Clinically, a force ranging from 150 to 200 g per molar is used when molar intrusion is performed.[10–18]

LEVELING WITH ORTHODONTIC IMPLANTS

Determination of the vertical dimension

The problem-oriented approach to diagnosis and treatment planning is summarized in chapter 4. This approach is also applied to treat vertical discrepancies. The vertical relationship should be carefully evaluated, and all possible solutions should be considered. With the introduction of orthodontic mini-implants and proper protocols described in chapter 4, vertical control through posterior intrusion can become a routine practice.

Overall general vertical dimension

For patients with vertical excess in whom orthognathic surgery has been ruled out as a treatment option, the parameters of the overall vertical dimension, including length, angle, proportion, and the mandibular relationship, should all be evaluated[56–59]:

1. The anterior facial height, chin point position, and overall vertical relationship between soft tissue and hard tissue at rest and during facial animation should be evaluated (Figs 7-19 and 7-20).
2. The local vertical relationship between soft tissue and hard tissue should be evaluated. The static and dynamic vertical relationships should also be evaluated. These parameters include the upper and lower lip length at rest and during function and the amount of exposure of the maxillary and mandibular anterior teeth at rest and during function (Figs 7-21 and 7-22).

Fig 7-19 Normal vertical relationships. *(a)* Skeletally, the proportion of the anterior facial height to posterior facial height *(red arrows)* is 1:0.65, and that of nasion–anterior nasal spine to anterior nasal spine–menton *(blue arrows)* is approximately 1:1. *(b)* The length from glabella to subnasale is similar to that from the subnasale to soft tissue menton *(blue arrows)*. In the mandibular facial height, the proportion of the vertical length of the upper lip to the vertical length of the lower lip *(red arrows)* is approximately 1:1.8 to 1:2.

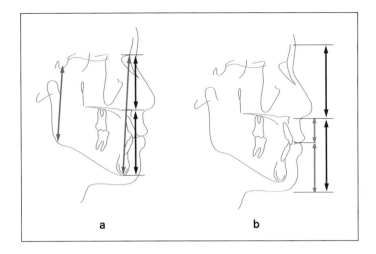

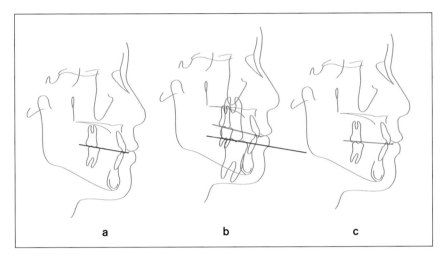

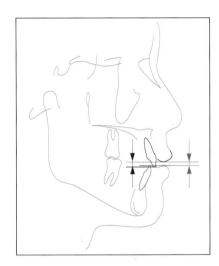

Fig 7-20 *(a)* Normal occlusal plane inclination *(blue)*. *(b)* If an occlusal plane is too steep *(red)*, occlusal interferences in anterior guidance are likely to occur, to say nothing of the unesthetic smile line. *(c)* If the occlusal plane is excessively flat *(red)*, an unesthetic, flat smile line results.

Fig 7-21 Normal relationship between the lips and teeth in a static state. The interlabial gap should be about 2 mm in centric occlusion. The maxillary incisors should be exposed by 2 to 3 mm in the resting state, while the mandibular central incisors should not be exposed, because they are as high as the lower lip. In the resting state, if the interlabial gap is more than 4 mm, this is generally regarded as lip incompetence. The amount of tooth exposure in females tends to be greater than that in males. Furthermore, the older the patient, the lesser the exposure of the maxillary teeth and the greater the exposure of the mandibular teeth. That is, deficient exposure of the maxillary anterior teeth and excessive exposure of the mandibular anterior teeth are characteristics of an older appearance.

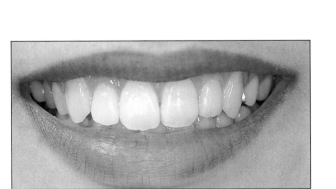

Fig 7-22 Normal relationship between the lips and teeth in a dynamic functional state. When the patient is smiling, it is recommended that the incisal edges of the maxillary anterior teeth take the shape of a "V" and be parallel to the lower lip line, because the upper lip is located 0 to 2 mm above the gingival margin of the maxillary central incisor.

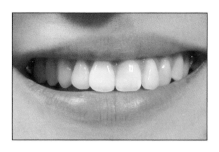

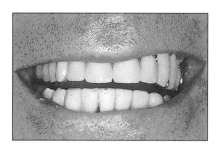

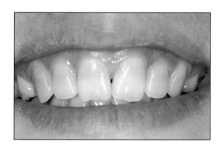

Fig 7-23a The vertical position of the molars plays a crucial role in the shaping of the smile line. A flat smile is caused by relative extrusion of the maxillary posterior teeth compared to the anterior teeth.

Fig 7-23b Typical appearance of a mouth with dentures. An older-looking smile is characterized by deficient exposure of the maxillary anterior teeth, excessive exposure of the mandibular anterior teeth, and a flat smile line.

Fig 7-23c The patient's smile displays an excessive amount of the maxillary gingiva, and the smile arc is flat.

Figs 7-24a to 7-24e Characteristics of patients with relatively excessive anterior facial height.

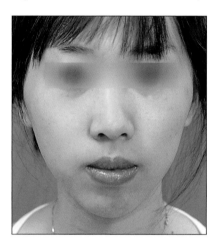

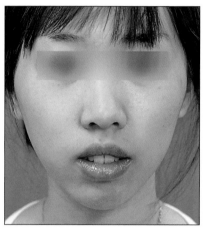

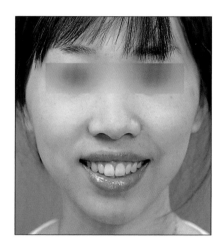

Fig 7-24a The mentalis muscle strains with lip closure.

Fig 7-24b The patient demonstrates lip incompetency at rest.

Fig 7-24c With a social smile (when one smiles consciously), there is little gingival display.

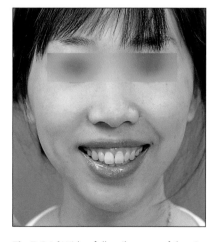

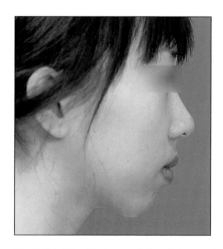

Fig 7-24d With a full smile, more of the gingiva is displayed.

Fig 7-24e The chin is retruded and the anterior face is relatively long. Esthetic improvement is expected from intrusion of the entire maxillary dentition.

Figs 7-25a to 7-25d Characteristics of patients with relatively excessive anterior facial height.

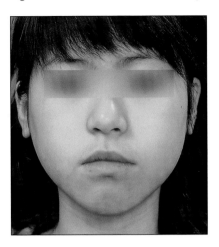

Fig 7-25a Although the overall facial look appears similar to that seen in Fig 7-24a, this facial type gives the impression of an older appearance.

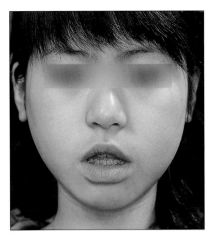

Fig 7-25b There is excessive show of the mandibular anterior teeth when the individual is resting, speaking, or smiling.

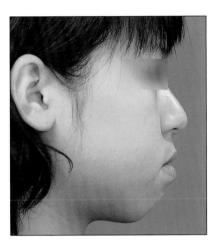

Fig 7-25c The patient has a retruded chin and a lower anterior face height that is long, similar to that seen in Fig 7-24e.

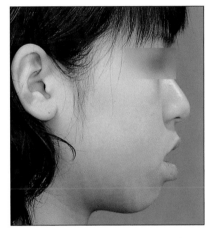

Fig 7-25d The patient demonstrates lip incompetency at rest. Esthetic improvement is anticipated from intrusion of the mandibular dentition.

3. The smile should be evaluated. The amount of incisal and gingival display, the transverse dimension of the smile, and the smile arc should be analyzed[57–59] (Fig 7-23).

The aforementioned parameters should be evaluated both at rest and during facial animation, and changes with age should also be considered. Based on the diagnosis, the anterior facial height should be considered during the planning of treatment objectives (Figs 7-24 and 7-25). Based on the anterior facial height as a treatment objective, the vertical positions of the anterior teeth and posterior teeth should be planned (Fig 7-26). Then, the VTO derived from this process should be reevaluated. If necessary, this process should be repeated until a satisfactory VTO is obtained. It is important to periodically reevaluate and verify VTO during treatment.

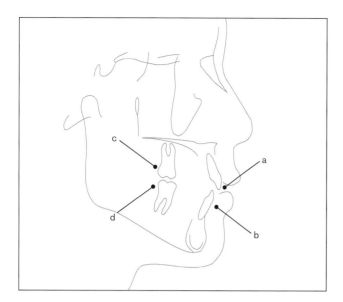

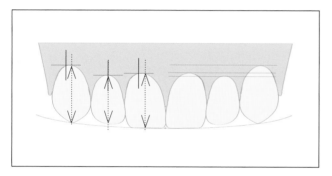

Fig 7-27 Relationships among the maxillary anterior teeth. The six maxillary anterior teeth can be esthetic only if they show suitable inclination, angulation, vertical height, and gingival relationships. The gingival level of the maxillary central incisors, lateral incisors, and canines has a pattern of high-low-high *(arrows)*. The crown of the lateral incisor is shorter than that of the central incisor by approximately 0.5 mm.

Fig 7-26 Process of creating the VTO for the vertical dimension. *(a)* First, the anteroposterior position of the maxillary anterior teeth is determined, while the upper lip esthetics are taken into consideration. Then, the vertical position of the maxillary anterior teeth is determined, with consideration of the vertical relationships at rest and during a smile. *(b)* The mandibular position for harmonious facial esthetics is determined. *(c)* The vertical position of the maxillary posterior teeth is determined; the smile line and planned anterior facial height must be considered. *(d)* The vertical positions of the mandibular anterior teeth and posterior teeth are determined according to the planned position of the mandible. The vertical positions of the mandibular anterior teeth at rest and during speech are determined. At this point, the tentative VTO is completed and should be verified again. The final VTO is completed through trial and error.

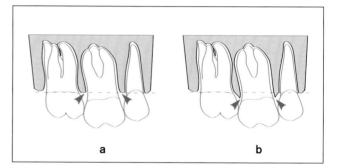

Fig 7-28 Determination of the vertical position. First, the periodontal condition, including the alveolar bone level and the position of furcation, should be considered when the vertical position of the molar is determined. Even periapical radiographs are not capable of providing enough information, because the interdental space becomes narrow if the tooth is extruded. Bone probing under local anesthestic may be helpful for examining the bone condition. The bone level and the position of furcation can be improved by intrusion. *(a)* If the tooth is extruded with a flat alveolar bone level *(arrows)*, the furcation is sufficiently located apically, and the teeth are nonvital, occlusal reduction is a better option. *(b)* If the tooth is extruded with an angular alveolar bone level *(arrows)*, intrusion may be recommended.

Local vertical dimension

Evaluation of the local vertical dimension should incorporate the following considerations:

1. For anterior teeth, an esthetic gingival line relationship should be considered in addition to the occlusal relationship and a functional alveolar bone relationship (Fig 7-27).[60]
2. For posterior teeth, a functional alveolar bone relationship should be considered before the occlusal relationship in treatment planning for vertical positioning (Fig 7-28). Occlusal reduction may be necessary to establish a normal alveolar bone relationship.

Conventional concepts of leveling

Classically, through the leveling stage, all treatment objectives anatomically and periodontally should be achieved from the point of vertical control. This includes leveling for the occlusion, leveling for the gingival margin, and leveling of the alveolar bone.

Figs 7-29a and 7-29b A high-positioned canine was brought into occlusion through the leveling procedure.

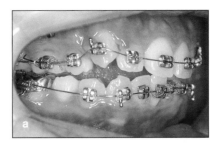 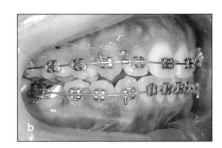

Fig 7-30a The incisal edges of the maxillary central incisors are aligned. However, the gingival margins *(arrows)* do not coincide because the crown lengths are different.

Fig 7-30b The gingival margins *(arrows)* have been leveled by rebracketing. Esthetic grinding of the crown has also been performed.

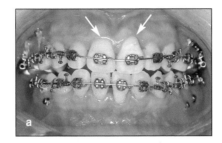 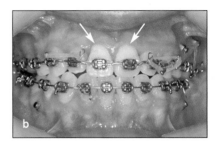

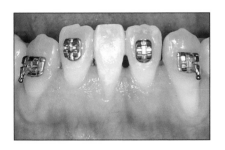 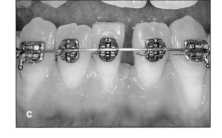

Fig 7-31a The mandibular central incisor has insufficient attached gingiva because of recession and is bypassed during intrusion.

Figs 7-31b and 7-31c After intrusion of the lateral incisors is completed, incisal reduction is performed on the central incisor.

Figs 7-32a and 7-32b The incisal edges of the central incisors have been aligned via intrusion of the maxillary left central incisor, but a vertical bone defect has formed. Periodontal inflammation has occurred with signs of bleeding on probing. From the perspective of periodontal health, incisal reduction of the maxillary left central incisor may be a better option. **(a)** Clinical situation prior to intrusion. **(b)** Result after intrusion.

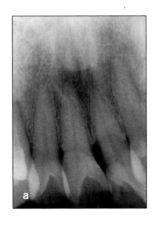 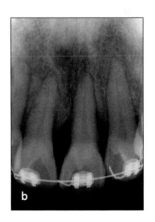

Leveling for occlusion

Through leveling, the incisal edges or occlusal surfaces of the teeth should be properly positioned in the vertical dimension and should be in occlusion (Fig 7-29).

Leveling for the gingival margin

Leveling should be used to form an esthetic gingival margin (see Fig 7-27). This can improve the overall esthetics by moving the teeth vertically (Figs 7-30 and 7-31).

Leveling for alveolar bone

After leveling, alveolar bone should have a healthy and functional bone level (Figs 7-32 to 7-34).

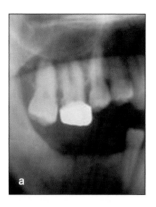
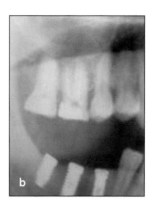

Fig 7-33a There is no space for prosthodontic restorations because the maxillary molars have extruded in response to the lack of opposing teeth.

Fig 7-33b Occlusal reduction has been performed, which has added vertical space for prosthodontics but has not improved the undesirable alveolar bone level resulting from extrusion.

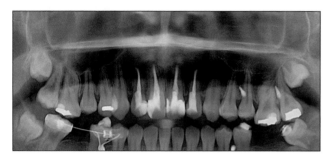

Fig 7-34a The maxillary first molars are extruded because the opposing teeth are missing. Consequently, the alveolar bone level has also changed.

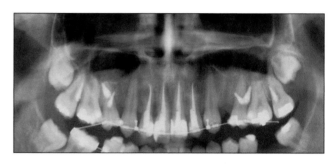

Fig 7-34b The alveolar bone is also leveled through the intrusion of the maxillary first molars.

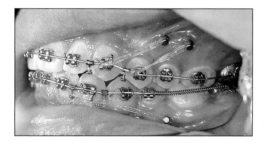

Fig 7-35a Leveling for the occlusal plane. The dual occlusal plane causes an unesthetic smile.

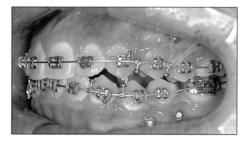

Fig 7-35b The level of the occlusal plane, and hence the smile, has been improved by intrusion of the premolars and tipping back of the posterior segments.

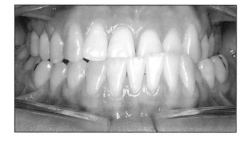

Fig 7-36a Leveling for the occlusal plane. The mandibular anterior occlusal plane is canted.

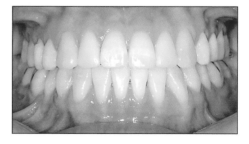

Fig 7-36b The cant of the occlusal plane has been improved by asymmetric intrusion.

Fig 7-37a Leveling for the harmonious lip. The vertical relationship between the maxillary anterior teeth and the upper lip when the patient smiles allows excessive show of gingiva.

Fig 7-37b The "gummy" smile has been improved nonsurgically through intrusion of the maxillary dentition.

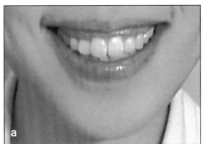
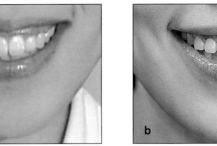

Fig 7-38a Leveling for the harmonious lip. The vertical relationship between the maxillary posterior teeth and the upper lip when the patient smiles creates a reverse smile line.

Fig 7-38b The smile has been improved nonsurgically through intrusion of the maxillary posterior teeth.

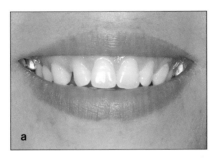
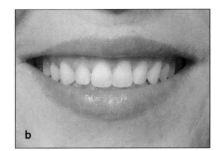

Fig 7-39a Leveling for the harmonious face. The patient has a long face and a retruded chin.

Fig 7-39b The skeletal relationships have been improved nonsurgically through maxillary and mandibular intrusion.

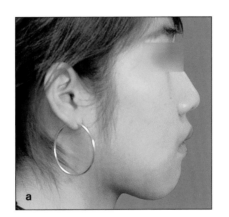
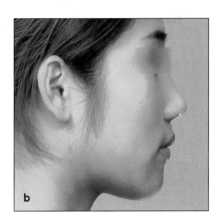

New concept of leveling: Improvement of the vertical relationships

Molar intrusion becomes possible through the use of orthodontic mini-implants. The mandibular position can be changed indirectly by molar intrusion achieved with mechanotherapy. Based on the mini-implant type of anchorage, an efficient technique, and utilizing a treatment paradigm, a total concept for leveling is proposed.

Leveling for the harmonious occlusal plane

The posterior occlusal plane on the left and right sides should be level and on the same plane as the anterior occlusal plane (Figs 7-35 and 7-36). Canting should also be corrected.

Leveling for the harmonious lip

An esthetic vertical relationship should be obtained between the anterior teeth and the lips when the patient smiles, both in the resting state and in facial animation (Figs 7-37 and 7-38). The occlusal plane should bisect the corners of the mouth.

Leveling for the harmonious face

If necessary, anterior facial height and chin point should be controlled by posterior intrusion for a more vertically harmonious face (Fig 7-39).

CASE REPORTS

The potential intrusive mechanics allowed by orthodontic mini-implants changed orthodontic treatment concepts, as demonstrated through the following case reports:

1. Case 7-1 illustrates leveling for the harmonious face. The patient's long face and retruded chin were improved nonsurgically by maxillary and mandibular intrusion.
2. Case 7-2 demonstrates leveling for the harmonious lip. The vertical relationship between the maxillary anterior teeth and the upper lip when the patient was smiling (a "gummy smile") was improved nonsurgically by intrusion of the entire dentition. The patient's long face and retruded chin were also improved.
3. Case 7-3 demonstrates leveling for the occlusal plane. Asymmetry and occlusal canting were corrected nonsurgically by three-dimensional tooth movement.

Case 7-1

A 23-year-old woman was referred from a local clinic for orthognathic surgery. She displayed a typical long-faced appearance: a long lower face, lip incompetence, extreme lip and mentalis strain on lip closure, and a retruded chin. She was unaccustomed to smiling, and her smile appeared very unnatural. An anterior open bite, Angle Class I molar relationship, and mild crowding were observed (Figs 7-40a to 7-40c). Cephalometric analysis confirmed anterior vertical excess, although the posterior facial height and the gonial angle were within normal range. That is, the mandibular position was not favorable, but the shape of the mandible was normal.

The treatment objectives consisted of the improvement of facial esthetics, improvement of smile esthetics, and establishment of normal anterior occlusion. Surgical correction may have been an option, but it did not seem to have any additional benefits compared to nonsurgical correction with mini-implants because the mandibular shape was normal. Therefore, it was decided that the maxillary and mandibular molars would be intruded and distalized with mini-implants.

Eight ORLUS mini-implants (Ortholution), 1.6 mm in diameter and 7.0 mm in length, were placed in the maxillary and mandibular buccal areas. Additional 1.6 × 8.0-mm ORLUS mini-implants were placed in the palatal interdental area between the molars. Anterior intrusion was not planned, so the anterior teeth were bypassed. Initially, 0.018 × 0.025-inch Bioforce nickel-titanium (NiTi) wires (GAC) were placed in the maxillary arch, and a 0.016 × 0.022-inch titanium-molybdenum alloy (TMA) wire (Ormco) with a constriction bend and a second-order bend was placed in the mandibular arch. Intrusive and distalizing forces were applied to crimpable hooks on the wires.

After 1 month of treatment, the maxillary posterior teeth were aligned, and a 0.017 × 0.025-inch TMA wire with a constriction bend and a second-order bend was placed in the maxillary arch. Palatal intrusive forces from the implants were applied 7 weeks into treatment.

Four months after the start of treatment, the anterior vertical relationships improved, and brackets were then bonded to the anterior teeth. At that time, 0.018 × 0.025-inch Bioforce NiTi wires were placed in the maxillary arch and 0.014-inch NiTi wires were overlaid with 0.016 × 0.022-inch TMA wires in the mandibular arch (Figs 7-40d to 7-40f). Intrusive and distalizing forces were applied continuously.

Following 7 months of treatment, the mandibular main wire was changed to a 0.016 × 0.022-inch Bioforce NiTi wire. After 12 months of treatment, 0.016 × 0.022-inch stainless steel wires were placed in the maxillary and mandibular arches to control the arch forms and occlusal plane (Figs 7-40g to 7-40i). Maxillomandibular elastics were also used for occlusal seating.

Active treatment to the planned position was completed after 14 months. Fixed retainers extending from first premolar to first premolar were used in the maxilla and mandible (Figs 7-40j to 7-40l). A circumferential retainer with tongue crib in the maxillary arch was worn full time for the first 6 months following treatment and only at night thereafter.

After 10 months of posttreatment follow-up, the results were well maintained (Figs 7-40m to 7-40o).

Case 7-1   Leveling for harmonious facial esthetics.

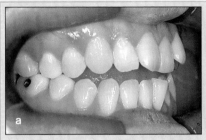
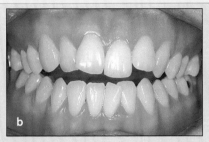
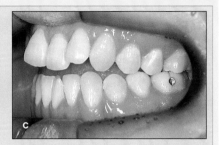

Figs 7-40a to 7-40c Clinical situation prior to treatment.

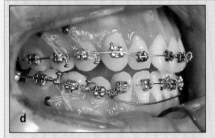
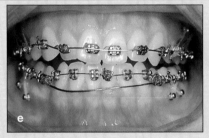
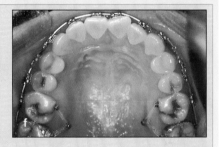

Figs 7-40d to 7-40f At 4 months of treatment.

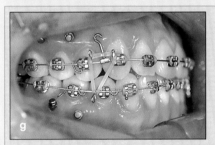
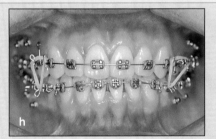
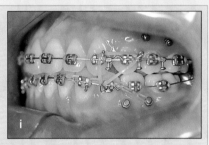

Figs 7-40g to 7-40i At 7 months of treatment.

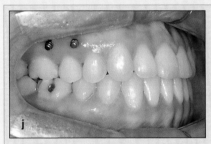
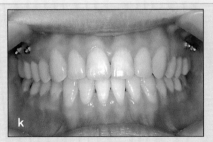
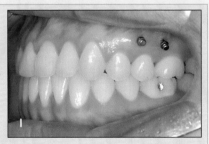

Figs 7-40j to 7-40l Result at completion of active treatment.

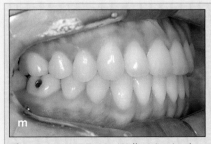
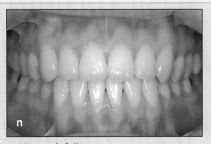
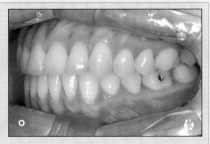

Figs 7-40m to 7-40o Well-maintained result at 10-month follow-up.

Case 7-1   *(cont)*

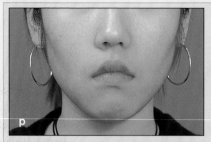
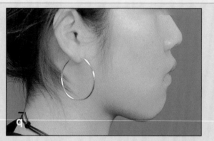
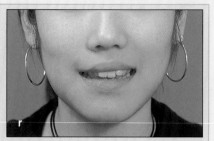

Figs 7-40p to 7-40r Facial views prior to treatment.

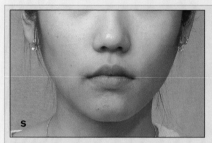
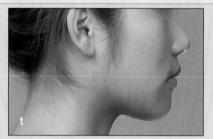
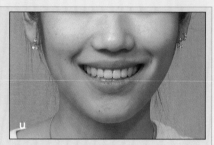

Figs 7-40s to 7-40u Facial views at the completion of active treatment.

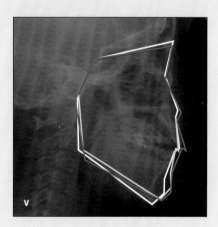

Fig 7-40v Cephalometric analysis prior to treatment. *(white)* Patient; *(green)* normal template; *(yellow)* VTO.

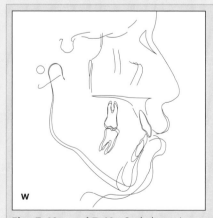
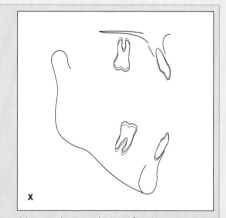

Figs 7-40w and 7-40x Cephalometric superimpositions at the completion of active treatment. *(black)* Prior to treatment; *(red)* at the completion of active treatment.

Case 7-2

The patient was a 23-year-old woman whose chief complaint was protrusion of the lips. She exhibited good occlusion and a nice social or posed smile (Figs 7-41a to 7-41c). However, the smile examination using videocameras revealed that she had excessive gingival exposure when she smiled fully (see Fig 7-41s). She also showed lip incompetence. Lateral cephalometry revealed that her facial disharmony was the result of vertical disharmony rather than anteroposterior problems.

The treatment objectives included the improvement of facial esthetics and smile esthetics through the correction of vertical relationships. Therefore, the decision was made to intrude and distalize the entire dentition using mini-implants.

ORLUS mini-implants of 1.8 mm in diameter and 8.0 mm in length were placed in the maxillary arch and 1.8 mm in diameter and 7.0 mm in length were placed in the mandibular arch. Two implants were placed in each quadrant for en masse intrusion and distalization of the entire dentition. The 0.018-inch slot preadjusted appliances with Roth prescriptions were bonded to four maxillary anterior teeth while 0.022-inch slot preadjusted appliances were used for the other teeth. The 0.018 × 0.025-inch Bioforce NiTi wires were placed as initial wires (Figs 7-41d to 7-41f). Intrusive and distalizing forces were applied to hooks on the wire, and approximately 250 g of force was applied to each implant. To control the rotation of the mandibular central incisors, a couple were applied using lingual buttons.

Because only buccal interdental implants were used, wire bends for three-dimensional control were applied; that is, constriction bends, second-order bends, and third-order bends were created for control of the arch form, occlusal plane, and posterior torque.

After 5 months of treatment, 0.017 × 0.025-inch TMA wires with the first-, second-, and third-order bends were engaged (Figs 7-41g to 7-41i). The occlusion did not seem to change, but the facial view changed significantly as a result of intrusion and distalization of the entire dentition.

At 11 months, treatment was completed (Figs 7-41j to 7-41l). Fixed retainers extending from canine to canine were bonded in the maxilla and mandible. A maxillary circumferential retainer was also worn at night.

At the 6-month follow-up examination, the results were well maintained (Figs 7-41m to 7-41o).

Case 7-2   Leveling for the harmonious lip.

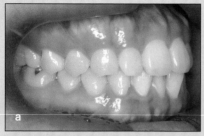
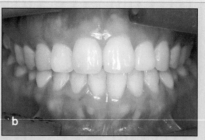
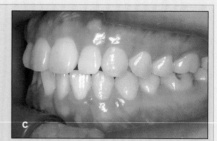

Figs 7-41a to 7-41c Clinical situation prior to treatment.

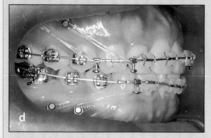
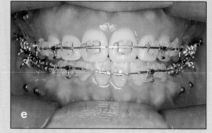
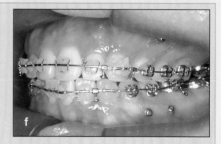

Figs 7-41d to 7-41f Initial appliances.

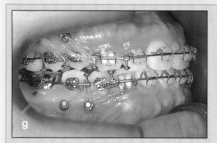
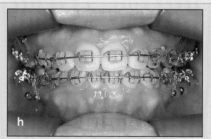
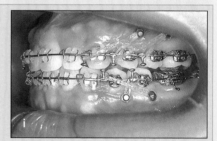

Figs 7-41g to 7-41i At 5 months of treatment.

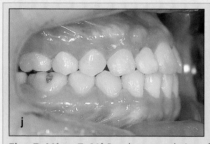
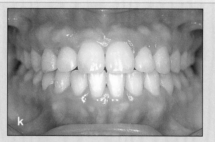
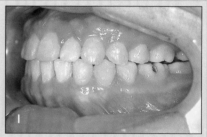

Figs 7-41j to 7-41l Result at completion of active treatment.

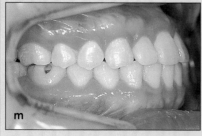
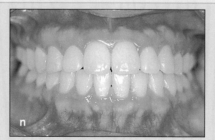
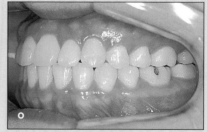

Figs 7-41m to 7-41o Well-maintained result at 6-month follow-up.

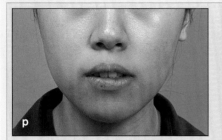
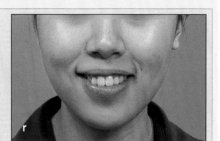
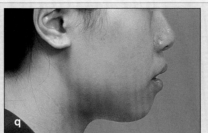
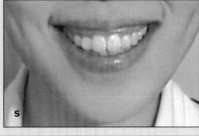
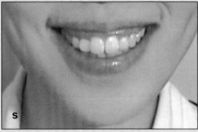

Figs 7-41p to 7-41s Facial views prior to treatment.

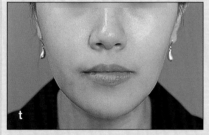
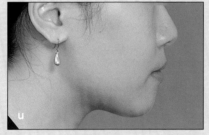
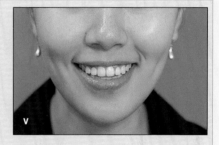

Figs 7-41t to 7-41v Facial views at the completion of active treatment.

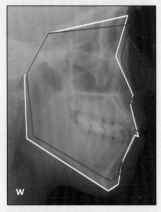
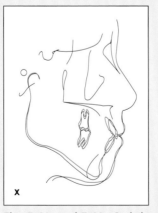
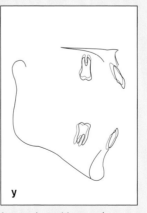
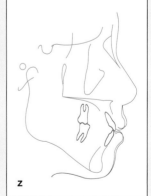

Fig 7-41w Cephalometric analysis prior to treatment. *(white)* Patient; *(green)* normal template.

Figs 7-41x and 7-41y Cephalometric superimpositions at the completion of active treatment. *(black)* Prior to treatment; *(red)* at the completion of active treatment.

Fig 7-41z Cephalometric superimposition at follow-up. *(red)* At the completion of active treatment; *(green)* at 18-month follow-up after completion of treatment.

Case 7-3

The patient was a 26-year-old woman whose chief complaints were an anterior cross bite and asymmetric exposure of the mandibular incisors during function (Figs 7-42a to 7-42c). She had a Class III short-faced appearance. She could position her incisors edge-to-edge in centric relation but had a significant anterior slide from centric relation to maximum intercuspation. She had also had an occasional clicking sound from the right temporomandibular joint, and, furthermore, the chin deviated to the right during mouth opening. She had no history of temporomandibular joint pain.

The facial examination revealed that the chin deviated to the left, the maxilla was canted downward on the right, and the interpupillary line canted downward to the left. The intraoral examination revealed an anterior crossbite with canting of the mandibular anterior occlusal plane and a relatively narrow maxillary dentition. Radiographic examination confirmed the pattern of a skeletal Class III relationship with short face and asymmetry.

Surgical correction was required to correct the retrusive maxilla and short anterior facial height, but the patient desired nonsurgical correction. In fact, surgical correction of the anterior canting would not have been easy. The treatment objectives were the improvement of facial esthetics, the improvement of smile esthetics, and the establishment of a normal anterior occlusion. The treatment plan was to distalize the mandibular dentition and to correct anterior canting with the use of mini-implants. Orthodontic expansion was also planned to correct the maxillary transverse deficiency.

Six weeks after treatment started, 0.016 × 0.022-inch Bioforce NiTi wires were placed in the maxillary and mandibular arches. In the mandibular arch, distalizing and intrusive forces were applied from two ORLUS mini-implants, 1.8 mm in diameter and 7.0 mm in length, on each side. The posterior occlusion was raised using resin for core buildup to prevent traumatic occlusion during anterior bite correction.

After 4 months of treatment, a 0.017 × 0.025-inch TMA wire with an expansion curve was placed in the maxillary arch for maxillary expansion (Figs 7-42d to 7-42f). The 0.016 × 0.022-inch Bioforce NiTi wires were used continuously for leveling and retraction. To improve facial esthetics by increasing the vertical dimension, extrusion of the premolar area was attempted using crossbite elastics. After 4 weeks, a 0.017 × 0.025-inch TMA wire was placed in the mandibular arch as well.

Following 8 months of treatment, the anterior crossbite and canting were improved. For correction of posterior canting, maxillomandibular elastics were used with consideration of the short face and the smile arc relationship (Figs 7-42g to 7-42i). For further extrusion of the left side, maxillomandibular elastics were used from both the buccal and palatal sides of the maxilla, and intrusive forces from mini-implants were used to hold the mandibular arch for anchorage control.

At the 15-month mark, compliance of the patient was not sufficient. Therefore, one ORLUS mini-implant (1.6 mm in diameter and 7.0 mm in length) was placed on the right, and then an extrusion spring made of 0.018-inch TMA wire was positioned to extrude the right posterior teeth. The spring was applied to the main wire by point contact to increase efficiency. Maxillomandibular elastics were also continuously used from the lingual side (Figs 7-42j and 7-42k).

At 17 months, active treatment was completed and a fixed retainer was used (Figs 7-42l to 7-42n). A circumferential retainer in the maxillary arch was worn full time for the first 6 months following treatment to maintain the transverse dimension. It was then worn only at night.

At the 10-month follow-up after the completion of treatment, the results were well maintained (Figs 7-42o to 7-42q).

Case 7-3 Leveling for the occlusal plane.

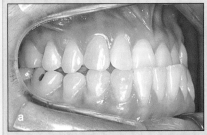
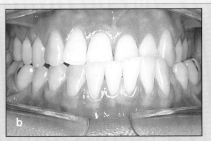
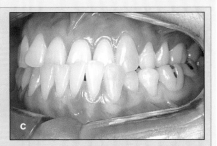

Figs 7-42a to 7-42c Clinical situation prior to treatment.

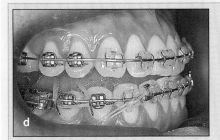
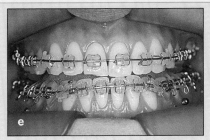
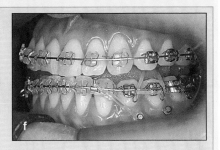

Figs 7-42d to 7-42f At 4 months of treatment.

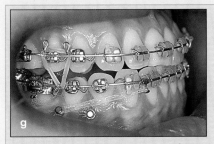
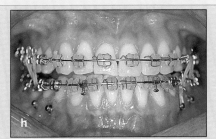
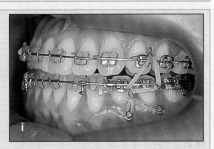

Figs 7-42g to 7-42i At 8 months of treatment.

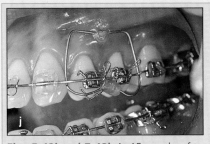
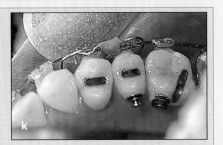

Figs 7-42j and 7-42k At 15 months of treatment.

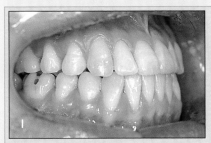
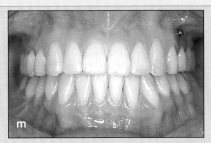
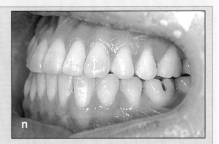

Figs 7-42l to 7-42n Result after completion of active treatment.

(cont)

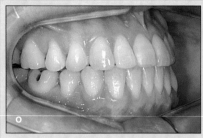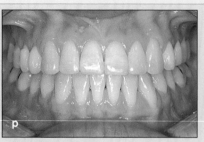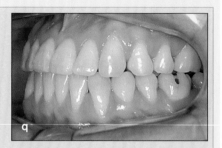

Figs 7-42o to 7-42q Well-maintained result at 10-month follow-up.

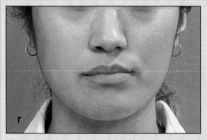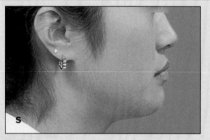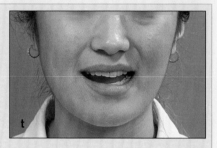

Figs 7-42r to 7-42t Facial views prior to treatment.

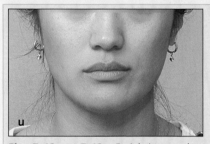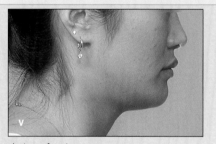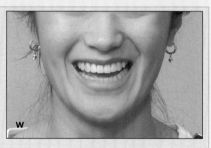

Figs 7-42u to 7-42w Facial views at the completion of active treatment.

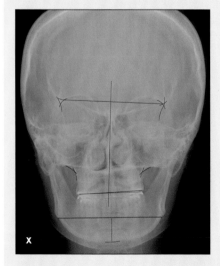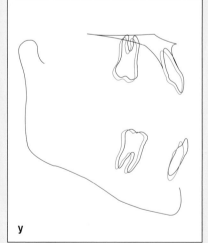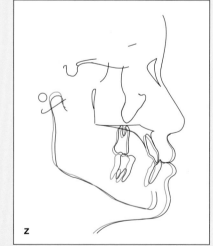

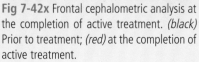

Fig 7-42x Frontal cephalometric analysis at the completion of active treatment. *(black)* Prior to treatment; *(red)* at the completion of active treatment.

Figs 7-42y and 7-42z Cephalometric superimpositions at the completion of active treatment. *(black)* Prior to treatment; *(red)* at the completion of active treatment.

SUMMARY

Traditionally, the paradigm for orthodontic mechanotherapy has been restricted within the biomechanical limitations of anchorage control. Molar intrusion has been regarded as clinically impossible because it is not possible to secure enough anchorage from the dentition. However, with the development of a stable anchorage system, loss of anchorage is no longer a concern.

The most outstanding characteristic of orthodontic treatment with implants is the ability to achieve intrusion of molars and nonsurgical control of the vertical dimension. Orthodontic mini-implants can be used for intrusion of overerupted teeth, improvement of angular bone level, nonsurgical correction of anterior open bite in patients with skeletal open bite, nonsurgical correction of excess anterior facial height, and improvement of the smile line. Orthodontic mini-implants will accelerate the paradigm shift to a new, treatment objective–oriented soft tissue paradigm.

REFERENCES

1. Ackerman JL, Proffit WR, Sarver DM. The emerging soft tissue paradigm in orthodontic diagnosis and treatment planning. Clin Orthod Res 1999;2:49–52.
2. Proffit WR, White RP, Sarver DM. Contemporary Treatment of Dentofacial Deformity Orthodontics. St Louis: Mosby, 2003:92–94.
3. Ackerman JL, Proffit WR. Soft tissue limitations in orthodontics: Treatment planning guidelines. Angle Orthod 1997;67:327–336.
4. Ricketts RM. The wisdom of the bioprogressive philosophy. Semin Orthod 1998;4:201–209.
5. Graber TM, Vanarsdall RL, Vig KWL. Orthodontics: Current Principles and Techniques. St Louis: Elsevier Mosby, 2005.
6. Proffit WR. Contemporary Orthodontics, ed 2. St Louis: Mosby-Yearbook, 1993:307.
7. Proffit WR. Contemporary Orthodontics, ed 3. St Louis: Mosby, 2000.
8. Burstone CJ. The segmented arch approach to space closure. Am J Orthod 1982;82:361–378.
9. Nanda R. Correction of deep overbite in adults. Dent Clin North Am 1997;41:67–87.
10. Sugawara J, Baik UB, Umemori M, et al. Treatment and posttreatment dentoalveolar changes following intrusion of mandibular molars with application of a skeletal anchorage system (SAS) for open bite correction. Int J Adult Orthodon Orthognath Surg 2002;17:243–253.
11. Sugawara J. Dr Junji Sugawara on the skeletal anchorage system. Interview by Dr Larry W. White. J Clin Orthod 1999;33:689–696.
12. Sherwood KH, Burch JG, Thompson WJ. Closing anterior open bites by intruding molars with titanium miniplate anchorage. Am J Orthod Dentofacial Orthop 2002;122:593–600.
13. Park YC, Lee SY, Kim DH, Jee SH. Intrusion of posterior teeth using mini-screw implants. Am J Orthod Dentofacial Orthop 2003;123:690–694.
14. Erverdi N, Keles A, Nanda R. The use of skeletal anchorage in open bite treatment: A cephalometric evaluation. Angle Orthod 2004;74:381–390.
15. Yao CC, Wu CB, Wu HY, Kok SH, Chang HF, Chen YJ. Intrusion of the overerupted upper left first and second molars by mini-implants with partial-fixed orthodontic appliances: A case report. Angle Orthod 2004;74:550–557.
16. Kuroda S, Katayama A, Takano-Yamamoto T. Severe anterior open-bite case treated using titanium screw anchorage. Angle Orthod 2004;74:558–567.
17. Lee JS, Kim DH, Park YC, Kyung SH, Kim TK. The efficient use of midpalatal miniscrew implants. Angle Orthod 2004;74:711–714.
18. Yao CC, Lee JJ, Chen HY, Chang ZC, Chang HF, Chen YJ. Maxillary molar intrusion with fixed appliances and mini-implant anchorage studied in three dimensions. Angle Orthod 2005;75:754–760.
19. Murakami T, Yokota S, Takahama Y. Periodontal changes after experimentally induced intrusion of the upper incisors in Macaca fuscata monkeys. Am J Orthod Dentofacial Orthop 1989;95:115–126.
20. Daimaruya T. Basic researches on molar intrusion treatment using SAS. Pre-conference: The 4th Asian Implant Orthodontic Conference, Seoul, Korea, December 3, 2005.
21. Ari-Demirkaya A, Masry MA, Erverdi N. Apical root resorption of maxillary first molars after intrusion with zygomatic skeletal anchorage. Angle Orthod 2005;75:761–767.
22. Melsen B, Agerbaek N, Markenstam G. Intrusion of incisors in adult patients with marginal bone loss. Am J Orthod Dentofacial Orthop 1989;96:232–241.
23. Daimaruya T, Takahashi I, Nagasaka H, Umemori M, Sugawara J, Mitani H. Effects of maxillary molar intrusion on the nasal floor and tooth root using the skeletal anchorage system in dogs. Angle Orthod 2003;73:158–166.
24. Daimaruya T, Nagasaka H, Umemori M, Sugawara J, Mitani H. The influences of molar intrusion on the inferior alveolar neurovascular bundle and root using the skeletal anchorage system in dogs. Angle Orthod 2001;71:60–70.
25. Lee JS. Development of Orthodontic Mini-Implant Anchorage System. Pre-Conference: Basic Researches on Implant Orthodontics. The 4th Asian Implant Orthodontics Conference, Seoul, Korea, December 3–4, 2005.
26. Ainamo J, Talari A. The increase with age of the width of attached gingiva. J Periodontal Res 1976;11:182–188.
27. Lee DY, Bailey LJ, Proffit WR. Soft tissue changes after superior repositioning of the maxilla with Le Fort I osteotomy: 5-year follow-up. Int J Adult Orthodon Orthognath Surg 1996;11:301–311.
28. Wessberg GA, O'Ryan FS, Washburn MC, Epker BN. Neuromuscular adaptation to surgical superior repositioning of the maxilla. J Maxillofac Surg 1981;9:117–122.
29. Wessberg GA, Washburn MC, LaBanc JP, Epker BN. Autorotation of the mandible: Effect of surgical superior repositioning of the maxilla on mandibular resting posture. Am J Orthod 1982;81:465–472.
30. Proffit WR, White RP, Sarver DM. Contemporary Treatment of Dentofacial Deformity Orthodontics, ed 1. St Louis: Mosby, 2003:197–199, 480–482.
31. Proffit WR, Phillips C, Turvey TA. Stability following superior repositioning of the maxilla by Le Fort I osteotomy. Am J Orthod Dentofacial Orthop 1987;92:151–161.
32. Proffit WR, Turvey TA, Fields HW, Phillips C. The effect of orthognathic surgery on occlusal force. J Oral Maxillofac Surg 1989;47:457–463.

33. Zarrinkelk HM, Throckmorton GS, Ellis E 3rd, Sinn DP. Functional and morphologic alterations secondary to superior repositioning of the maxilla. J Oral Maxillofac Surg 1995;53:1258–1267.

34. O'Ryan F, Epker BN. Surgical orthodontics and the temporomandibular joint. I. Superior repositioning of the maxilla. Am J Orthod 1983;83:408–417.

35. Proffit WR, Phillips C. Adaptations in lip posture and pressure following orthognathic surgery. Am J Orthod Dentofacial Orthop 1988;93:294–302.

36. Graber TM, Vanarsdall RL, Vig KWL. Orthodontics: Current Principles and Techniques. St Louis: Elsevier Mosby, 2005:180–182.

37. Denison TF, Kokich VG, Shapiro PA. Stability of maxillary surgery in openbite versus nonopenbite malocclusions. Angle Orthod 1989;59:5–10.

38. Bailey LJ, Phillips C, Proffit WR, Turvey TA. Stability following superior repositioning of the maxilla by Le Fort I osteotomy: Five-year follow-up. Int J Adult Orthodon Orthognath Surg 1994;9:163–173.

39. Proffit WR, Bailey LJ, Phillips C, Turvey TA. Long-term stability of surgical open-bite correction by Le Fort I osteotomy. Angle Orthod 2000;70:112–117.

40. Lopez-Gavito G, Wallen TR, Little RM, Joondeph DR. Anterior open-bite malocclusion: A longitudinal 10-year postretention evaluation of orthodontically treated patients. Am J Orthod 1985;87:175–186.

41. Kim YH, Han UK, Lim DD, Serraon ML. Stability of anterior openbite correction with multiloop edgewise archwire therapy: A cephalometric follow-up study. Am J Orthod Dentofacial Orthop 2000;118:43–54.

42. Huang GJ. Long-term stability of anterior open-bite therapy: A review. Semin Orthod 2002;8:162–172.

43. Janson G, Valarelli FP, Henriques JF, de Freitas MR, Cancado RH. Stability of anterior open bite nonextraction treatment in the permanent dentition. Am J Orthod Dentofacial Orthop 2003;124:265–276.

44. de Freitas MR, Beltrao RT, Janson G, Henriques JF, Cancado RH. Long-term stability of anterior open bite extraction treatment in the permanent dentition. Am J Orthod Dentofacial Orthop 2004;125:78–87.

45. Janson G, Valarelli FP, Beltrao RT, de Freitas MR, Henriques JF. Stability of anterior open-bite extraction and nonextraction treatment in the permanent dentition. Am J Orthod Dentofacial Orthop 2006;129:768–774.

46. Kawamura M, Nojima K, Nishii Y, Yamaguchi H. A cineradiographic study of deglutitive tongue movement in patients with anterior open bite. Bull Tokyo Dent Coll 2003;44:133–139.

47. Yamaguchi H, Sueishi K. Malocclusion associated with abnormal posture. Bull Tokyo Dent Coll 2003;44:43–54.

48. Huang GJ, Justus R, Kennedy DB, Kokich VG. Stability of anterior openbite treated with crib therapy. Angle Orthod 1990;60:17–24.

49. Proffit WR, Phillips C, Turvey TA. Stability following superior repositioning of the maxilla by Le Fort I osteotomy. Am J Orthod Dentofacial Orthop 1987;92:151–161.

50. Proffit WR, Turvey TA, Phillips C. Orthognathic surgery: A hierarchy of stability. Int J Adult Orthodon Orthognath Surg 1996;11:191–204.

51. Lindhe J, Karring T, Lang, NP. Clinical Periodontology and Implant Dentistry, ed 3. Copenhagen: Munksgaard, 1997:760–765.

52. Bondevik O. Tissue changes in the rat molar periodontium following application of intrusive forces. Eur J Orthod 1980;2:41–49.

53. Mostafa YA, Weaks-Dybvig M, Osdoby P. Orchestration of tooth movement. Am J Orthod 1983;83:245–250.

54. Proffit WR. Contemporary Orthodontics, ed 3. St Louis: Mosby, 2000.

55. Melsen B. Tissue reaction to orthodontic tooth movement—A new paradigm. Eur J Orthod 2001;23:671–681.

56. Sarver, DM. Esthetic Orthodontics and Orthognathic Surgery. St Louis: Mosby, 1998.

57. Sarver DM, Ackerman MB. Dynamic smile visualization and quantification: Part 1. Evolution of the concept and dynamic records for smile capture. Am J Orthod Dentofacial Orthop 2001;124:4–12.

58. Sarver DM, Ackerman MB. Dynamic smile visualization and quantification: Part 2. Smile analysis and treatment strategies. Am J Orthod Dentofacial Orthop 2003;124:116–127.

59. Graber TM, Vanarsdall RL, Vig KWL. Orthodontics: Current Principles and Techniques. St Louis: Elsevier Mosby, 2005:28–52.

60. Kokich VG, Nappen DL, Shapiro PA. Gingival contour and clinical crown length: Their effect on the esthetic appearance of maxillary anterior teeth. Am J Orthod 1984;86:89–94.

ANTERIOR-POSTERIOR CONTROL 8

ANTERIOR RETRACTION

Treatment planning, biomechanics, and mechanics

Based on a proper diagnosis and detailed treatment plan, mechanics should be designed to achieve the force system required[1-6] (Figs 8-1 to 8-3). Biomechanically, the retraction of anterior teeth to the proper position should be performed with anterior torque control, canine axis control, and vertical control of the anterior teeth. Because of the availability of orthodontic mini-implants, anteroposterior anchorage control no longer poses an anchorage problem.

Specifically, with extraction treatment, in addition to the selection of mechanics, the selection of the bracket prescription should be considered when a preadjusted appliance is used. When mini-implants are used as anchorage, the length of time in which a retractive force is delivered to the molar can be shortened, and utilization of excessive offsets for antirotation of molars may not be appropriate.

As with other edgewise mechanics, with mini-implants consideration should be given to anterior torque. Depending on the planned amount of retraction, an anterior bracket prescription with additional labial crown torque may be desirable. The general principles for extraction treatment with a conventional edgewise technique are also important to consider for extraction treatment with mini-implants.

Control of anchorage and line of action

Anchorage is necessary for maximum retraction of anterior teeth, anterior torque control, and canine axis control (Figs 8-4 and 8-5). Orthodontic mini-implants can provide more rigid or absolute anchorage, and with the placement of implants in specific positions and the adjustment of the length of lever arms, the line of action can be controlled to achieve the treatment objectives[7,8] (Figs 8-6 to 8-8).

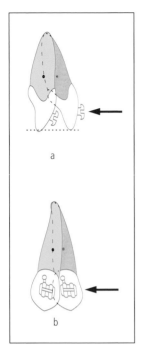

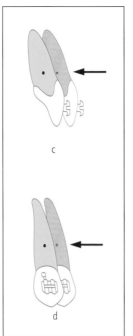

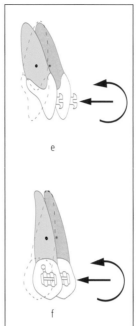

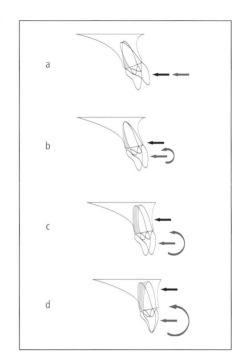

Fig 8-1 *(a and b)* For incisor and canine retraction, bodily movement is required in most cases; if force is applied to the bracket, uncontrolled tipping occurs. For bodily movement, it is necessary that *(c and d)* force be applied through the center of resistance or *(e and f)* force be applied to the bracket with a moment for root control. The moment-force ratio for bodily movement is approximately 10:1, although this may vary depending on the root length, shape, and alveolar bone condition. In other words, when one force is applied to the bracket, 10 moments must be delivered together to the bracket to produce bodily movement.

Fig 8-2 Depending on the specific treatment objectives for the anterior teeth, *(a)* uncontrolled tipping, *(b)* controlled tipping, *(c)* bodily movement, and *(d)* root movement should occur. Increased anchorage and a longer treatment period are required with increasing amounts of alveolar bone reactions. *(red)* Alveolar bone reaction required for movement; *(blue arrow)* line of action required for the movement; *(green arrow)* equivalent force system required on the bracket.

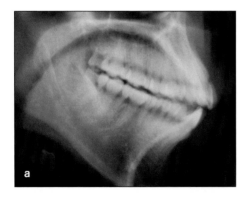

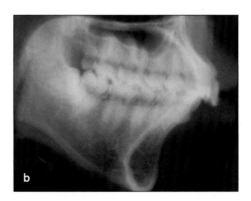

Figs 8-3a and 8-3b It is critical that the available amount of alveolar bone and root shapes be evaluated on the cephalometric radiograph before anterior retraction. The relationship between the root apex and the lingual cortical bone should be considered, and the planned treatment positions of the root apices should be checked in advance to determine whether a sufficient amount of alveolar bone is present at the apical area. Even with the same amount and shape of anterior protrusion, the volume of alveolar bone lingual to the apices of the maxillary anterior teeth can differ. **(a)** If sufficient alveolar bone is present near the apex, the chances of root resorption are reduced even with an extensive amount of anterior retraction. **(b)** If the quantity of alveolar bone is insufficient, there is a greater chance of root resorption with the same amount of anterior retraction.

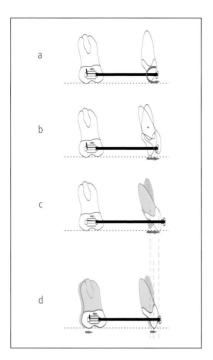

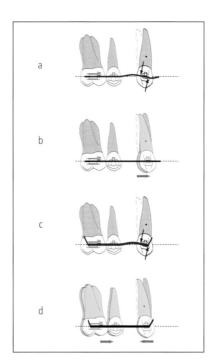

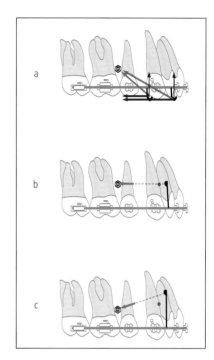

Fig 8-4 Loss of anchorage during anterior torque control. *(a)* A moment causes the incisor to rotate. When the moment (torque) is delivered to the anterior tooth, *(b)* rotation of the anterior tooth occurs around its center of resistance. *(c)* As a consequence, the incisal edge moves anteriorly; because of this tendency, a space may form distal to the incisors, or, *(d)* in cases in which the dentition is cinched back, the molar moves forward. For root movement of the anterior teeth, the incisal edges of the anterior teeth should be at their original positions; to accomplish this, anchorage should be reinforced in the same manner as when anterior teeth are retracted.

Fig 8-5 Loss of anchorage during canine axis control. In cases in which the distally tipped canine undergoes mesial tipping, loss of anchorage occurs. *(a)* When the moment is delivered to the canine by archwire for leveling and alignment, rotation of the canine occurs around the center of resistance. *(b)* In cases where the archwire can be sliding freely, the canine tip moves anteriorly. *(c)* Even in cases in which the dentition is linked by cinch-back, the moment on the canine makes the canine tip move anteriorly. *(d)* As a consequence, the canine tip and molar move anteriorly according to their anchorage value.

Fig 8-6 Changing the insertion sites and hook positions can control the line of action. In this way, the type of tooth movement can be managed in anterior retraction, and the intrusive force vector *(a)* can be increased for anterior intrusion. The long lever arms can move the line of action to the occlusal plane and induce *(b)* bodily movements or *(c)* root movements.

Fig 8-7a The line of action can be moved occlusally for anterior torque control through the use of long lever arms.

Fig 8-7b Labial space is limited in the vestibule, and labial lever arms may cause discomfort and an unesthetic appearance. Space is abundant in the palatal area, so palatal lever arms can be applied in the desired directions. (Figs 8-7a and 8-7b courtesy of Dr BS Yoon, Seoul, Korea.)

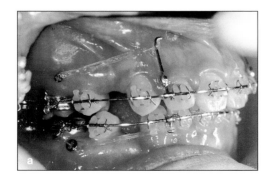

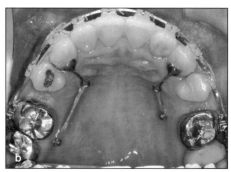

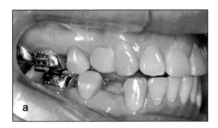

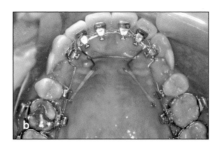

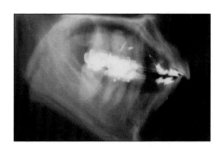

Figs 8-8a and 8-8b To reduce lip protrusion, four premolars were extracted. Ormco 0.018-inch lingual brackets are used for esthetics, and palatal interdental mini-implants are used for maximum anterior retraction. Palatal lever arms provide anterior torque control by managing the line of action. The line of action for space closure has been moved apically to achieve bodily retraction.

Fig 8-8c Cephalometric radiograph before space closure.

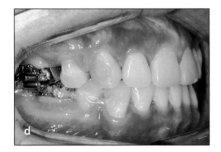

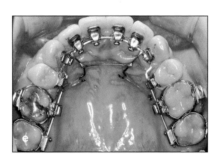

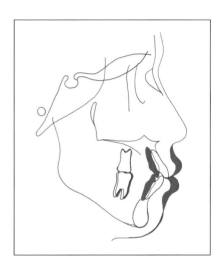

Figs 8-8d and 8-8e After 9 months, space closure has been accomplished. (Courtesy of Dr JK Lim, Seoul, Korea.)

Fig 8-8f Cephalometric superimposition before and after space closure. *(blue)* Prior to space closure; *(red)* after space closure. The anterior teeth are being retracted with translation.

Control of anterior torque

Generally, sliding mechanics using a 0.022-inch slot preadjusted appliance with additional labial crown torque and a 0.019 × 0.025-inch stainless steel (SS) wire are suggested. Edgewise brackets provide weak torque control (Fig 8-9). For cases requiring critical anterior torque control, a 0.018-inch slot preadjusted appliance with additional labial crown torque for the four anterior teeth and a 0.018 × 0.025-inch SS wire are useful for space closure, because play between the wire and brackets is reduced on the anterior teeth (Fig 8-10).

Anterior intrusion can also facilitate anterior torque control. The intrusive force has effects on anterior torque, and these effects should be considered in the selection of the anterior bracket prescription and the mechanics.

Special attention is needed to prevent exacerbation of anterior torque during the leveling and alignment stage; the anterior torque must be sufficiently established prior to the initiation of anterior retraction. During space closure, torque must be continuously monitored to prevent exacerbation in comparison with the stage preceding space closure. If the torque appears to have been lost, it is best to decrease the retractive force or to add more moment on the anterior teeth. Additionally, the strategy used to control the anterior torque at the finishing stage after space closure is no longer desirable because anteroposterior anchorage control during space closure is no longer an issue (Fig 8-11).

Fig 8-9 The edgewise bracket is advantageous for second-order control. However, it is disadvantageous for third-order control. There are four ways to apply a moment to anterior teeth: *(a)* by twisting a rectangular wire; *(b)* by using high-torque brackets (brackets that have a prescription for large amounts of labial crown torque); *(c)* by applying intrusive force; and *(d)* by modulating the line of action. When anchorage is under control, the use of high-torque brackets and memory wires, such as copper-nickel-titanium wires and titanium-molybdenum alloy (TMA) wires, is simple and effective.

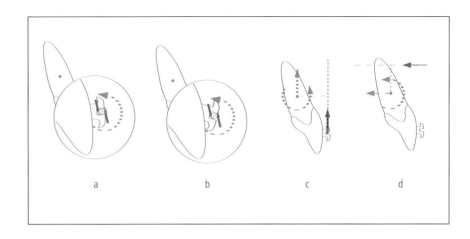

a   b   c   d

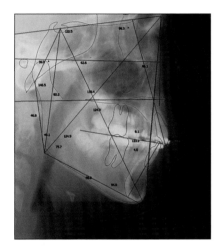

Fig 8-10a Torque was lost during anterior retraction.

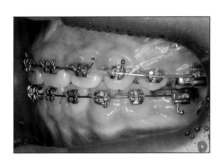

Fig 8-10b A 0.019 × 0.025-inch TMA wire with a compensating curve is placed in the anterior 0.018-inch Roth bracket to increase the torque.

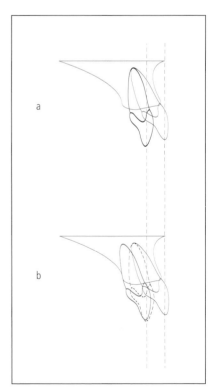

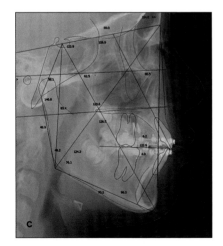

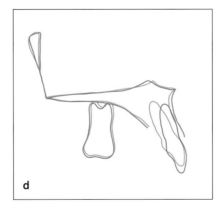

Figs 8-10c and 8-10d Torque has been improved. The sagittal position of the anterior teeth is maintained by the use of a mini-implant. *(purple)* Before torque control; *(orange)* after torque control.

Fig 8-11 A classic strategy for anterior torque control during space closure is first *(a)* tipping and then *(b)* uprighting. It is advantageous to preserve anchorage but not efficient in regard to the treatment time.

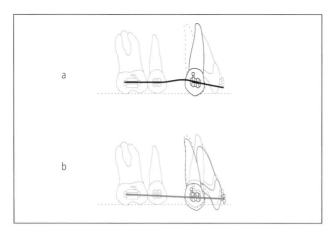

Fig 8-12 If the canine is tipped distally, *(a)* the canine axis should be corrected before the alignment of the anterior teeth. *(b)* If the main archwire is engaged in the brackets of the anterior teeth and distally tipped canine, the anterior teeth will be extruded before the canine axis is controlled. During space closure, axis control of the canine is also important for occlusal plane control.

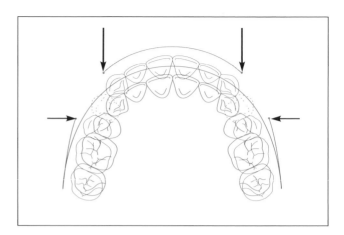

Fig 8-13 In premolar extraction cases, the arch form should be altered according to the amount of retraction. If more retraction is necessary, a greater change in the arch form is also necessary. *(red)* As the extraction space closes, the premolar area should be constricted. *(arrows)* Direction of retraction and constriction.

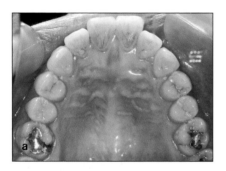
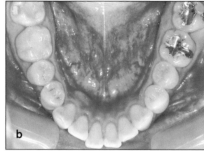

Figs 8-14a and 8-14b Occlusal views prior to first premolar extraction and anterior retraction. (Figs 8-14a to 8-14g courtesy of Dr JK Lim, Seoul, Korea.)

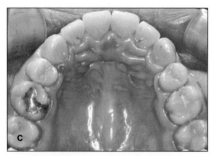
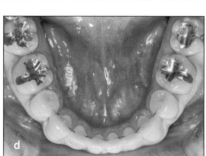

Figs 8-14c and 8-14d Occlusal views after closure of the extraction spaces.

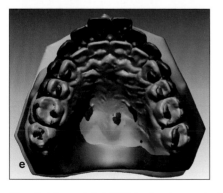
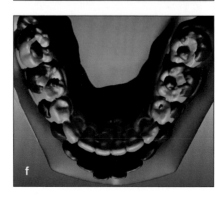
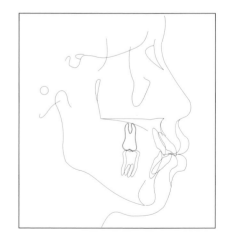

Figs 8-14e and 8-14f Note the changes in the arch form of the **(e)** maxilla and **(f)** mandible after maximum anterior retraction. As the extraction space is closed by the anterior retraction, the premolar areas are constricted. *(gray)* Prior to treatment; *(green)* at the completion of treatment.

Fig 8-14g Cephalometric superimposition at the end of treatment. *(black)* Prior to treatment; *(red)* at the end of active treatment.

Figs 8-15a to 8-15d Arch form skewing. In dentitions requiring extensive retraction, lingual tipping of the canine (loss of canine torque) easily occurs, and the intercanine distance becomes narrower. The arch form is easily skewed from a U shape to a V shape. When an implant is used, the entire extraction space can be used for anterior retraction, and thus it is more important to control the arch form and canine torque. The use of sliding mechanics in a rigid SS wire heavier than 0.017 × 0.025-inch with a moderate rate of space closure serves as a satisfactory method for solving such problems. **(a)** Pretreatment maxillary occlusal view. **(b)** Pretreatment mandibular occlusal view; **(c)** Posttreatment maxillary occlusal view; **(d)** Posttreatment mandibular occlusal view.

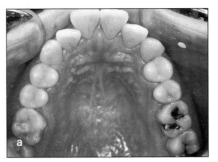
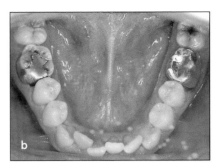
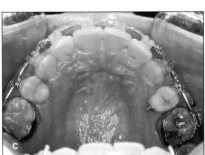
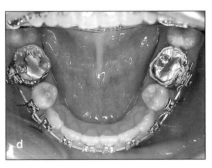

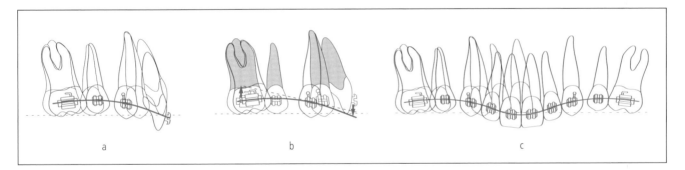

Fig 8-16 Vertical bowing can occur while a light wire is used. *(a)* As a molar is tipped mesially and a canine is tipped distally with retractive force, the main archwire will deflect. *(b)* Consequently, premolars will be tipped mesially and anterior teeth will be extruded. Vertical bowing will result because of this tipping during space closure; therefore, vertical bowing can be prevented by canine and molar axis control during space closure. *(c)* Because this phenomenon looks from the anterior view like the teeth are cars in a roller coaster, this has been known as the *roller coaster effect.*

Control of the canine axis

The canine has a large root-surface area. Therefore, it can negatively influence other teeth if its position is unfavorable[9] (Fig 8-12). The distal tipping of the canine not only worsens the vertical positions of the anterior teeth but also exacerbates the torque by twisting the rectangular wire with lingual crown torque. Distal tipping of the canine exacerbates the side effects caused by the intrusive force of the implant.

Control of arch form

In extraction treatment, the arch width at the premolars should be altered in accordance with the amount of anterior retraction. The more the anterior teeth are retracted,

the more the arch form should be changed (Figs 8-13 and 8-14).

With increasing amounts of anterior retraction, significant attention should be given to arch form. Control of arch form is also related to the canine torque and axis control. With lingual and distal tipping of the canine, the intercanine width decreases and the arch form is altered to a V shape rather than a U shape (Fig 8-15).

Control of bowing

Tipping into the extraction site causes vertical and transverse bowing (Figs 8-16 to 8-20). Mini-implants alone cannot prevent tipping of canines. Extensive force vector may exacerbate the bowing tendency.

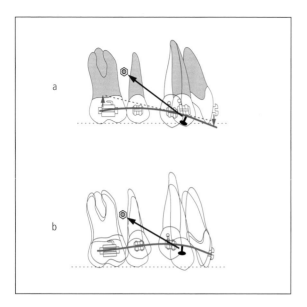

Fig 8-17 Vertical bowing can occur even with mini-implants. *(a)* As a canine is tipped distally with a retractive force, the main archwire will deflect. *(b)* Consequently, the premolars are tipped mesially and intruded. Anterior torque is worsened by the deflection of the archwire, particularly with a rectangular main archwire. There is no bite deepening with the bowing effect caused by the mini-implant because of the intrusive force vector, and this is different from the outcome with the conventional vertical bowing.

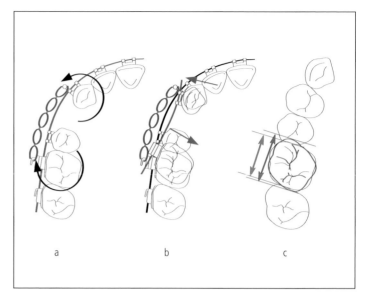

Fig 8-18 Transverse bowing can occur with a light archwire. The situation in the occlusal dimension occurs in the same manner as vertical bowing. *(a)* When the canines are retracted with light archwire, the force is applied facial to the center of resistance and the teeth are rotated. *(b)* As the first molars are rotated mesially and canines are rotated distally, the main light archwire deflects. Consequently, the arch form becomes skewed and there is a lack or an excess of buccal overjet in the posterior region. *(c)* In addition, the mesially rotated first molars occupy more space *(red arrow)* than properly positioned first molars *(grey arrow)*. As the result, the ideal anterior relationship is lost in a Class I molar relationship.

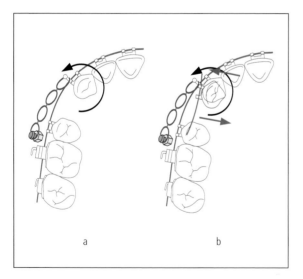

Fig 8-19 Transverse bowing can occur even with mini-implants. *(a)* As the canine is rotated distally by the retraction force, *(b)* the molar can be rotated mesially by deflection of the archwire.

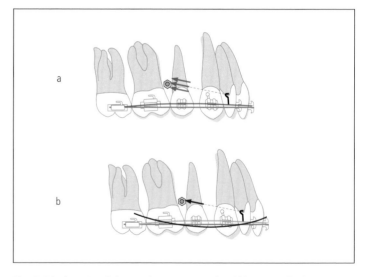

Fig 8-20 The axis of the tooth or rotation should be controlled to prevent even slight tipping. In addition, the intrusive force vector should be controlled. *(a)* Basically, bowing results from an insufficient moment-to-force ratio that causes tipping instead of translation, frequently with excessive retraction force. *(b)* Bowing can be avoided by using a stiffer archwire, providing additional bends for moments, and by reducing the retraction force. *(red arrow)* Excessive retraction force; *(blue arrow)* reduced retraction force; *(red wire)* wire deflected by vertical bowing; *(blue wire)* wire bonded to create sufficient moment.

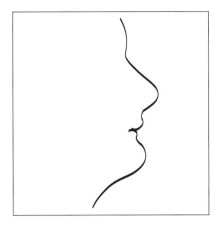

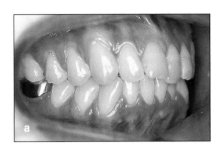

Figs 8-22a and 8-22b The chief complaint of the patient is anterior crowding. (a) Pretreatment right lateral intraoral view. (b) Pretreatment right lateral facial view.

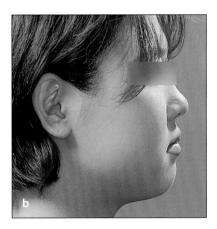

Fig 8-21 Improper extraction treatment can induce unfavorable changes. When the anterior teeth are retracted excessively after premolar extraction, the lips become depressed, resulting in an older overall appearance. The anterior guidance also becomes deeper and steeper, which may have functionally adverse effects on the temporomandibular joint. Premolar extraction treatment does not always induce such problems. However, in patients who undergo excessive retraction of the anterior teeth based on strong anchorage, there is an increased risk of the development of such problems.

Figs 8-22c and 8-22d After extraction of the maxillary and mandibular first premolars, treatment has been completed. (c) However, the anterior teeth appear to have been overretracted. (d) If the lips are retracted excessively, the nasolabial fold deepens, forming a shadow, and the lips look thin, creating an older facial appearance.

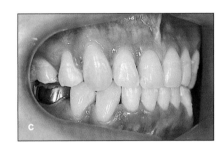

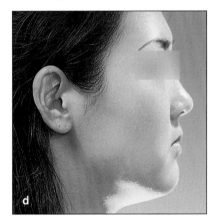

Special considerations and monitoring

There are differences between conventional extraction mechanics and extraction mechanics with mini-implants. When extraction mechanics are used with mini-implants, the following concepts should be considered:

1. Too much retraction is as detrimental as too little. When strong anchorage is present, the amount of retraction can increase. A flat lip caused by too much retraction is unattractive and gives the patient an older appearance. The more the anterior teeth are retracted, the higher the risk of root resorption.
2. Intrusive force is not always positive. In conventional mechanics, intrusive force is difficult to achieve. With apically located interdental mini-implants, intrusive forces are easily produced but can cause unwanted side effects, including iatrogenic canting. Therefore, any intrusive force vector should be carefully controlled.
3. Strong anchorage makes every tooth movement possible. On the other hand, tooth movement should be maintained within biologic limitations. Additionally, with a greater range of tooth movement, the risk of root resorption or periodontal breakdown also increases.

Amount of retraction

Excess retraction may cause a patient to exhibit an older facial appearance (Figs 8-21 and 8-22), and this problem will be exacerbated as the patient ages. Excessive retraction is worse than insufficient retraction (Fig 8-23).

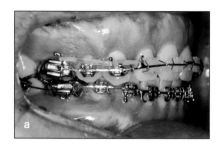
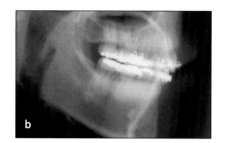
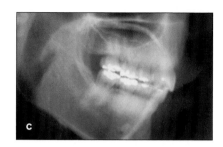

Figs 8-23a to 8-23c (a and b) A patient concerned about overuprighting of the anterior teeth. **(c)** The patient returned on a second visit months later concerning excessive retraction of the anterior teeth. Anterior torque was controlled well, but unfortunately the root apices are palatal to the alveolar trough.

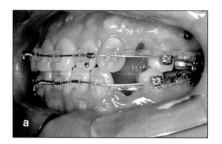
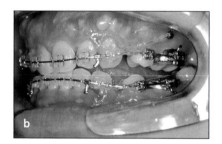
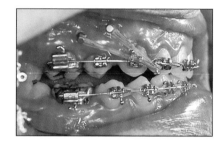

Figs 8-24a and 8-24b (a) Left intraoral view. A 0.018-inch Roth prescription and a 0.017 × 0.025-inch TMA wire with a compensating curve is being used for anterior retraction. **(b)** As the canine has tipped distally, a lingual crown torque has been produced by deflection of the wire. Because of the intrusive force vector from the implants, the vertical positions of the anterior teeth have been maintained, the bite has not deepened, and the torque of the four anterior teeth has worsened. Additionally, however, the posterior occlusion has been opened by the intrusive force from the deflected main archwire.

Fig 8-25 Side effects from intrusive mechanics can develop even when a stiff wire is used. Intrusive force vectors cause buccal tipping and intrusion of the maxillary first molar, and it has led to greater vertical and transverse discrepancies with the second molar.

Intrusive force

Adverse effects may develop because of intrusive force (Figs 8-24 and 8-25). Distal tipping of the canine and an open bite at the first molar area may develop. Particularly when the second molar is not included in the full appliance, the first molar is likely to be intruded. If the retractive force has an intrusive force vector, vertical control is important during space closure. Depending on the case, an intrusive force vector may cause the anterior teeth to exhibit labial flaring instead of lingual tipping. This labial flaring may increase the risk of root resorption.

Canting of the occlusal plane

If the intrusion progresses more quickly on one side, occlusal plane canting may be induced (Fig 8-26). This results in a canted smile line from a frontal view that is very difficult to correct.

Root resorption

When a greater amount of tooth movement is required, the risk of root resorption is increased,[10-12] in particular during anterior root movement (Fig 8-27). Systematic risk management may be required to help prevent root resorption.[10,11]

Rate of space closure

During space closure in which mini-implants are used as anchorage, the extraction space may fail to close, particularly in adolescent patients or patients with curved main archwires (Fig 8-28). This does not reflect a lack of movement of adjacent teeth but rather the distalization of the posterior teeth as a result of retractive force from the implants. This phenomenon can be assessed with an examination of the interarch relationship and evaluation with a cephalometric superimposition. Because the implant is

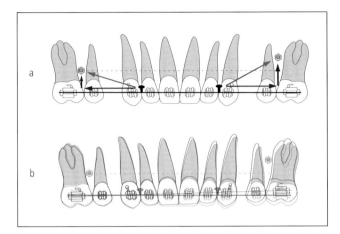

Fig 8-26 *(a)* Different vertical positions of implants or different retractive forces cause discrepancies in the intrusive forces on the right and left sides, and *(b)* these may cause iatrogenic occlusal canting on the frontal plane.

Pretreatment
- Periapical radiographic examination
- Informed consent
- Evaluation of family history

During treatment
- Semiannual periapical radiographic examination
- Periodontal control
- Avoidance of heavy and intermittent forces
- Discontinuation of orthodontic force in the event of root resorption

Posttreatment
- Occlusal adjustment
- Systematic oral hygiene control for periodontal health

Fig 8-27 Protocols for prevention of root resorption.

Fig 8-28a Left lateral view before space closure.

Fig 8-28b During space closure, the mandibular space has been closed while the maxillary space remains the same. In contrast to the initial Class 1 molar relationship, the molar relationship has changed to a Class III relationship.

Figs 8-28c and 8-28d The cephalometric superimposition confirms distalization of the maxillary posterior teeth. Monitoring the relationship between the implant and the teeth can reveal such problems. *(blue)* Prior to space closure; *(red)* during space closure. (Figs 8-28a to 8-28d courtesy of Dr JK Lim, Seoul, Korea.)

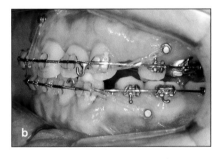
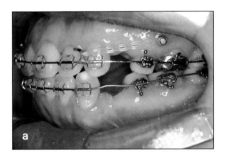
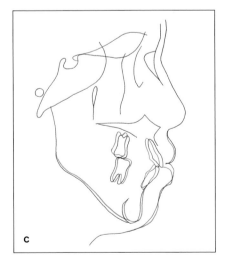
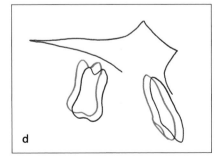

not moving as long as it is stable, the change in distance between the implant and adjacent teeth becomes a useful landmark for monitoring tooth movement. The solution for failure of space closure is simple: Elastics can be hooked or placed onto the molars instead of the implants to move both anterior teeth and posterior teeth at the same time, as in conventional treatment.

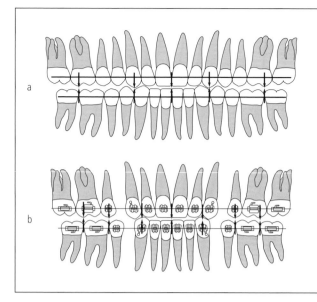

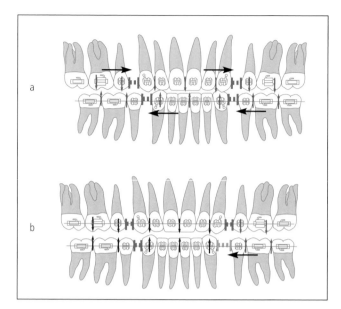

Fig 8-29 *(a)* If there is no tooth size disharmony and the maxillary and mandibular arches are well balanced, the molars and the canines can have a bilateral Class I relationship and the ideal midline and anterior tooth relationships can be achieved in the normal dentition. *(b)* In Class I cases, there should be no discrepancy in the bilateral molar and canine relationship, the maxillary and mandibular midlines, the arch forms, or the anterior relationship during space closure. In addition, there should be no discrepancy in the residual space. Special attention is required for the normal relationships of all factors during space closure.

Fig 8-30 *(a)* If the dental midlines deviate *(red arrows)*, the bilateral sagittal relationship usually is not symmetric. *(b)* If the dental midlines coincide *(blue arrows)* and if there is a symmetric sagittal relationship, there should be a different amount of space *(dashed orange line)*, or tooth size discrepancies.

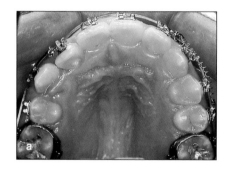

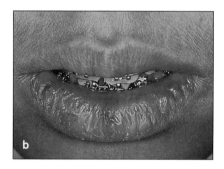

Fig 8-31a Because of unilateral premolar extraction on the right side, the anteroposterior positions of the maxillary right and left canines are different.

Fig 8-31b As a result of the varied canine positions, the dental midlines did not coincide.

Midline and interarch relationships

To correct midline deviation, the diagnosis is of the utmost importance.[13,14] This deviation usually occurs as a result of skeletal asymmetry. However, in this discussion, midline deviation will be discussed only with regard to orthodontic correction.

The midline is strongly associated with the interarch relationship (Fig 8-29). For the improvement of the midline and interarch relationships, space is required. Hence, progression toward the improvement of the interarch relationship and midline correction should be accomplished simultaneously with space closure.

Anterior midline deviation accompanies anteroposterior problems (Fig 8-30). More specifically, there is a discrep-

ancy in the anteroposterior position of the canine. Particularly in asymmetric extraction, the anteroposterior positions of the canines can easily differ, and thus the arch form may be skewed accordingly (Fig 8-31). To correct the anterior midline deviation through orthodontic tooth movement,[13] the molar and the canine must be in the proper anteroposterior position and must have a proper arch form. Four anterior teeth must also be translated laterally (Figs 8-32 and 8-33). The orthodontic mechanics for the correction of the anterior midline deviation are used to create the space for the proper positioning of canines and molars, to translate canines and molars, to coordinate the arch form, and to translate anterior teeth laterally (Fig 8-34). The mechanics used to obtain space and to translate teeth are explained in detail in this chapter.

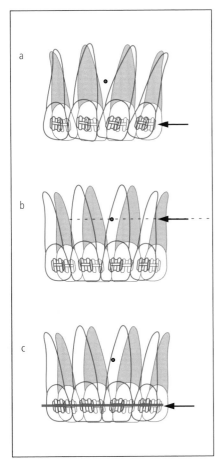

Fig 8-32 *(a)* Lateral force on the bracket causes uncontrolled tipping rather than translation. *(b)* To translate laterally, an appropriate moment to control the root position or force through the center of resistance is necessary. *(c)* With the proper rate of movement, twin brackets can easily control roots in the second-order dimension, if the play between wires and brackets is not excessive. *(blue arrows)* Line of action.

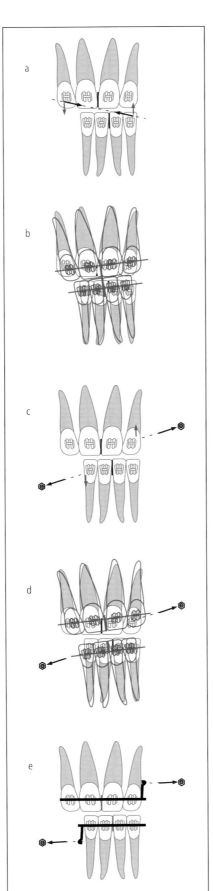

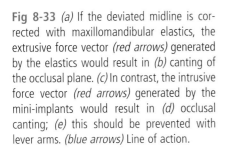

Fig 8-33 *(a)* If the deviated midline is corrected with maxillomandibular elastics, the extrusive force vector *(red arrows)* generated by the elastics would result in *(b)* canting of the occlusal plane. *(c)* In contrast, the intrusive force vector *(red arrows)* generated by the mini-implants would result in *(d)* occlusal canting; *(e)* this should be prevented with lever arms. *(blue arrows)* Line of action.

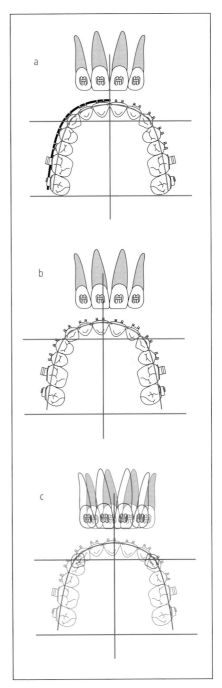

Fig 8-34 *(a)* Normally, a midline is in alignment with a proper arch form and proper anteroposterior positions of canines and molars. *(b)* In a case of midline deviation in which a premolar is lost on only one side and the arch form of the mandible is normal, the anteroposterior positions of the right and left canines also deviate. To correct the midline deviation, lateral bodily movement of the anterior teeth and anteroposterior repositioning of the canines is required. *(c)* To correct canine positions, anteroposterior bodily movement of the canine, premolar, and molar is required.

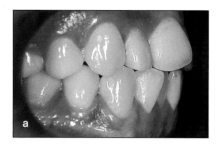
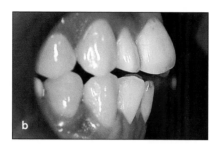

Figs 8-35a and 8-35b There is a centric occlusion–centric relation discrepancy between (a) the right lateral view in centric occlusion and (b) the right lateral view in centric relation. If a centric occlusion–centric relation discrepancy exists, the amount of planned distalization should be increased. Centric occlusion–centric relation discrepancies must not only be assessed during diagnosis and treatment planning but also must be monitored during treatment.

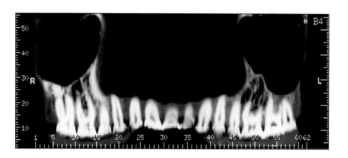

Fig 8-36 The distal limits of the hard tissue are the posterior border of the maxillary tuberosity.

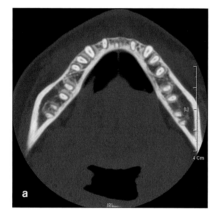
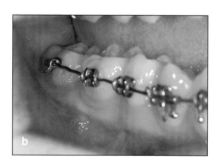

Figa 8-37a and 8-37b In the mandible, distalization is limited by (a) the cortical bone of the mandibular ramus and (b) the soft tissue condition of the distobuccal side of the second molar.

After the positions of the canine and the molar are controlled, and 0.017 × 0.025-inch titanium-molybdenum alloy (TMA) wire and 0.017 × 0.025-inch SS wire are used sequentially, the arch form can be well controlled. Additionally, if a sufficiently stiff wire close to the full bracket slot size is used, such as 0.019 × 0.025-inch wire for a 0.022-inch slot or 0.017 × 0.025-inch wire for a 0.018-inch slot, the axes of the anterior teeth can also be controlled well and can easily be translated laterally.

A midline deviation accompanying three-dimensional canting, which contains a deviation of the right and left vertical positions of a tooth, is difficult to correct. The discrepancies of the right and left vertical molar positions should be improved first. Correction of vertical discrepancies is discussed in detail in chapter 9.

POSTERIOR DISTALIZATION

Treatment planning

The most important factor in the success of molar distalization is to decide whether or not the molar should be distalized, and this should be decided based on an adequate database of information about the patient (Fig 8-35), including the required space determined from the visual treatment objective and the anatomic conditions that allow for distalization.

If more than 3 mm of space per side is required, premolar extraction is preferred because of the efficiency of

Figs 8-38a and 8-38b It is important to assess whether sufficient space is available for molar distalization. The tooth bud of the third molar *(arrow)* occupies a space in the maxilla, leaving insufficient space for distalization and impeding tooth movement.

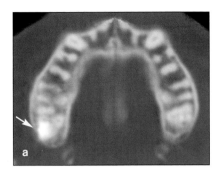
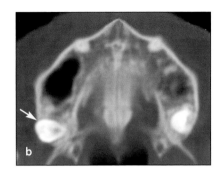

Figs 8-39a to 8-39e In a 15-year-old boy, the entire mandibular dentition is distalized to correct protrusion of the anterior teeth. Attention should be given to the condition of the third molars. **(a and b)** Cephalometric films prior to treatment and after distalization of mandibular dentition. **(c and d)** Panoramic films pretreatment and after distalization. **(e)** Left occlusal view after distalization.

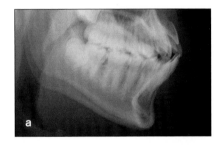
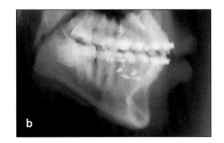
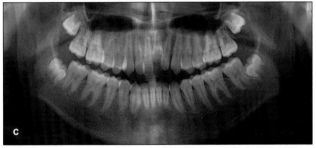
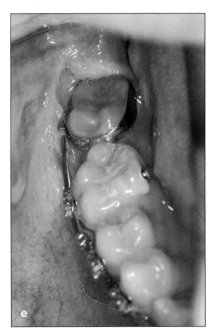
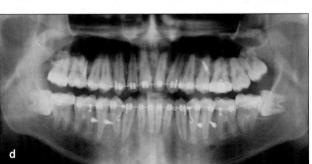

treatment. For patients in whom the premolars have been extracted, distalization of more than 3 mm may be inevitable.

Tooth movement should be limited to remain within the alveolar trough.[4–6,15] As is the case with any type of tooth movement, there also must be enough space for distalization. Specifically, the most posterior cortical bone in the maxilla, the tuberosity (Fig 8-36), and the most pos-terior lingual cortical bone in the mandible (Fig 8-37) are the posterior limitations of distalization.[16]

The availability of space for posterior movement of the molar must be evaluated prior to distalization (Figs 8-38 to 8-40). The third molar should always be extracted first to secure the space for distalization (see Fig 8-38). With mini-implant anchorage, the resistance from the third

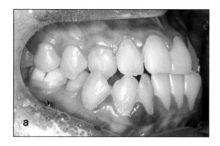

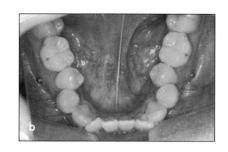

Figs 8-40a and 8-40b A 22-year-old woman with anterior crowding exhibits a skeletal Class III malocclusion and midfacial deficiency. The treatment plan normally would be orthognathic surgery with maxillary advancement to improve facial esthetics. However, the patient refused surgical correction and requested only orthodontic treatment. If the mandibular molar were to be extracted, the resulting molar relationship would be Class III with unstable one-to-one contact in the mandibular first molar area. To avoid a Class III molar relationship, mandibular molar distalization was planned.

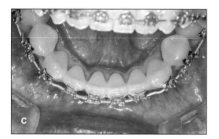

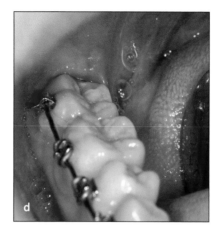

Figs 8-40c to 8-40f Satisfactory anterior and posterior occlusion has been obtained through mandibular molar distalization. The patient has requested additional anterior tooth retraction. Although the mandibular right and left second molars appear to be embedded in the bone of the retromolar area in a panoramic radiograph and cephalometric film, there does not seem to be any major problems, and the periodontal condition, including the attached gingiva, appears good.

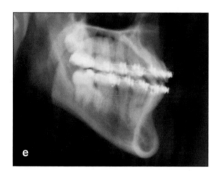

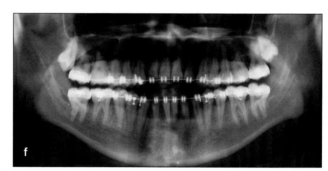

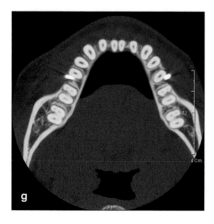

Fig 8-40g Computed tomographic view reveals the roots of the mandibular right and left second molars to be in contact with the cortical bone of the mandible. Considering the anatomic condition, further distal movement of the dentition would be inappropriate.

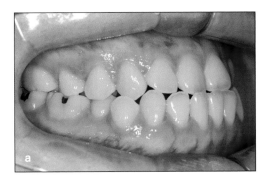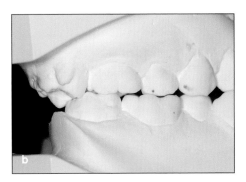

Figs 8-41a and 8-41b Particularly in a patient with an Angle Class III malocclusion, the maxillary second molar may interfere with distalization of mandibular molars. **(a)** Right intraoral view. **(b)** Casts exhibiting extruded second molar.

molar can be disregarded. Although an existing third molar may not always be a limitation, the third molar occupies space. Therefore, it may restrict the amount of space available for the distalization of other molars, possibly posing a critical obstacle regardless of the developmental stage. Moreover, distalization increases the possibility of third molar impaction[17,18] and makes the extraction of the third molar more difficult. Thus, considering the availability of space for movement and the possibility of third molar impaction, the necessity of third molar extraction should be determined prior to other procedures.

If third molar extraction is not feasible because of accessibility, the use of molar distalization should be reconsidered. The second molar may be extracted if the third molar appears to be of normal shape and size, especially in the maxilla.

In addition to the limiting factor of the hard tissue, there is also a limiting factor of the soft tissue, the attached gingiva (see Fig 8-37b). For the maintenance of oral hygiene, it is essential that attached gingiva exist on the distobuccal side after molar distalization, especially in the mandible. The second molar may be jeopardized if there is movable tissue on the buccal aspect. This condition increases the chance of furcation involvement. In other words, whether healthier periodontal tissues will be present on the most distal tooth of the dentition after distalization must be evaluated. If not, molar distalization should be reconsidered and premolar extraction may be preferable.

Occlusal forces resulting from abnormal functions such as bruxism or clenching can act to prevent or reduce molar distalization (Fig 8-41). Molars receive relatively more occlusal force than other teeth, and in the case of bruxism or clenching, the second molar receives especially strong occlusal forces that must be taken into consideration for treatment efficiency.

If the limiting factors of hard and soft tissues are controlled, molar distalization of 2.5 mm is very predictable.

Biomechanics

For bodily movement to occur, distal force should be applied three dimensionally through the center of resistance of the molars. Clinically, however, this is impossible. When viewed three dimensionally, the force can be delivered away from the center of resistance so that the teeth rotate three dimensionally, thus making control of the second molar imperative. Furthermore, the root surfaces of the first and second molars are very wide and difficult to control, which affects the other teeth.

The second molar should be distalized first, via either one-by-one or en masse distalization. That is, distalization forces should be efficiently delivered to the second molars rather than to any other teeth. From a biomechanical viewpoint, three-dimensional control of the second molar is crucial. Anteroposterior, vertical, and arch form control are also required.

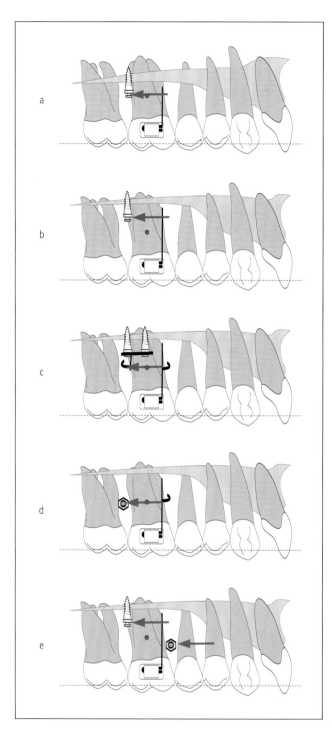

Fig 8-42 *(a)* The system using one implant in the midpalatal suture area and a transpalatal arch is simple and effective, but it cannot be applied in all cases. With shallow palatal vaults, distalization forces from an implant travel through the center of resistance of the molar, which causes translation to occur. *(b)* However, with deep palatal vaults, distalization forces from the implants are exerted apically over the center of resistance of the molar, causing root movement to occur. Such problems can be resolved by *(c)* changing the line of action through use of an attachment on the implant, *(d)* use of a buccal interdental implant, or *(e)* use of a combination of a midpalatal implant and buccal implants.

Selection of implant location

Midpalatal implants

Because the stability of buccal implants was less reliable in the past, midpalatal implants were attractive because of good primary stability obtained from the utilization of cortical bone. However, through the development of an improved design of orthodontic implants, the stability of the buccal implant has been improved. There is no longer a significant difference in the stability of midpalatal implants and buccal implants in patients 15 years and older.[19]

Distalizing mechanics that incorporate midpalatal implants possess a number of advantages. Midpalatal implants never impede tooth movement and do not limit the amount of distalization. There is abundant palatal space, so the line of action can be regulated according to the type of tooth movement needed[7] (Figs 8-42 to 8-46). Another advantage is that primary stability can be readily obtained, even in patients younger than 15 years of age, who might have decreased buccal alveolar bone quality (see chapter 4).

The disadvantages of midpalatal implants include the increased discomfort patients experience from palatal appliances and the additional laboratory time required for the making of appliances for these implants.

Palatal interdental implants

Use of palatal interdental implants presents advantages such as the use of palatal space to regulate the line of action and the presence of more available interdental space than in the case of buccal interdental implants (Fig 8-47; see chapter 4). However, the shortcomings of palatal interdental implants are the possibilities that the movement of adjacent teeth may be impeded and a transpalatal arch may be required. The surgical procedure involved is also more difficult than the procedure for buccal implants.

Buccal interdental implants

Initially, the stability of maxillary buccal implants was questioned. With the development of new implants, there is no reason to refrain from the use of buccal implants in patients 15 and older.[19] Use of buccal implants is preferable because of their ease of implantation and simple application in treatment.

Buccal interdental implants have the potential limitation of hindering the movement of adjacent teeth. If properly positioned, however, with 2 to 3 mm of distal move-

Figs 8-43a to 8-43d The distalizing mechanics created with an implant and a transpalatal arch are simple and efficient in the case of a shallow palatal vault, which is a common characteristic of growing patients. On cephalometric radiographs the direction of the distalizing force through the center of resistance of the first molar is confirmed. **(a and b)** Before distalization. **(c and d)** After distalization.

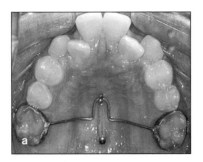
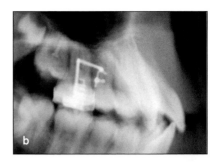
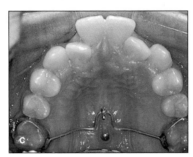
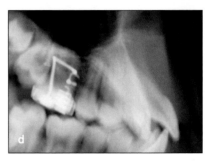

Figs 8-44a and 8-44b Implants in the parasagittal area may be used for distalization to prevent injury at growing sites. It is also efficient to generate the distalizing forces from two points. **(a)** Pretreatment occlusal view. **(b)** Postdistalization occlusal view.

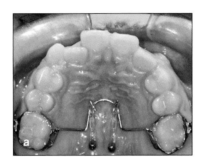
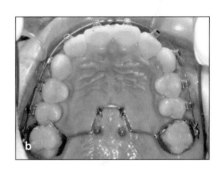

Figs 8-45a and 8-45b For patients with deep palates, an attachment on a midpalatal implant may be required to control the line of force. The distalizing force vector should pass through the center of resistance, which is located around the furcation area. **(a)** Occlusal view. **(b)** Cephalometric view.

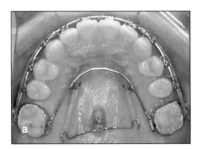
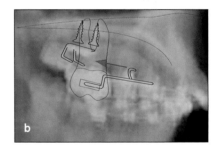

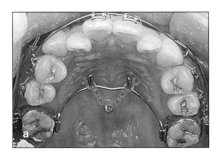
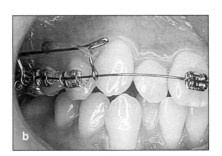
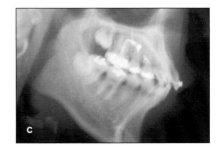

Figs 8-46a to 8-46c Additional implants on the buccal side can solve the problem shown in Fig 8-42 *(b)*. Specifically, a midpalatal implant induces root movement, and buccal implants with a sliding yoke induce crown movement. **(a)** Occlusal view. **(b)** Right lateral view. **(c)** Cephalometric view.

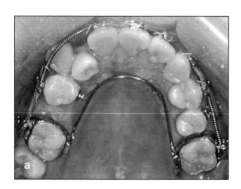

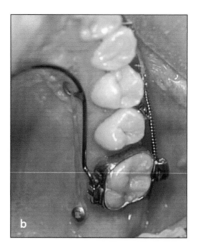

Figs 8-47a and 8-47b When interdental palatal implants are used in deep palatal vaults, it is advantageous to deliver orthodontic force through the center of resistance of the molar. (a) Occlusal view. (b) Closeup view of the palatal mini-implant.

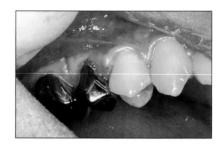

Fig 8-48 It is also important to secure enough space for distalization that the position of the insertion site should be 1.0 to 1.5 mm distal to the gingival vertical reference line between two adjacent teeth. If the protocol for the prevention of root damage is followed, the possibility of root damage is minimized.

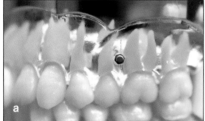

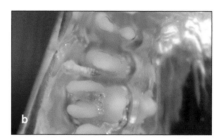

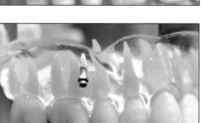

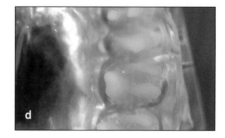

Figs 8-49a to 8-49d (a and b) In implantation parallel to the occlusal plane, the apical end of the implant becomes located deep between the teeth, significantly increasing the possibility that the movement of adjacent teeth will be hindered. (c and d) In implantation oblique to the occlusal plane, the apical end of the implant becomes more apically and buccally located, and a wider interdental and buccal space can be used. This decreases the possibility that the movement of adjacent teeth will be hindered.

ment on either side, there is little to no possibility that tooth movement will be restricted (Figs 8-48 and 8-49). More strictly speaking, the buccal alveolar bone is being used rather than the interdental alveolar bone (Fig 8-50). If buccal space is used with accurate implant positioning, movement of at least a half-cusp width is possible. Depending on the case, more space may be utilized (Fig 8-51).

Types of mechanics

Generally, the buccal space is the position of choice. Broadly speaking, distalizing mechanics can be classified into *direct anchorage type* or *indirect anchorage type*,

according to how the implants are used. Mechanics may also be classified into the *one-by-one type* and the *en masse type*, according to how molars are distalized. In addition, mechanics can also be classified into mechanics using buccal implants, palatal implants, or a combination of these two. In all cases, distalizing mechanics can control the anteroposterior relationship, vertical relationship, and arch form.

Direct versus indirect anchorage

The indirect anchorage type is more stable and fail-safe, while the direct anchorage type provides more efficient progression of treatment. In cases in which asymmetric movement or large amounts of tooth movement are

Figs 8-50a and 8-50b Implants were initially positioned closer to the distal side than to the middle of the interproximal area. As the teeth underwent distalization, the implants seemed to move toward the mesial side rather than toward the middle of the interproximal space. If properly positioned, buccal implants are likely to achieve a half-cusp width of distalization on either side. **(a)** Lateral view. **(b)** Occlusal view.

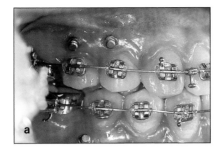

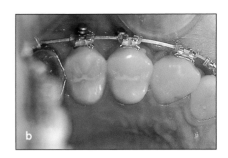

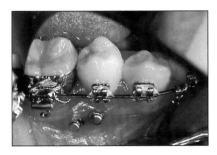

Fig 8-51 Even in cases requiring more than a half-cusp width of tooth movement, a buccal implant may be used. Distalization has been performed according to the treatment plan, but the patient desires more retraction of the anterior teeth. Therefore, with the consent of the patient, an additional implant has been placed distal to the first. At the start of distalization, the first implant had been positioned closer to the distal side than to the middle of the interproximal area. With distalization, the first implant is located mesial to the midline. The second implant is placed closer to the first molar than to the middle of the interdental space.

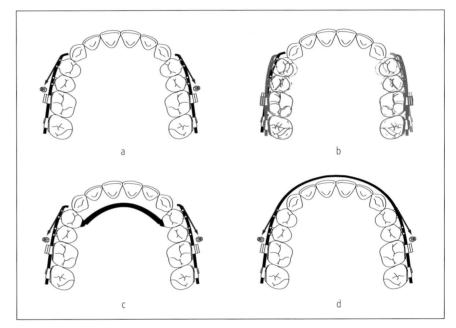

Fig 8-52 *(a)* When the posterior segments are divided and distalizing force is delivered to the segments, *(b)* the risk of rotation of each segment is high. Consequently, the arch in the premolar area is widened. Use of *(c)* crossarch splinting or *(d)* continuous arch mechanics is advisable because both of these methods are easy to control.

required, the indirect anchorage type is recommended because of its superior stability.

One-by-one versus en masse movement

The one-by-one type of movement of each tooth is easier to control than the en masse type, although the en masse type with groups of teeth results in more efficient progression of treatment. For asymmetric distalization, the one-by-one type of tooth movement is recommended until a symmetric molar position is achieved.

Sectional archwire mechanics

Although it is advantageous that brackets are not needed on the anterior teeth, arch form is more difficult to control during distalization of posterior segments (Fig 8-52a, b). There is also a risk that the premolar area will widen. Therefore, when sectional mechanics are used, it is preferable that crossarch splinting (Fig 8-52c) or continuous arch mechanics (Fig 8-52d) should be applied; if not, use of indirect anchorage or limited application is advisable.

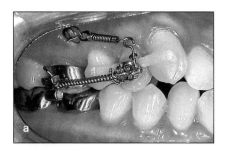
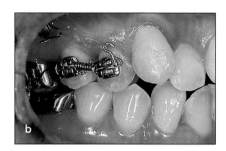

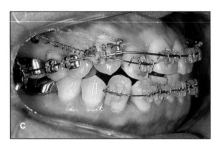
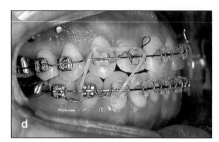

Figs 8-53a to 8-53d The molars will be distalized to relieve the crowding. **(a)** First, the canine and two premolars are splinted into one unit using fiber-reinforced resin composite, and a bracket is bonded to the unit. Then a distalizing force is applied to the first molar using open coil springs, and retractive force from mini-implants is also applied to hold the anterior unit. **(b)** After molar distalization, brackets are bonded to premolars, which are distalized with open coil springs and retractive force from the mini-implant. **(c)** After premolar distalization, brackets are also bonded to the anterior teeth, **(d)** and the anterior teeth are aligned.

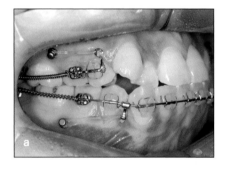
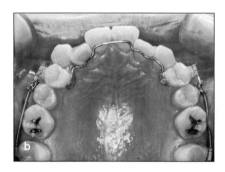

Figs 8-54a and 8-54b Sectional mechanics with lingual crossarch splinting is effective and esthetic for the treatment of crowding. **(a)** Right lateral view. **(b)** Occlusal view.

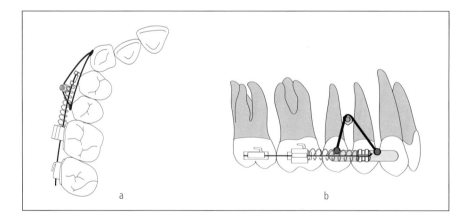

Fig 8-55 Molar distalization method I, using buccal implants. Sectional mechanics with indirect anchorage is three-dimensionally stable, so it is preferred in the case of asymmetric distalization. However, the anchorage unit, including the teeth and implants, can be moved approximately 1 mm; thus, overloading should be avoided. *(a)* Occlusal view. *(b)* Lateral view.

Continuous archwire mechanics

Arch form control is considered more predictable with continuous full archwire mechanics than it is with sectional mechanics. Simultaneous distalization and intrusion of the molars is possible with continuous full archwire mechanics.

Mechanics with one-by-one distalization

With mechanics for one-by-one distalization of each tooth (Figs 8-53 to 8-55), the molars are moved individually. The second molar is moved first, and then the first molar is moved. Other teeth are moved subsequently. This can be achieved either with indirect anchorage or with direct

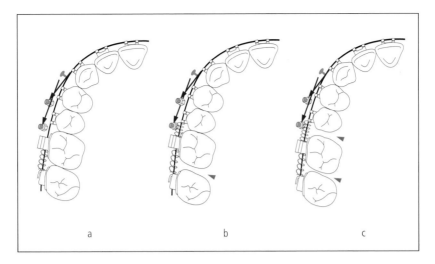

Fig 8-56 Molar distalization method II, using buccal implants. For the distalization of the entire dentition, about 500 g of orthodontic force per side is needed, so the use of two implants per side is recommended. Even in the distalization of the entire dentition, control of the second molar is key; control of the first molar is also important. *(a)* In the first step, an open coil spring is inserted between the maxillary first and second molars to induce distal driving of the second molar. *(b)* After the second molar is moved about 1 mm *(arrowhead)*, an open coil spring is inserted between the first and second molars. An open coil spring is also inserted passively or actively 1 to 2 mm between the first and second molars in an opened condition. *(c)* With all of these procedures, retractive force is delivered to the entire dentition by hooks on the main wire. Arch form control is important, especially in cases in which distalizing force is applied to the entire dentition. (*Arrowheads* indicate space opening.)

Fig 8-57 Modification of molar distalization method II, using buccal implants. *(a)* To decrease the load-deflection ratio by increasing the length of an open coil spring, the second premolar can be bypassed until initiation of the distal movement of molars. *(b)* In the treatment of crowding, anterior teeth can be bypassed until space for anterior alignment is secured. Retractive force is delivered to the canine, the premolar, and the hooks on archwire.

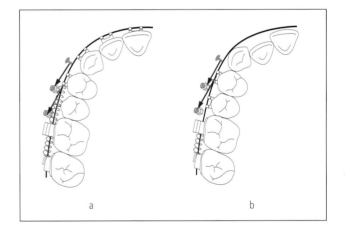

anchorage. Indirect anchorage is recommended for patients requiring asymmetric distalization or a large amount of tooth movement, because indirect anchorage is more stable three dimensionally.

Mechanics with en masse distalization

The second molar, the first molar, and the other premolars can be distalized en masse because of the increased anchorage supplied by mini-implants (Figs 8-56 to 8-59). However, en masse distalization of the entire dentition is more difficult for the following reasons: *(1)* all of the teeth should be monitored simultaneously and *(2)* the anterior teeth are easier to move than posterior teeth. Therefore, the retractive forces are also easily concentrated on the anterior teeth instead of the posterior teeth, and arch expansion occurs more easily than distalization.

These problems should always be considered in the planning and monitoring of the tooth movement when utilizing en masse distalization. Control of the second molar is of critical importance in all distalization mechanics, and the distalizing force should mainly be delivered to the second molar, even in en masse movement.

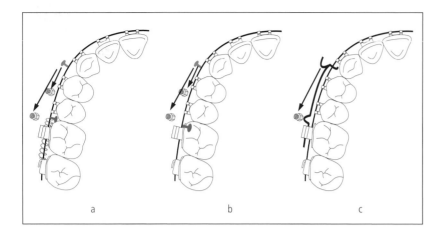

Fig 8-58 Molar distalization method III. To deliver distalizing force to the molar efficiently, crimpable hooks or omega stops are used. For arch form control, it is recommended that stiff wire be used as the main wire. *(a)* Using crimpable hooks and open coil spring; *(b)* using a crimpable hook, and *(c)* using a sliding yoke.

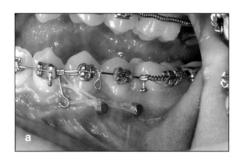

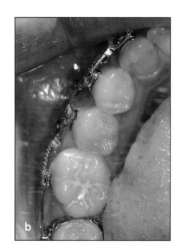

Figs 8-59a and 8-59b If a crimpable hook or an omega loop is used to place a stop anterior to the molar, retractive force can be delivered effectively to the molar.

Selection of mechanics

During selection of mechanics, the following concepts should be considered:

1. The degree of difficulty of the mechanics. En masse distalization may reduce the treatment time, but its progression is more difficult. The progression of one-by-one distalization is less complicated.
2. The treatment positions of the anterior teeth. If the positions of the anterior teeth are not to be changed, sectional mechanics with lingual crossarch splinting is preferable to minimize unnecessary forces on the anterior teeth.
3. The treatment positions of the posterior teeth. If asymmetric distal movement is needed, symmetric molar positions should be achieved first. If intrusion of the posterior teeth is needed, the mechanics for posterior intrusion should be utilized first. If intrusion and distalization of the entire dentition are required, en masse mechanics with a continuous arch is preferred.

Mechanics using mini-implants and headgear

In classic mechanics for distalization, the more difficult problem does not concern moving the molars distally but rather moving the remaining teeth distally after distal movement of the molars. Mini-implants can solve such problems. An effective method is to use classic mechanics, such as headgear and a Cetlin removable appliance, to move the molars distally and then to use mini-implant anchorage to move the other teeth distally (Fig 8-60). This sequence of mechanics is especially useful when the permanent teeth are not erupted fully because full bonding is not necessary during molar distalization.

Special considerations and monitoring

Second molar

Three-dimensional control of the second molar is of primary importance for successful distalization (Figs 8-61 to 8-65).

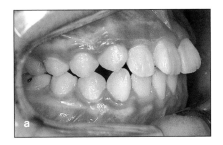
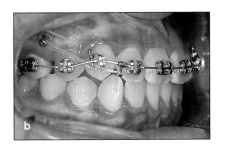
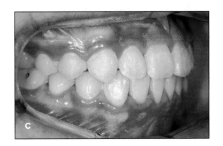

Figs 8-60a to 8-60c (a) A 13-year-old girl with protruded maxillary teeth and maxillary crowding has an Angle Class II canine relationship and excessive overjet. The canines are not fully erupted; therefore cervical headgear and a removable appliance with a distal finger spring are to be used for distalization of the maxillary molars according to the Hwang protocol. The distal finger spring on the first molar is activated 1.5 to 2.0 mm for the daytime, and cervical headgear is used at night. This protocol is effective for molar distalization and prevents mesial movement of anterior teeth. **(b)** After molar distalization, implants are placed between the second premolar and the first molar. The other teeth are retracted simultaneously through the use of mini-implants. **(c)** The active treatment is completed after 11 months.

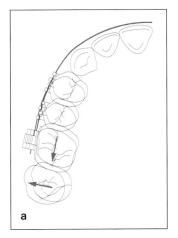
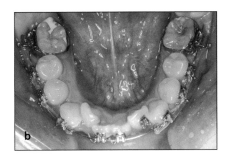

Figs 8-61a and 8-61b During distalization, **(a)** the maxillary second molar can easily be tipped to the buccal side, while **(b)** the mandibular molar can easily be tipped to the lingual side because of the anatomic structure. Therefore, the appliance should always include the teeth up to the second molar.

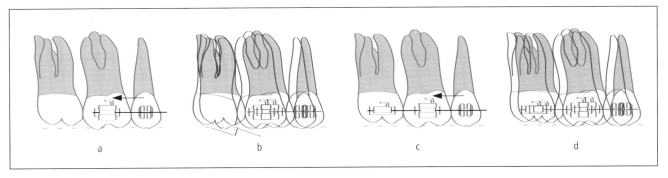

Fig 8-62 *(a)* If the appliance is not attached to the second molar, the second molar may be tipped back by distal movement of the first molar. *(b)* As a consequence, marginal ridge discrepancies appear. *(c and d)* Therefore, it is imperative that the appliance include the second molar for control.

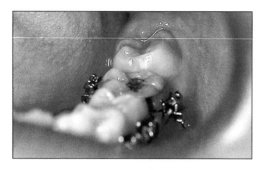

Fig 8-63 The second molar did not erupt fully; hence, distalization of the mandibular dentition was performed, but the second molar was uncontrolled. As a result, the second molar has tipped distally. For control of a partially erupted molar, a minitube is effective.

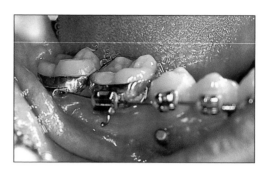

Fig 8-64 Even if the appliance is attached to the second molar, bodily movement is difficult to attain, because the molar has a large root and because the force is away from the center of resistance. In this situation, there is a greater tendency for tipping, particularly in the mandible. The cardinal signs of tipping are marginal ridge discrepancies with high mesial marginal ridges.

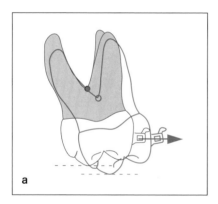

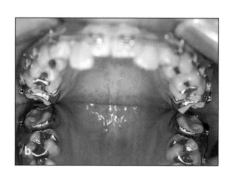

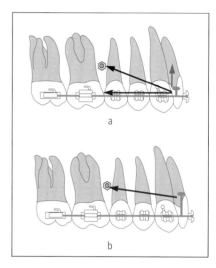

Figs 8-65a and 8-65b (a) If the second molar is tipped buccally *(red)*, the palatal cusps move occlusally. **(b)** Occlusal view. Observe that the torque of the second molar worsens as a result.

Fig 8-66 *(a)* Because the implant is apically located, the distalizing force from implants includes an intrusive force vector *(red arrow)*. *(b)* An intrusive force vector may cause side effects and can be minimized by lengthening of the lever arm.

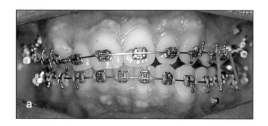

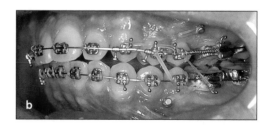

Figs 8-67a and 8-67b When side effects of the intrusive force develop unilaterally, correction is extremely difficult. Control of the intrusive force vector is necessary for prevention. **(a)** Frontal view. **(b)** Left lateral view.

Figs 8-68a and 8-68b Intrusive force vectors cause bowing accompanied by anterior bite opening. Such problems may be alleviated by the use of a stiff wire, lowering of the lever arm, and the use of maxillomandibular elastics.

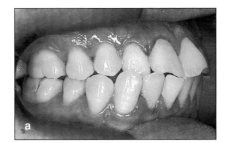
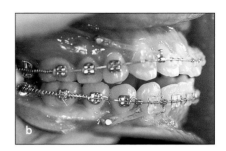

Figs 8-69a and 8-69b Note the axis of the canines. The combination of an intrusive force vector and distal tipping of a canine may cause bite opening to occur in the premolar area. This problem is likely to occur with a light wire, such as the 0.017 × 0.025-inch TMA wire. **(a)** Right lateral view; **(b)** left lateral view.

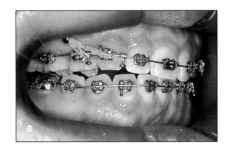
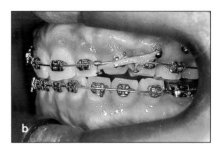

Fig 8-70 Even during distalization, bowing may appear. *(a)* The combination of an intrusive force vector and distal tipping of a canine may cause bite opening in the premolar area, and this causes deformation of the main archwire. *(b)* An intrusive force may develop from the deflection of the wire and act on the molars.

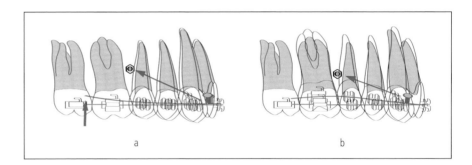

Intrusive force vector

Because the implant is located in the apical interdental area, if a retractive force is derived from implants, an adverse intrusive force vector may develop. This factor may induce canting (Figs 8-66 and 8-67) of the occlusal plane.

Bowing

In both extraction treatment and nonextraction treatment with distalization, bowing may occur because of three-dimensional rotation of teeth (Figs 8-68 to 8-70)

Arch form

The mechanics applied for distalization of the molars with buccal implants can easily expand the arch (Figs 8-71 to 8-74). The classic prescription for extraction treatment of the first maxillary molar includes additional offset for over-

correction to prevent mesial rotation of the first molar. This may be beneficial in conventional extraction treatment, but it may not be beneficial in treatment with implants, because orthodontic force is not applied to the first molar for a significant period of time. Excessive offset of the first molar can alter the horizontal position of the second molar and, consequently, the arch form will be skewed.

Periodontal considerations

Soft tissue problems from excess gingival tissue can easily occur in the area distal to the second molar (Figs 8-75 and 8-76). After distalization, attached gingiva should remain at the distobuccal side of the second molar for better maintenance of periodontal health and to help prevent possible furcation involvement.

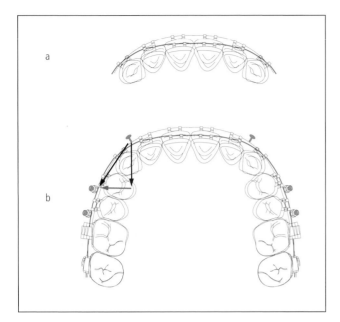

Fig 8-71 Depending on the geometric positions of an implant and a hook, the distalizing force between them may have a horizontal force vector. Furthermore, the root area of the molar is large and more difficult to move than that of the anterior teeth. *(a)* In other words, under the same conditions, anterior teeth move more quickly. *(b)* Because of this, arch expansion is more likely to occur than distalization. Anterior retraction may result from arch expansion, not from distalization.

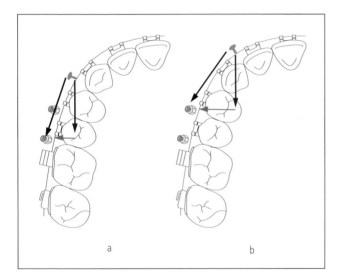

Fig 8-72 A hook between *(a)* a canine and a premolar is better at reducing a horizontal force vector than is a hook between *(b)* a lateral incisor and a canine. The hook between a canine and a premolar *(a)* can also reduce the possibility of soft tissue irritations.

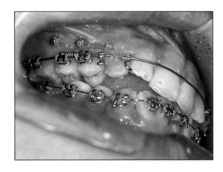

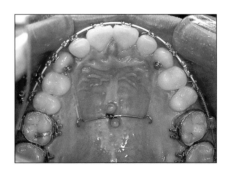

Fig 8-73 A horizontal force vector from the distalizing force has made the premolar tip buccally and increased the arch width; an intrusive force vector has made the canine intrude on the main arch of the 0.017 × 0.025-inch TMA wire. The clinical sign of arch expansion is increased buccal overjet in the premolar area. Use of a stiff wire can help resolve such problems.

Fig 8-74 In a situation in which a midpalatal implant is used, the arch form should also be controlled. Because of the position of force application, the distalizing force included a constrictive force vector in the canine area, and the intercanine width has decreased. Depending on the force system of distalizing mechanics, the arch form is likely to either be expanded or constricted.

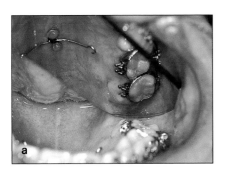
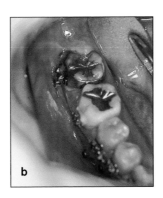
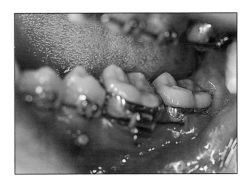

Figs 8-75a and 8-75b As the second molar moves distally, the adjacent soft tissues are compressed. Because the remodeling of gingival tissues takes a long time, additional periodontal surgery may be required after treatment. **(a)** The maxillary palatal gingiva is thick, meaning that much time is needed for remodeling. **(b)** Because the molar can be readily tipped back, the distal area is buried more deeply with movement. This causes plaque control to become more difficult, which only worsens the overall problems.

Fig 8-76 As the molar is tipped back, supragingival plaque is conducive to formation of subgingival plaque. Particularly when a band is used and the tube is positioned toward the gingival side of the band, inflammatory gingivitis with gingival hyperplasia may develop with improper oral hygiene.

Fig 8-77 In canine or premolar retraction, the retractive force is transmitted to the anterior teeth through the wire via friction resistance. This retractive force may cause uncontrolled tipping of the four anterior teeth and loss of anterior torque, depending on the condition of the main archwire. For example, canine retraction on the round wire exacerbates the anterior torque if the wire is engaged in the anterior teeth. (*red arrow*) Retraction force to anterior teeth caused by friction; (*blue arrow*) Retraction force to canine.

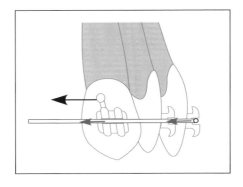

Anterior torque

If anterior retraction is required to any extent, the considerations for anterior torque control should be addressed in the same manner as they are during extraction treatment (Fig 8-77).

MOLAR PROTRACTION

Treatment planning

Molar protraction is more difficult in the mandible.[20,21] It also becomes less predictable when *(a)* the molar is moving into an edentulous area in the mandible and significant time has passed since tooth loss, and the alveolar bone has narrowed or resorbed; *(b)* the molar is moving into an atrophic edentulous area with reduced alveolar ridge height; and *(c)* where the protracted molar is fully developed with complete root formation.

The most significant risk factor is the periodontal condition of the molar that is to be protracted. Alveolar bone loss, gingival recession, and dehiscence may occur during protraction.[22-24] Therefore, the treatment plan should be based upon a thorough clinical evaluation of the periodontal condition of the molar to be protracted, surrounding bone conditions, and the age of the patient. Bone is remodeled more rapidly in the maxilla than in the mandible.

At the University of Pennsylvania, teeth have been moved into defects, with the patients' contralateral side serving as the control. Radiographs revealed that loss of attachment occurred when a tooth was moved into a defect in an edentulous area.[22] The tooth can move away from a defect and, with sufficient eruption, a bony defect can be reduced or eliminated; this usually is the treatment of choice to improve osseous architecture.[22]

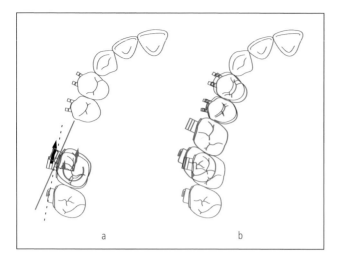

Fig 8-78 *(a)* Protractive force on a labial hook *(black arrow)* leads to mesial rotation *(red arrows)*. *(b)* As a result, the arch form is disrupted and buccal overjet increases in the second molar area.

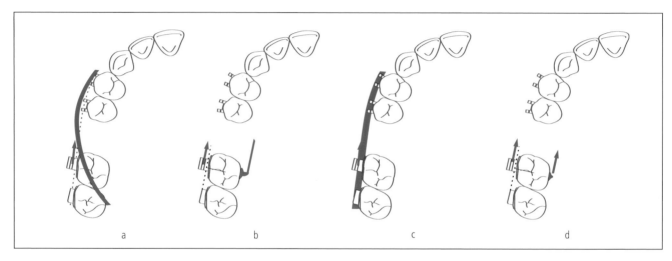

Fig 8-79 The following recommendations can be useful for first-order rotation control. For a large amount of protraction, it is recommended that the methods in *(c)* and *(d)* be used together. *(a)* Creation of a toe-in compensating curve on a resilient wire such as 0.017 × 0.025-inch TMA wire can offset the tendency for mesial rotation. However, this method is technique sensitive, difficult to control, and, in short, is not fail-safe. *(b)* Crossarch splinting methods, such as transpalatal arch and lingual arch, are reliable for maintaining the arch form and controlling molar rotation. Patient discomfort is relatively high with these methods, and crossarch splinting cannot be used in cases of unilateral protraction. *(c)* Use of a stiff wire heavier than 0.017 × 0.025-inch SS as a main archwire works to a certain degree. For this method, it is important to use minimal protractive force and to use a tube rather than a bracket for biomechanical efficiency. Fine control is difficult with this method, and it may not be suitable for patients requiring long treatment periods. *(d)* Use of a lingual button is simple and effective. In first-order rotation control, the use of a couple of lingual buttons is most effective.

A study involving closure of edentulous spaces in the mandible was done on a group of patients ranging in age from 11 to 17 years, and the results were compared with those from a group of patients ages 23 to 46 years.[23] The results indicated that the older adults had more loss of crestal bone and greater root resorption than the younger patients.[23]

Biomechanics and mechanics

As with molar distalization, the force is applied to the teeth away from their center of resistance, and therefore rotation of molars may occur three-dimensionally. This can cause treatment time for protraction to be prolonged, particularly in the mandible, and therefore the risk of side

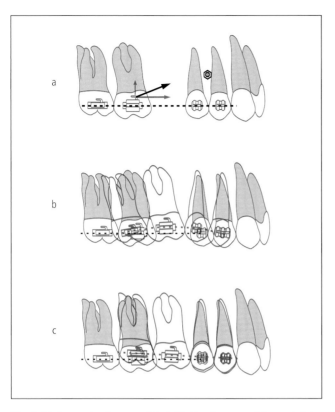

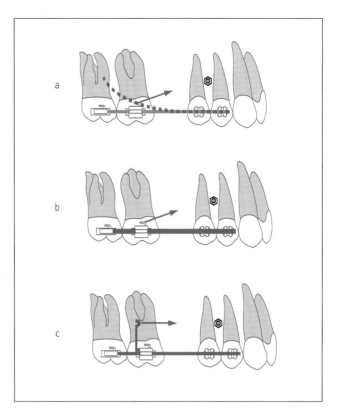

Fig 8-80 Protractive force on *(a)* a labial hook causes *(b)* a mesial tipping tendency. Generally, mini-implants are positioned apically; protractive force has an intrusive force vector, so intrusion of posterior teeth may occur. *(c)* If intrusion occurs on only one side, occlusal canting develops.

Fig 8-81 Tipping control and vertical control are necessary. *(a)* A compensating curve can offset the mesial tipping tendency. With this method, however, vertical control is impossible. *(b)* With the use of a stiff wire heavier than 0.017 × 0.025-inch SS, the side effects of mesial tipping and intrusion can be minimized. This is not completely effective in preventing unwanted intrusion, especially if protraction is prolonged and delicate control is impossible. *(c)* A lever arm engaged in an auxiliary tube of the first molar can resolve both problems effectively.

Figs 8-82a and 8-82b As the molar has been rotated distally by protractive force, the arch form has expanded unilaterally. Note the rotation and buccolingual position of the mandibular right first molar.

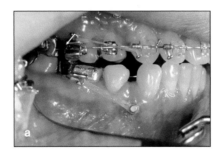

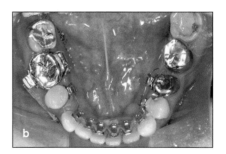

effects increases. For successful protraction, molars must be controlled three-dimensionally (Figs 8-78 to 8-82).

The protraction mechanics must provide components that can control the molar three-dimensionally to allow for first-order rotation, second-order rotation, third-order ro-

tation, and vertical position (Figs 8-83 to 8-88). If movement lasts for a long period of time, a large amount of movement and asymmetric movement are required, and the use of indirect anchorage is advisable because of its superior stability.

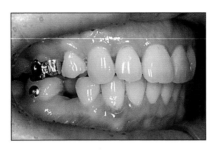

Fig 8-83a The patient has been referred for treatment because of an open mandibular extraction space that cannot be closed.

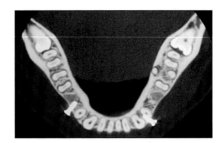

Fig 8-83b The computed tomogram reveals that the mandibular molar has three roots, all surrounded by cortical bone.

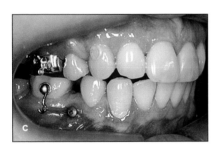

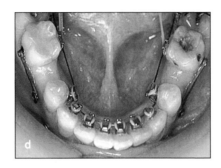

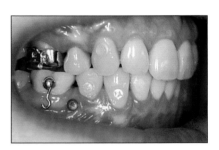

Figs 8-83c and 8-83d A mini-implant is used as anchorage for protraction, while a lever arm provides axis control and vertical control of the molar. The appliance is attached to the second molar for rotation and arch form control. Protraction is achieved with a 0.016 × 0.022-inch SS archwire.

Fig 8-83e Intraoral view after space closure.

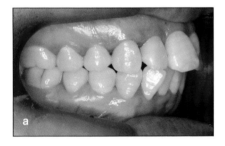

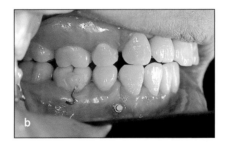

Fig 8-84a Right intraoral view of a patient with a chief complaint of protrusion of the lips.

Figs 8-84b and 8-84c Four first premolars were extracted, and treatment was conducted with Ormco lingual appliances. Anchorage has been lost in the maxilla, while the anterior teeth have been excessively retracted in the mandible; thus, the maxillomandibular relationship has worsened.

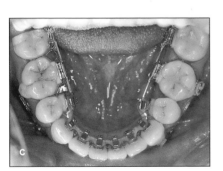

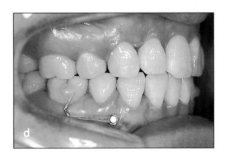

Fig 8-84d An implant is inserted between the mandibular canine and premolar, and the molars are protracted to improve the maxillomandibular relationship.

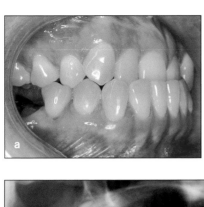
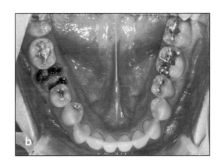
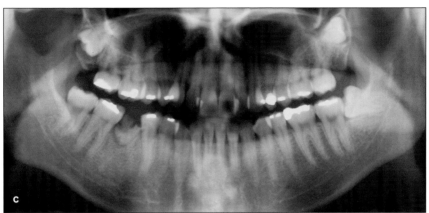
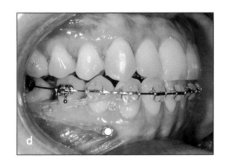
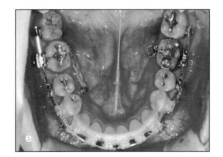
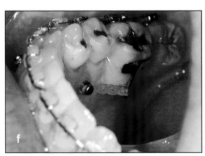
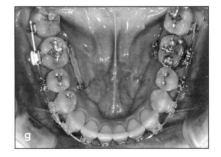

Figs 8-85a to 8-85g A 24-year-old woman has anterior crossbite and a severely damaged mandibular right first molar, so the second and third molars will be protracted. For treatment efficiency and rotation control, a buccal mini-implant and a lingual mini-implant are used. To control the arch form, the third molar is included in the appliance and 0.017 × 0.025-inch SS archwire is used as the main wire. The lingual lever arm is used for axis and vertical control. **(a to c)** Pretreatment clinical situation. **(d to f)** During protraction. **(g)** Result after protraction. (Courtesy of Dr BS Yoon, Seoul, Korea.)

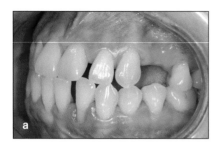
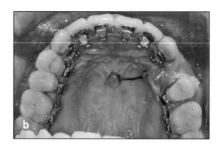
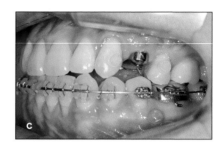

Figs 8-86a to 8-86c A lever arm bonded to the implant is used to control the line of action. **(a)** Pretreatment clinical situation. **(b)** During protraction. **(c)** Result after protraction; molar relationship is improved. (Courtesy of Dr BS Yoon, Seoul, Korea.)

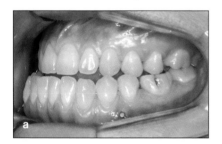
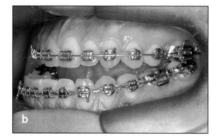
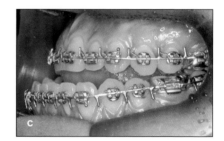

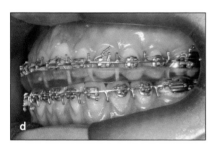
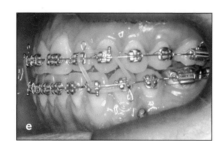

Figs 8-87a to 8-87e For the proper decompensation of presurgical orthodontics, the entire dentition is protracted with the aid of mini-implants. As a result, sufficient mandibular setback can be achieved surgically. **(a)** Pretreatment clinical situation. **(b)** During protraction of the entire dentition. **(c)** After dental decompensation, surgical archwires are engaged. **(d)** Immediate result after orthognathic surgery. **(e)** During finishing, the surgical splint is removed.

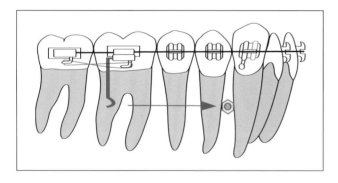

Fig 8-88 For protraction of the entire dentition, the axis of the molar, the vertical dimension, and the arch form must be controlled. To avoid tipping of the teeth and unwanted intrusive force, the lever arm should be adjusted toward the occlusal plane and the protractive force should be placed on the first molars and not the second molars. *(green arrow)* Line of action for protraction.

Special considerations and monitoring

Arch form

In cases of molar protraction, mesial rotation occurs, the arch form is skewed, and the buccal overjet is increased in the second molar area. The arch form may skew readily as distal rotation of the molar occurs.

Occlusal plane canting

Even a very light force may cause adverse side effects if treatment is prolonged. If the treatment period is long, particularly for unilateral protraction of the molar, occlusal plane canting may readily occur even under the influence of slight forces.

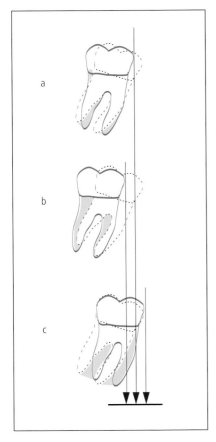

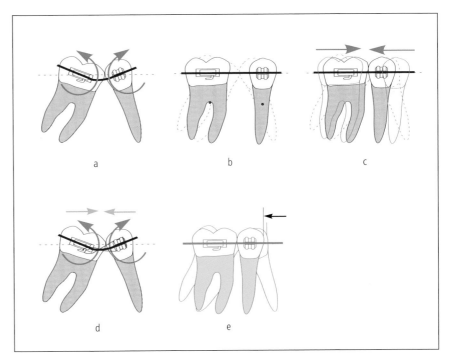

Fig 8-89 The axis control of a single molar can largely be classified into three types: *(a)* axis control by rotation around the center of resistance of a molar; *(b)* axis control by rotation around the distal root apex of a center of resistance of a molar; and *(c)* axis control by root movement. Among these three types, axis control by root movement requires the largest number of alveolar bone reactions and, therefore, requires more anchorage and longer treatment time. (*Shaded area* indicates reaction of alveolar bone required for movement.)

Fig 8-90 Rowboat effect. *(a)* The insertion of a wire into tipped teeth generates moments in the opposite directions; because of these moments, the tooth rotates around the center of resistance. *(b)* Consequently, a space between the teeth is generated. *(c)* If the retractive force is delivered mutually until space closure occurs, anteroposterior movement will take place, depending on the anchorage value (the root surface area). In other words, if the generation of the space *(a)* is prevented by *(d)* rope tie, this is equivalent to the delivery of a retractive force on each other; therefore, it is much like performing *(a)* and *(c)* simultaneously, so that *(e)* uprighting of the tooth and retraction of the premolar occur together. In summary, through the rowboat effect, axis control results in a change of the anteroposterior tooth position.

Periodontal considerations

Because gingival remodeling is much slower than alveolar remodeling, space closure is usually accompanied by problems of soft tissue bunching or excess. Treatment of problems related to gingival excess after space closure and additional surgical excisions might be needed.

Moreover, as gingival tissue is folded, accessibility is decreased and oral hygiene control becomes difficult. Close monitoring should be continuous throughout the treatment, particularly at the mesial side of protracted molars.

MOLAR AXIS CONTROL

Treatment planning and biomechanics

Broadly speaking, molar axis control can be classified into three types according to the treatment objective (Fig 8-89). The force system for each type, the required period of treatment time, and the degree of difficulty differ accordingly (Fig 8-90).

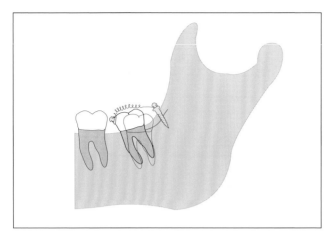

Fig 8-91 For tooth movement like that shown in Fig 8-89*a*, a single force is sufficient. If enough space is available distal to the last molar, the molar can be uprighted effortlessly by placing an implant in the retromolar area and applying a single force.

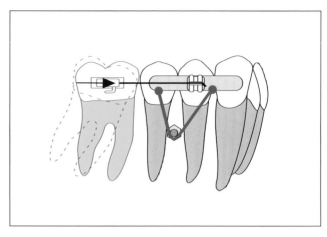

Fig 8-92 If a substantial amount of mesial movement of the root is required, particularly in the mandible, more stable, indirect application is advisable.

Root movement is the most difficult problem to control; it should be considered similar to molar protraction, which, as mentioned, is one of the more unpredictable types of tooth movement, especially in a mandible with a narrowed, atrophic edentulous ridge.

Mechanics

The mechanics for root movement should also have forces and moments that will control the molar three-dimensionally in the same manner as the mechanics for molar protraction (Fig 8-91). If a long period of treatment is needed, the use of indirect application is advisable (Fig 8-92).

Special considerations and monitoring

Treatment period
The fact that root movement takes a significant amount of time must be taken into consideration, especially in narrowed, atrophic edentulous areas of the mandible.

Traumatic occlusion
When the teeth are uprighted, trauma from occlusion and parafunction may occur, making continuous occlusal ad-

justment necessary. Traumatic occlusion may exacerbate an existing periodontal condition.

Periodontal considerations
Periodontal maintenance is required, especially on the mesial and distal sides of the teeth. Generally, the periodontal health of teeth requiring uprighting may be compromised; therefore, special care with regard to periodontal health is crucial for successful molar uprighting. Movement toward the narrowed, atrophic ridge has to be closely monitored because of the risk of buccal recession dehiscence and loss of attachment.[22–24]

SUMMARY

Because of the availability of orthodontic mini-implants, anteroposterior anchorage control no longer poses a problem. Anterior retraction, posterior distalization, and molar protraction, once considered difficult or impossible to achieve, can be performed predictably and efficiently. Treatment planning and design of the biomechanics and mechanics involves careful clinical examination of patients, establishment of obtainable treatment objectives, and consideration of the biologic and treatment limitations of tooth movement. During treatment, periodontal conditions, torque, and arch form must be monitored carefully along with the progression of tooth movement to prevent adverse side effects, which can include gingival recession, unwanted intrusive forces, occlusal canting, and excessive retraction.

REFERENCES

1. Burstone CJ, Koenig HA. Optimizing anterior and canine retraction. Am J Orthod 1976;70:1–19.
2. Burstone CJ. The segmented arch approach to space closure. Am J Orthod 1982;82:361–378.
3. Kusy RP, Tulloch JF. Analysis of moment/force ratios in the mechanics of tooth movement. Am J Orthod Dentofacial Orthop 1986;90:127–131.
4. Handelman CS. The anterior alveolus: Its importance in limiting orthodontic treatment and its influence on the occurrence of iatrogenic sequelae. Angle Orthod 1996;66:95–109 [erratum 1996:246].
5. Wehrbein H, Bauer W, Diedrich P. Mandibular incisors, alveolar bone, and symphysis after orthodontic treatment. A retrospective study. Am J Orthod Dentofacial Orthop 1996;110:239–246.
6. Sarikaya S, Haydar B, Ciger S, Ariyurek M. Changes in alveolar bone thickness due to retraction of anterior teeth. Am J Orthod Dentofacial Orthop 2002;122:15–26.
7. Park YC, Choy K, Lee JS, Kim TK. Lever-arm mechanics in lingual orthodontics. J Clin Orthod 2000;34:601–605.
8. Choy K, Pae EK, Kim KH, Park YC, Burstone CJ. Controlled space closure with a statically determinate retraction system. Angle Orthod 2002;72:191–198.
9. Park YC, Lee JS. Atlas of Contemporary Orthodontics, vol I. Seoul: Shinhung, 2001:107–110.
10. Brezniak N, Wasserstein A. Orthodontically induced inflammatory root resorption. Part II: The clinical aspects. Angle Orthod 2002;72:180–184.
11. Brezniak N, Wasserstein A. Root resorption after orthodontic treatment: Part 2. Literature review. Am J Orthod Dentofacial Orthop 1993;103:138–146.
12. Baumrind S, Korn EL, Boyd RL. Apical root resorption in orthodontically treated adults. Am J Orthod Dentofacial Orthop 1996;110:311–320.
13. Bishara SE, Burkey PS, Kharouf JG. Dental and facial asymmetries: A review. Angle Orthod 1994;64:89–98.
14. Burstone CJ. Diagnosis and treatment planning of patients with asymmetries. Semin Orthod 1998;4:153–164.
15. Engelking G, Zachrisson BU. Effects of incisor repositioning on monkey periodontium after expansion through the cortical plate. Am J Orthod 1982;82:23–32.
16. Sugawara J, Daimaruya T, Umemori M, et al. Distal movement of mandibular molars in adult patients with the skeletal anchorage system. Am J Orthod Dentofacial Orthop 2004;125:130–138.
17. Kim TW, Artun J, Behbehani F, Artese F. Prevalence of third molar impaction in orthodontic patients treated nonextraction and with extraction of four premolars. Am J Orthod Dentofacial Orthop 2003; 123:138–145.
18. Kandasamy S, Woods MG. Is orthodontic treatment without premolar extractions always non-extraction treatment? Aust Dent J 2005;50:146–151.
19. Lee JS. Development of orthodontic mini implant anchorage system. Pre-Conference: Basic Researches on Implant Orthodontics. The 4th Asian Implant Orthodontics Conference, Seoul, Korea, December 3–4, 2005.
20. Roberts WE, Arbuckle GR, Analoui M. Rate of mesial translation of mandibular molars using implant-anchored mechanics. Angle Orthod 1996;66:331–338.
21. Roberts WE, Marshall KJ, Mozsary PG. Rigid endosseous implant utilized as anchorage to protract molars and close an atrophic extraction site. Angle Orthod 1990;60:135–152.
22. Graber TM, Vanarsdall RL, Vig KWL. Orthodontics: Current Principles and Techniques. St Louis: Mosby, 2005:914–915.
23. Stepovich ML. A clinical study on closing edentulous spaces in the mandible. Angle Orthod 1979;49:227–233.
24. Gunduz E, Rodriguez-Torres C, Gahleitner A, Heissenberger G, Bantleon HP. Bone regeneration by bodily tooth movement: Dental computed tomography examination of a patient. Am J Orthod Dentofacial Orthop 2004;125:100–106.

VERTICAL CONTROL 9

ANTERIOR INTRUSION

Treatment planning and biomechanics

In general, intrusion is more difficult to achieve than extrusion[1] (Fig 9-1), and basic biomechanics should be understood to allow for monitoring and adjustment of successful vertical correction. Force-driven appliances and use of light continuous force are desirable for efficient and successful intrusion[1-5] (Figs 9-2 to 9-4; Table 9-1). The axis and anteroposterior position of incisal edges should be controlled along with the vertical position of the incisal edge. The guidelines for selection of mechanics are described in chapter 6.

Treatment objectives should be planned three-dimensionally.[1,3,5] For treatment planning, a thorough periodontal evaluation,[6,7] vertical control, axis control, and anteroposterior control of the incisal edge should be considered (Figs 9-5 to 9-8).

Selection of mechanics

An intrusion spring is advantageous for efficient tooth movement, precise adjustment, and control.[1-3,5,6] Continuous full-arch mechanics are advantageous for convenience and simplicity of treatment but can have negative effects (Fig 9-9). Mini-implants are used to control the adverse side effects of each of the different types of mechanics (Fig 9-10).

A direct, single-force application from implants is simple and effective, but excessive force magnitude should never be used for intrusion. Adding a single-force component from implants can increase the treatment efficiency because intrusive force from an implant is relatively constant and unchanging, although force systems between the bracket and wire do change. When shape-driven mechanics and force-driven mechanics are combined, the combined mechanics have the advantages of both systems.

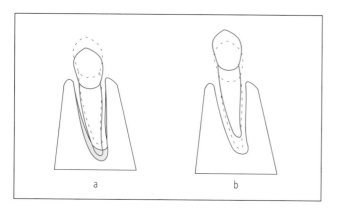

Fig 9-1 *(a)* To bring about the intrusion of teeth, orthodontic forces should resorb the alveolar bone *(shaded area)*, but *(b)* teeth can be extruded with the stretching of the periodontal ligament with minimal alveolar bone response. In other words, with the same amount of orthodontic force, extrusion can be achieved more easily than intrusion with alveolar bone response.

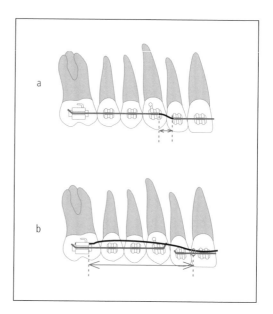

Fig 9-2 To maintain an optimal force level, the load-deflection ratio must be low. If it is too high, the orthodontic force decreases rapidly, even with slight tooth movement. *(a)* Full-arch mechanics have a high load-deflection ratio because of the short interbracket distance *(red arrow)*. *(b)* Sectional-arch mechanics have a low load-deflection ratio because of the greater interbracket distance *(red arrow)*.

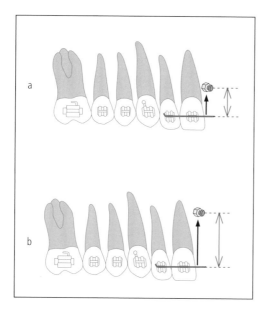

Fig 9-3 *(a)* If orthodontic force is applied from a nearby implant, the load-deflection ratio is likely to be high. *(b)* However, if orthodontic force is applied from a distant implant, the load-deflection ratio is likely to be low.

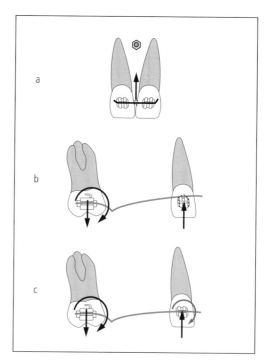

Fig 9-4 *(a and b)* Force-driven mechanics provide only a single force, which is more favorable for anterior intrusion than are *(c)* shape-driven mechanics with anterior archwires.

Table 9-1	Force values for anterior intrusion[1]	
Teeth	**Force per side (g)**	**Total force in midline (g)**
Maxillary		
Central incisors	25	50
Central and lateral incisors	50	100
Central and lateral incisors and canine	100	200
Mandibular		
Central and lateral incisors	20	40
Central and lateral incisors and canine	80	160

Fig 9-5 Treatment planning for anterior intrusion. Clinically, anterior intrusion can be roughly classified into four groups: *(a)* intrusion with lingual tipping, *(b)* intrusion with labial flaring, *(c)* intrusion with an unchanged axis, and *(d)* intrusion along the axis. Note the change in the anteroposterior position of the incisal edges and axes despite the fact that the same amount of bite opening occurs. Clinically, as is commonly seen, intrusion with lingual tipping is not necessary.

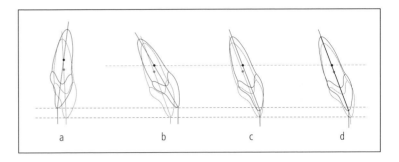

Fig 9-6 Treatment mechanics planning for anterior intrusion. Through intrusion, the anteroposterior position of the incisal edge and the long axis can be controlled by changing the point of application or by the addition of a retractive force. The control of the anteroposterior position of the incisal edges is also related to torque control (incisor axis control). *(a)* Intrusion with lingual tipping. If intrusive force is applied to uprighted incisors from lingual appliances, intrusion with lingual tipping occurs; this is generally undesirable. This type of movement rarely occurs with labial appliances. *(b)* Intru-

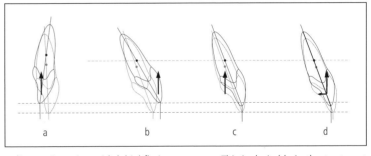

sion with labial flaring. If an intrusive force is applied to labial appliances, intrusion with labial flaring can occur. This is desirable in the treatment of Class II division 2 malocclusions but undesirable in patients with normal incisor long axes. *(c)* Intrusion with the incisor axis unchanged. If intrusive force is applied through the center of resistance, the teeth are intruded bodily. This is desirable in patients with normal incisor axes and normal overjets. *(d)* Intrusion along the axis. If intrusive force is applied with a small retractive force, intrusion occurs along the incisor axis. This is desirable in patients with normal axes and excessive overjets.

Fig 9-7 Even with the same point of application, different tooth movements occur depending on the axis of the incisor. *(a)* If an intrusive force is applied through the center of resistance, bodily movement occurs. *(b)* However, in the case of the lingually tipped incisor, even with the same point of force application, intrusion with lingual tipping occurs because the intrusive force is applied away from the center of resistance. Even with the same intrusive force applied to labial appliances, *(c)* incisors with normal axes exhibit less labial tipping than do *(d)* labially flared incisors, because the more labially flared the tooth is, the larger the moment that occurs.

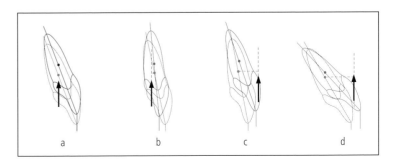

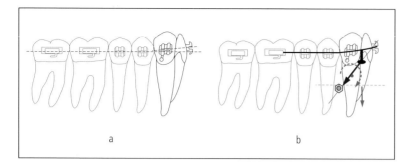

Fig 9-8 *(a)* When six mandibular anterior teeth are extruded, the canine is usually tipped distally. That is, for successful intrusion of six anterior teeth, axis control of the canine accompanies the intrusion. *(b)* For axis control of the canine, application of intrusive force to the mesial side of the canine is advantageous. Use of a second-order bend to produce moments for controlling the canine axis is also beneficial.

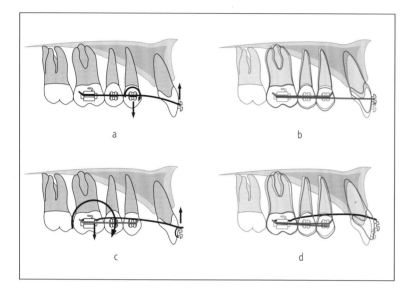

Fig 9-9 Intrusion with continuous arch mechanics may cause unwanted sequelae. With continuous arch mechanics, *(a)* extrusive force is easily concentrated on the canines and may result in *(b)* canting of the occlusal plane. With sectional-arch mechanics, *(c)* tip-back moments from an intrusion spring may cause *(d)* tipping back of posterior segments.

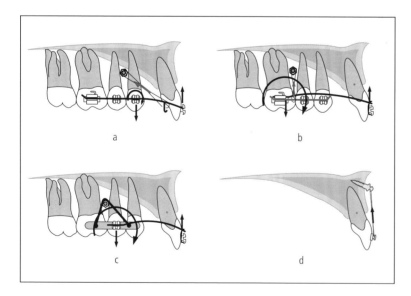

Fig 9-10 Orthodontic implants prevent unwanted movements in conventional intrusion mechanics. *(a and b)* The force system can be improved by implants, and *(c)* indirect anchorage can also be used for anchorage reinforcement. *(d)* A direct single force from an implant can also be used.

Single force from an implant

A single force from an implant is effective, but application of a single force causes uncontrolled tipping (Figs 9-11 to 9-13). Therefore, this type of mechanics should be selected with caution when the desired treatment posi- tions of root apices are considered. When anterior inter- dental implants are used, as anterior teeth are intruded and retracted, elastic chains and the implant may be cov- ered by the soft tissue.

Fig 9-11 Implant positions for applying intrusive forces directly from implants. *(a)* Implants placed between central incisors are favorable for applying intrusive force, and one implant is enough for intrusion. However, the force system generated by these mechanics is likely to cause labial flaring. *(b)* Implants located on the mesial side of canines are advantageous for intruding the six anterior teeth and for controlling the canine axis. *(c)* Implants located on the distal side of canines are advantageous for increasing the retractive force vector.

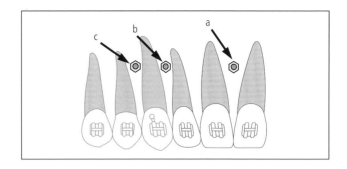

Figs 9-12a and 9-12b A 26-year-old woman, whose chief complaint is protrusion of maxillary teeth and crowding in the maxillary arch, has typical characteristics of Class II division 2 malocclusion: upright and extruded maxillary central incisors and a labially flared maxillary lateral incisor. To intrude and flare the maxillary incisors, intrusive force from mini-implants is applied to labial clear buttons.

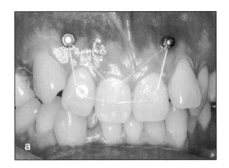
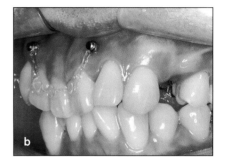

Fig 9-12c During intrusion, partial canine retraction is performed with 0.018-inch Ormco lingual brackets to secure space for alignment. The lingual brackets are not bonded to the maxillary incisors.

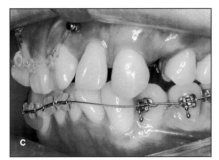
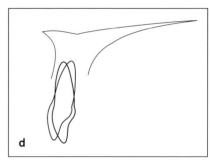

Fig 9-12d Superimposition of *(black)* pretreatment and *(blue)* postintrusion positions of the incisors. Through the use of only a single force, intrusion with uncontrolled tipping can be obtained. (Figs 9-12a to 9-12d courtesy of Dr JK Lim, Seoul, Korea.)

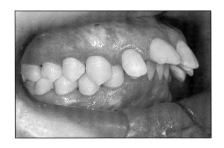
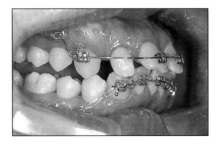
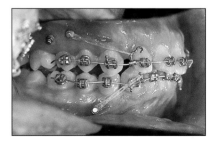

Fig 9-13a Clinical situation prior to treatment.

Fig 9-13b Implants have been placed between the mandibular premolars to intrude and retract the mandibular anterior teeth, and a single force is applied to the anterior sectional arch.

Fig 9-13c After bite opening, appliances are bonded to the other teeth and continuous arch mechanics are used for further intrusion and retraction. To increase the intrusive force vector, crimpable hooks are positioned toward the occlusal direction.

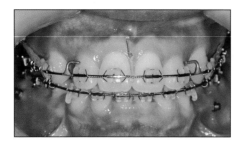

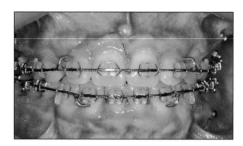

Fig 9-14a During space closure, the anterior bite deepened. An implant has been placed under the anterior nasal spine, and a single force is applied to the main archwire to intrude the anterior teeth. (Figs 9-14a and 9-14b courtesy of Dr JK Lim, Seoul, Korea.)

Fig 9-14b After 4 months of treatment, the anterior bite has opened. If implants are used, intrusion and retraction can be performed simultaneously. However, in such cases, the elastic chains and implant are likely to be buried in the soft tissue. Therefore, the closed technique was used.

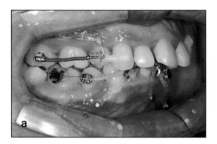

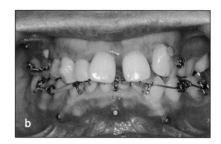

Figs 9-15a and 9-15b A 26-year-old woman, whose chief complaints are protruded maxillary incisors and spacing, exhibits a severe deep overbite and an excessive overjet. To enhance esthetics during treatment, Ormco 0.018-inch maxillary lingual appliances have been placed. A midsagittal interdental implant has been placed to intrude the mandibular incisors with maximum treatment efficiency, and two interdental implants have been placed to apply retractive force for torque control during intrusion. The mandibular canines have been bypassed to increase the load-deflection ratio and to prevent extrusion of the canine.

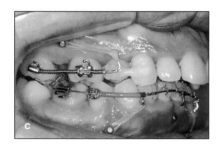

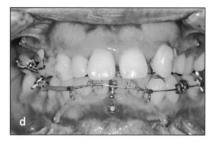

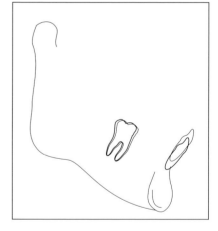

Figs 9-15c and 9-15d After 8 weeks of treatment, the mandibular anterior teeth are intruded.

Fig 9-15e Cephalometric superimposition. *(black)* Pretreatment; *(blue)* after 8 weeks of intrusion.

Intrusion arch with indirect anchorage

Precise control of the force system is possible through the use of an intrusion spring combined with an anchorage unit splinted with an implant. This is the ideal force system for anterior intrusion. Therefore, it is very useful where there is a high risk of root resorption. Indirect anchorage is discussed in more detail in chapter 11.

Continuous arch with orthodontic implants

A single force from implants can be incorporated into conventional continuous full-arch mechanics for intrusion, including reverse nickel-titanium (NiTi) wires or titanium-molybdenum alloy (TMA) wires. This can prevent the side effects of conventional continuous full-arch mechanics and increase treatment efficiency by adding

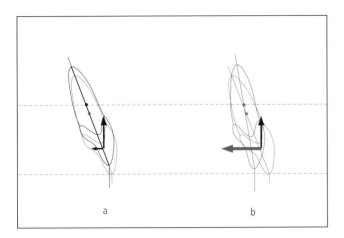

Fig 9-16 Excessive retractive force causes the loss of anterior torque. The amount of retractive force should be less than the amount of intrusive force. *(a)* Correct force system. *(b)* Incorrect force system with excessive retraction force *(red arrow).*

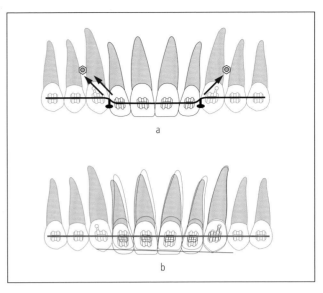

Fig 9-17 *(a)* Increased application of intrusive force on one side *(double arrows)* leads easily to asymmetric intrusion *(b).*

continuous single force (Figs 9-14 and 9-15). In addition, full-arch mechanics with orthodontic implants can move anterior and posterior teeth simultaneously, as well as anteroposteriorly and vertically. That is, the entire dentition can be intruded and distalized with this type of mechanics.

However, a force system cannot be calculated, and precise control is impossible because frictional mechanics and a statically indeterminate force system are involved. To prevent root resorption and uncontrolled tipping of anterior teeth, an excessive force should never be applied (Fig 9-16). For anterior vertical control, use of a light wire is necessary, but retraction on the light wire is likely to cause a loss of anterior torque.

Special considerations and monitoring

Periodontal control

Supragingival plaque is conducive to formation of subgingival plaque as teeth intrude.[7] Hence, periodontal control must precede orthodontic treatment to minimize inflammatory disease, particularly intrusion. Proper oral hygiene control, including periodic professional plaque control, is critical for successful treatment.

Root resorption

Risk factors for a predisposition to root resorption should be a part of screening at the commencement of treatment.[8–12] Periodic periapical radiographic examination at an interval of 4 to 6 months is suggested when predisposing clinical factors are found (eg, pipette-shaped roots, previous trauma, etc).

Arch form and canting

As intrusion proceeds, teeth should be closely monitored three-dimensionally. The arch form, the occlusal plane from the frontal view, and the anteroposterior or sagittal position of the incisal edges should all be monitored at each visit. If intrusion does not progress symmetrically and bilaterally, skewing of the arch form or canting of the occlusal plane from the frontal view may occur (Fig 9-17). The patient's profile should also be checked closely. In general, the facial appearance is more important than the intraoral view to patients.

Anterior torque

Anterior torque should be controlled appropriately.[3–5] Anterior torque may be lost when retraction is performed with intrusion on a light wire. A retraction force should not exceed the intrusive force (see Fig 9-16). During

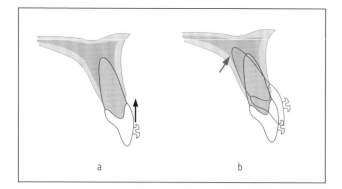

Fig 9-18 *(a)* If the buccolingual dimensions of the alveolar bone are narrow, *(b)* excessive labial flaring caused by an intrusive force at the labial brackets increases the risk of root resorption in lingual cortical bone.

intrusion, excessive labial tipping may also result from moments generated by an intrusive force vector. If so, the risk of root resorption can increase in the event of root contact with the lingual cortical bone (Fig 9-18).

Stability and retention

There must be enough time for reorganization after intrusion. It is beneficial to provide full-time retention with a fixed bonded lingual retainer.

ANTERIOR EXTRUSION

Biomechanics

Extrusion is easier to perform than intrusion, but extrusion accompanied by an increase in vertical dimension is more difficult to achieve than intrusion. Decreasing the facial vertical dimension causes relaxation of the soft tissue[13]; on the other hand, increasing the facial vertical dimension causes stretching of the soft tissue. Therefore, stability and maintenance are more difficult when the vertical dimension has been increased.

The biomechanical principles for anterior extrusion are similar to those for anterior intrusion[14,15] (Figs 9-19 to 9-21), in that teeth should be controlled three-dimensionally. The axis and anteroposterior position of incisal edges should be controlled along with the vertical position. Additionally, torque control is important. Conventional continuous full-arch leveling may result in extrusion with uncontrolled tipping, which aggravates the anteroposterior position of the root apices of the incisors.[15]

Selection of mechanics

The guidelines for selection of mechanics are described in chapter 6. Extrusion may be accompanied by periodontal soft tissue stretching, so biologic considerations may be more important than biomechanical considerations.

Leveling with a conventional continuous arch

Although the conventional continuous full-arch is disadvantageous for anterior torque control and anchorage control, it is simple and easy to use. When these mechanics are used, anterior torque and bite opening in premolar areas should be closely monitored (Fig 9-22).

Maxillomandibular elastics

Generally, the use of maxillomandibular elastics is regarded as mechanics that provide intermittent force. As long as patient cooperation is good, maxillomandibular elastics are effective in extrusion because they represent force-driven mechanics. Maxillomandibular elastics can be used directly or indirectly from implants. The directions of maxillomandibular elastics should be adjusted to control torque.

Cantilever springs (extrusion arch)

Although a cantilever spring may require more chair time, it is biomechanically ideal for extrusion, because it has an advantage over both anchorage control and adjustment during treatment by changing the point of force application (Figs 9-23 and 9-24). A small force is enough to perform extrusion of four anterior teeth; thus anchorage can be controlled by the use of minimum force, even without implants. About 40 to 50 g of force is enough for the extrusion of four anterior teeth.

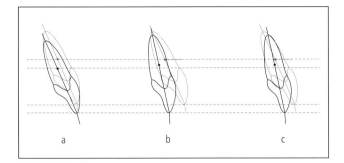

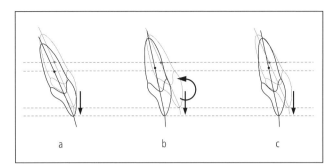

Fig 9-19 Treatment planning for anterior extrusion. Vertical control, axis control, and anteroposterior control of the incisal edge and root apex should be considered. Clinically, anterior extrusion can be classified roughly into three groups: *(a)* extrusion with bodily movement, *(b)* extrusion with controlled tipping, and *(c)* extrusion with uncontrolled tipping. Normally, extrusion with uncontrolled tipping is unfavorable. Note the change in the vertical positions of the center of resistance and the anteroposterior positions of the incisal edges, root apex, and axis, although the same amount of extrusion occurs.

Fig 9-20 Mechanics planning for anterior extrusion. Through extrusion, the axis can be controlled by changing the point of force application or by the addition of moments for root control. *(a)* Extrusion with bodily movement. If extrusive force is applied through the center of resistance, teeth are extruded bodily. This is possible with sectional mechanics. *(b)* Extrusion with controlled tipping. If extrusive force is applied near the center of resistance, teeth are extruded with controlled tipping. This is possible with sectional mechanics or continuous arch mechanics with lingual root torque. However, with continuous arch mechanics, precise adjustment through the addition of a moment to the bracket is difficult to accomplish. *(c)* Extrusion with uncontrolled tipping. If extrusive force is applied away from the center of resistance, teeth are extruded with uncontrolled tipping. In general, conventional continuous arch leveling with round wire causes this kind of extrusion, which is unfavorable for treatment.

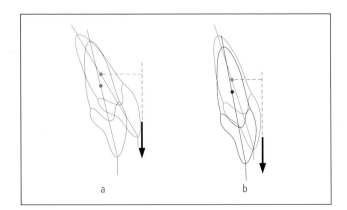

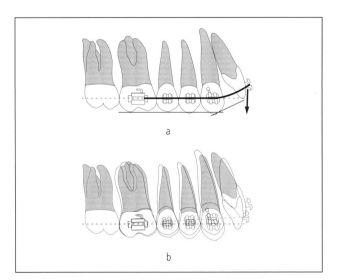

Fig 9-21 Mechanics planning for anterior extrusion. Even with the same point of force application, different tooth movement occurs, depending on the axis of the incisor. If extrusive force was equally applied to labial brackets, more lingual tipping would occur in *(a)* labially flared incisors than in *(b)* upright incisors, because the more labially flared the teeth, the larger the moment becomes. In many patients with an open bite, the anterior teeth are labially flared and undererupted because of abnormal tongue habits. Therefore, extrusion with uncontrolled tipping is likely to occur in patients with open bite.

Fig 9-22 In open bite patients with dual occlusal planes, *(a)* it is easy to extrude anterior teeth because conventional continuous arch leveling produces extrusive force at the labial brackets. *(b)* However, extrusion with uncontrolled tipping is likely to occur. As a result, anterior torque is reduced and the root apices of the incisors are protruded rather than retracted. This is generally unfavorable for treatment. Moreover, intrusive force is easily concentrated on the canines, so occlusal plane canting and bite opening may occur in the premolar area.

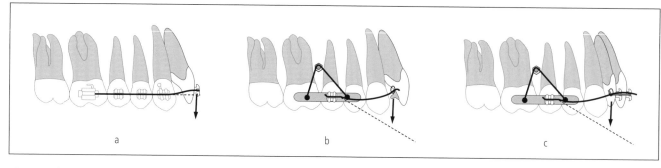

Fig 9-23 *(a)* Use of continuous arch mechanics is a simple and convenient way to perform extrusion of anterior teeth but not biomechanically efficient. *(b)* For extrusion, a lingual approach is better in terms of biomechanics and esthetics. *(b and c)* For precise control, use of a cantilever spring is more favorable. By controlling the point of force application, this type of mechanics controls extrusion.

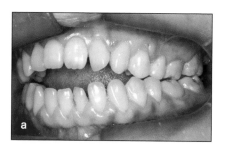
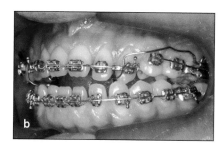
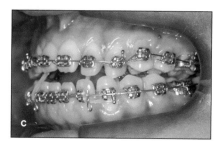
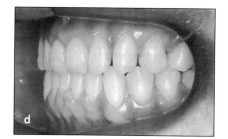

Figs 9-24a to 9-24d Even with the use of a sectional arch with an extrusion cantilever spring, loss of anchorage may occur. **(a)** Because of the insufficient exposure of the maxillary anterior teeth, the treatment plan is to extrude the maxillary anterior teeth. The occlusion in the posterior segments is adequate. Dual occlusal planes are present in the maxillary arch. **(b)** Although only extrusion of the maxillary anterior segment with an extrusion cantilever spring was planned, the posterior teeth have been intruded and tipped mesially because of the reaction of the extrusion spring. **(c)** Maxillomandibular elastics are used for extrusion, and lingual buttons are used for anterior torque control in the maxilla. **(d)** Treatment is completed. Even with force-driven mechanics, excessive extrusive forces cause side effects.

Indirect anchorage from implants and anchorage units splinted together with an implant (see chapter 11) are very useful for reinforcing anchorage. Additionally, with regard to biomechanics and control of the tongue-thrusting habit, the lingual approach may be more desirable.

Direct push mechanics from implants

It is possible to use direct push mechanics, a kind of spring, from implants. For biomechanical efficiency, active parts should be tied by a point contact to prevent the production of moments. If the spring is bonded to or inserted into brackets at both sides, moments are produced and the force system becomes a statically indeterminate force system, which diminishes efficiency.

Special considerations and monitoring

Torque

As mentioned previously, extrusive force on labial brackets produces moments of lingual crown torque (Fig 9-25).

Functional aspects

Open bites are generally accompanied by abnormal swallowing and improper tongue posture. Habit control is important not only during the retention period, for stability, but also during active treatment.[16] If tongue-thrust swallowing is not controlled, a jiggling force is applied to the anterior teeth during treatment, and this causes root resorption and alveolar bone loss (Fig 9-26); therefore,

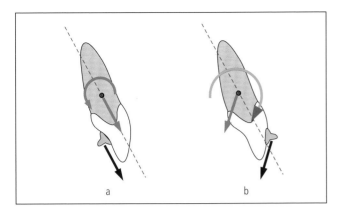

Fig 9-25 It is better to use *(a)* lingual buttons to control anterior torque than *(b)* labial buttons.

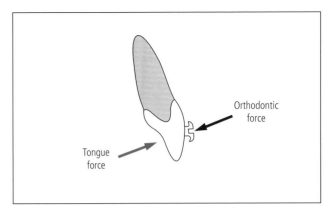

Fig 9-26 A jiggling force may be produced if abnormal tongue habits are not controlled. This may cause root resorption.

periodic periapical radiographic examination is required for monitoring.

Stability and retention

A moderate amount of extrusion can be stable long term.[17,18] Two aspects of stability should be considered: stability of the tooth movement itself and stability related to function. After extrusion, periodontal tissue and supragingival fibers are stretched; this may cause stress concentration in the gingival tissue.[19] Furthermore, the gingiva has a relatively slow turnover rate. Therefore, the gingiva needs more time for reorganization after extrusion than after intrusion.[20] Whenever possible, maintenance through a permanent fixed retainer is strongly recommended.

If functional problems from anterior open bite remain after treatment, they could contribute to relapse. The tongue should be positioned over the incisive papilla area. A tongue crib should be used at night for at least 1 year to control tongue position habits.

POSTERIOR INTRUSION

Treatment planning

Posterior intrusion is one of the most difficult tooth movements to accomplish because molars have multiple large roots and intrusion requires much alveolar bone reaction as well as a longer treatment time. The longer the period of treatment becomes, the more unwanted movements appear, because even a light force can make teeth move if applied for a long time. Treatment is prone to result in unwanted extrusion instead of planned intrusion.

Moreover, three-dimensional control is critical in molar intrusion; thus, a three-dimensional treatment plan is important for posterior intrusion (Figs 9-27 to 9-29). Besides the vertical position, the arch form, the tooth axes, the inclination of the occlusal plane, and the posterior torque should be planned as individual treatment objectives. Most of all, the long-term periodontal health should take precedence over the other considerations (see chapter 7).

Biomechanics

The biomechanical principles of posterior intrusion are similar to those of anterior intrusion. However, posterior intrusion requires more force and yet seems to exhibit a lower incidence of root resorption. Bodily movement is generally required, but the following difficulties exist:

1. Biomechanic efficiency is critical (Fig 9-30).
2. It is difficult to know the accurate location of the center of resistance of the teeth because there are individual differences in root shape and bone level, among other issues.
3. Clinically, it is also impossible to apply an orthodontic force three-dimensionally through the center of resistance.

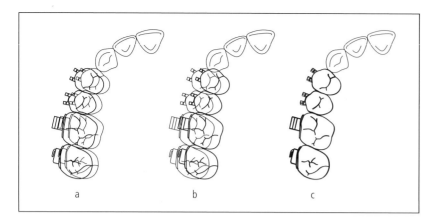

Fig 9-27 Treatment planning for posterior intrusion. Depending on the treatment objective, the arch should be *(a)* expanded, *(b)* constricted, or *(c)* maintained.

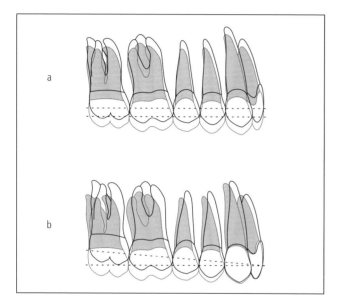

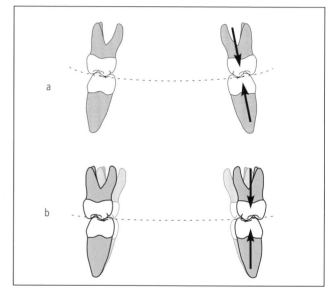

Fig 9-28 Treatment planning for the occlusal plane. Clinically, the change of an occlusal plane can roughly be classified into two groups. *(a)* Parallel intrusion means that the molars and premolars are intruded to the same degree. This is necessary for correction of a "gummy" smile or long face. *(b)* Nonparallel intrusion indicates that the second molar areas are intruded more than the premolar areas. The reverse may happen because of unwanted sequelae. Nonparallel intrusion is needed for the correction of an open bite, which is more difficult to achieve. Note the change in inclination of the posterior occlusal plane and the changes in the axes of individual posterior teeth. To create a steeper occlusal plane, individual posterior teeth should be tipped back.

Fig 9-29 Treatment planning for torque. Posterior torque should be obtained according to the relationship of the basal bone and posterior occlusion. *(a)* Normal posterior torque. *(b)* Camouflage treatment with posterior torque compensation.

4. The location of force application is usually limited because the locations for possible implant placement are limited. Implants cannot always be placed in the most desired positions.

5. Even if the force system is designed precisely for molar intrusion in the beginning, adjustment of the force system will be required depending on the changes with tooth movement during treatment.

6. Posterior intrusion is not just a matter of vertical control (Figs 9-31 to 9-34). For successful posterior intrusion, the arch form, tooth axis, inclination of the occlusal plane, and posterior torque must all be controlled in addition to the vertical dimension.[21–28]

A statically indeterminate system is not efficient for posterior intrusion because of continuous changes in the

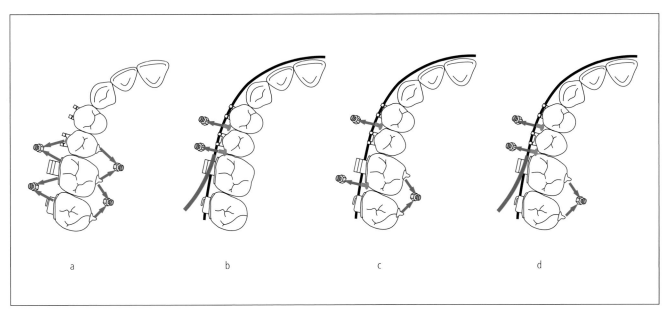

Fig 9-30 Biomechanical efficiency of posterior intrusion. *(a)* Use of a single force in posterior intrusion rather than brackets and wires is effective and efficient, so that intrusion progresses more quickly. However, it is not effective for controlling the arch form, tooth axis, or inclination of the occlusal plane or for detailed adjustment. *(b)* Intrusion through a second-order bend or step bend of the wire is advantageous for controlling the arch form, axis, and individual tooth positions but is less efficient from the viewpoint of vertical control because of the limitations of a statically indeterminate force system. *(c and d)* A combination of the two force systems mutually compensates for the disadvantages of each of the systems. In other words, from a buccal view, the posterior intrusion is a statically indeterminate force system, and from a palatal view, it is a statically determinate force system. Therefore, it is effective and efficient for controlling the vertical position, arch form, and other issues.

force system in the bracket with even slight movements. Because posterior teeth have a larger root-surface area, posterior intrusion is affected more by biomechanical efficiency than is anterior intrusion. In other words, the use of continuous full-arch mechanics via wires that are engaged in bracket slots is not effective or efficient for applying intrusive force to posterior teeth, and teeth intrude very slowly or extrusion occurs instead of intrusion. It is more effective and more efficient to use a single force and a statically determinate force system for vertical control of intrusion.

To use a statically determinate system and single forces, implants should be placed in appropriate positions. The selection of the insertion site may be limited by anatomy and accessibility. Furthermore, a greater number of implants are needed to deliver a single force, which is more efficient.

Additionally, the use of many single forces is disadvantageous for three-dimensional control, and detailed adjustment is required during the progression of treatment. The best way is to use brackets and wires for detailed adjustment. A continuous arch, which is a statically determinate force system, is advantageous for controlling the arch form, long axis, and individual tooth positions. A combination of the two force systems mutually compensates for the disadvantages of each individual system.

In posterior intrusion, control of the second molar area is more difficult, because the roots of a molar are bigger than those of a premolar and orthodontic implants are generally placed in premolar areas because of better accessibility. Therefore, excessive intrusion can occur in the premolar areas. Placement of implants in the area near the second molars or creation of a sufficient second-order bend may be useful.

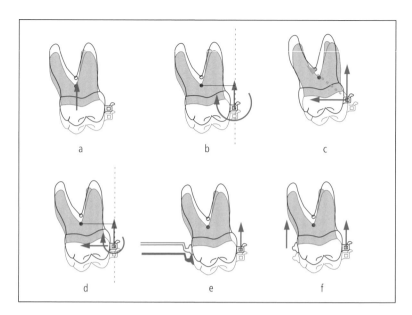

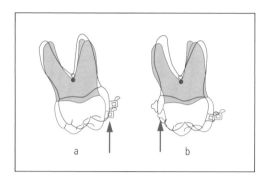

Fig 9-31 Biomechanical considerations for first- and third-order control. Rotation occurs if an intrusive force is applied away from the center of resistance. *(a)* When intrusive force is applied from the buccal side, buccal tipping occurs in addition to intrusion. Palatal cusps look fallen and the arch form is widened. *(b)* When the intrusive force is applied from the palatal side, palatal tipping occurs and the arch form becomes constricted. Similarly, control of posterior torque and control of arch form are related to each other.

Fig 9-32 Biomechanical considerations for first- and third-order control. Buccal intrusive forces cause buccal tipping. *(a)* Clinically, it is nearly impossible to apply orthodontic force three-dimensionally through the center of resistance. *(b)* For bodily intrusion, intrusive force and palatal crown torque are applied together, but this makes it difficult to provide the accurate amount of moment. Even if a precise force system is applied, a slight movement can change the force system, so it is biomechanically inefficient. *(c)* Buccal intrusive and constrictive forces can be applied simultaneously to reduce buccal tipping. The amount of constrictive force should be similar to that of intrusive force, but this system is also difficult to control precisely. *(d)* It is possible to use methods *(b)* and *(c)* at the same time, but accurate adjustment is also difficult. *(e)* It is very effective to use crossarch splinting to control arch form and torque. This is uncomfortable to patients and ineffective for unilateral intrusion. The biomechanical efficiency of treatment is also decreased by crossarch splinting. *(f)* A palatal point of force application is also needed, but intrusion with buccal and palatal force is preferred. This system is superior from all biomechanical points of view, except in that it is not fail-safe.

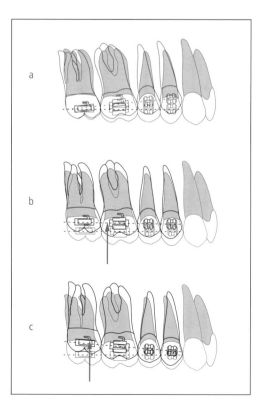

Fig 9-33 Biomechanical considerations for second-order control. Implants cannot be placed exactly where they are needed, and it may be difficult to design the line of action as needed. *(a)* Because molars have larger root surfaces, the premolar areas are intruded first, even with the same intrusive force. If intrusive forces are applied anterior to the center of resistance of the posterior segment, the mesial tipping tendency of the posterior segment increases. *(b and c)* For successful posterior intrusion, the vertical position and the axis of the second molar should be controlled properly. Axis control is related to occlusal plane control.

Fig 9-34 Biomechanical considerations for second-order control. There are two ways to control the inclination of the occlusal plane and the axis of the second molar in posterior intrusion: *(a)* change the point of force application and *(b)* use bends in the main wire. The fact that moments are necessary for control of rotation should be kept in mind. A single force cannot control the inclination of an occlusal plane, and it is necessary that *(c)* two forces or a *(d)* second-order bend be used to produce moments for rotation of the occlusal plane. An up-and-down bend or L-loop can also be added to the main wire to increase efficiency. A second-order bend needs precise adjustment and is not effective for controlling the inclination of the occlusal plane when a transpalatal appliance is used with rigid splinting.

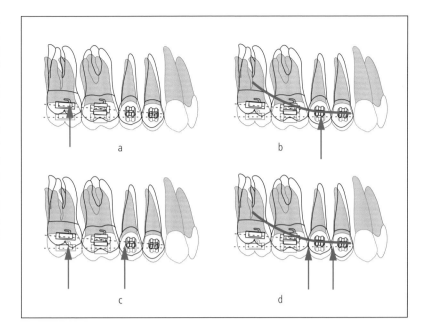

Selection of mechanics

Molar intrusion mechanics must have components to control the molars three-dimensionally. The mechanics for posterior intrusion should include control of the following components: the vertical position; the arch form (control of the buccolingual position of individual teeth); the torque of the individual teeth; the axis of the individual teeth; and the inclination of the occlusal plane.

Selection criteria

The following criteria should be considered:

1. Biomechanical efficiency. The use of force-driven mechanics, which have a statically determinate force system, is more efficient than the use of shape-driven mechanics, which have a statically indeterminate force system.[2]
2. Reliability. Continuous full-arch mechanics are more fail-safe.
3. Adjustability. The use of single forces is advantageous for major adjustment, while continuous full-arch mechanics are advantageous for minor detailing.

4. Technique sensitivity. Crossarch splinting is less technique sensitive with less adverse tooth-movement response.
5. Patient discomfort. The use of crossarch splinting or a transpalatal arch (TPA) is less comfortable for patients.

Strategies for intrusion of the maxillary dentition

The center of resistance of maxillary molars is located toward the palatal side. Therefore, palatal root control is more difficult and more important (Fig 9-35). A palatal point of force application is very helpful for controlling the palatal roots of the molars and for increasing biomechanical efficiency. The use of palatal interdental implants or midpalatal implants to apply intrusive force from the palatal side is strongly recommended. From the biomechanical point of view, for posterior segment intrusion, midpalatal implants with attachments are better than palatal interdental implants between the first molar and second molar, because the former can control the point of application via attachments. However, the palatal interdental implants are more comfortable for patients.

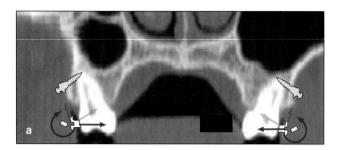
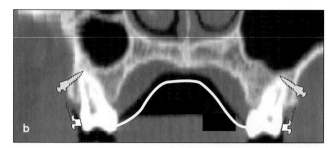
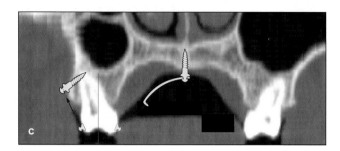
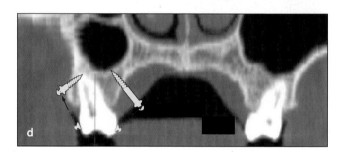

Figs 9-35a to 9-35d Palatal root control is key for maxillary molar intrusion. **(a)** It is possible to control torque by providing the moment with the twisted wire and the bracket slot. However, it is a statically indeterminate system, making accurate control difficult and efficiency low. It is also possible to control torque by applying a constriction force or by applying a combination of torque and constriction force. **(b)** However, the use of crossarch splinting would be more efficient. **(c and d)** Use of buccal and lingual intrusive forces together is the most effective protocol.

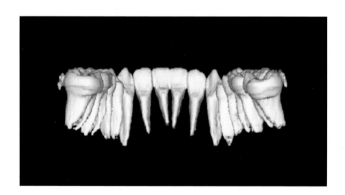

Fig 9-36 Normal root inclination of the mandibular molar. From a lingual view, three-dimensional computed tomographic reconstruction reveals that the lingual angulation of the roots of the posterior teeth increased. The mandibular second molar is tipped more lingually than the first molar.

Strategies for intrusion of the mandibular dentition

Intrusion of the mandibular dentition is more difficult than intrusion of the maxillary dentition because the mandible is made of high-density cortical bone, which has a slower rate of bone turnover. Clinically, it is difficult to place implants in the first and second molar area because of limited interproximal space buccally, much irritation from mastication, low accessibility, extremely moveable cheek muscle, and the hard cortical bone in this area that may compromise the stability of implants. Most of all, it is difficult to place implants in the lingual side. Therefore, the focus should be set on controlling the second- and third-order positions of mandibular molars from the beginning (Figs 9-36 to 9-40). Crossarch splinting is simple and effective for controlling the arch form and torques, although treatment eficiency may be compromised.

Intrusion of one or two teeth

Even for the intrusion of one or two teeth, three-dimensional controls are essential. Indirect anchorage, such as an anchorage unit splinted with an implant, is useful for intrusion of one or two teeth (see chapter 11).

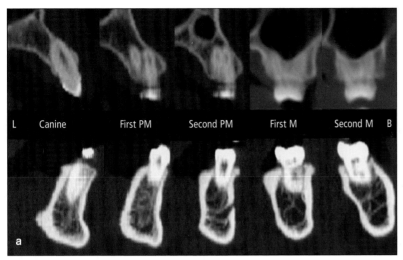
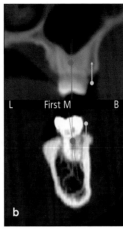
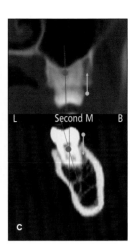

Figs 9-37a to 9-37c Note the difference in torque (root inclination) between the maxillary and mandibular teeth. **(a)** Mandibular molars have greater lingual inclination than maxillary molars, and thus buccal intrusive force produces less lingual crown torque in the mandible than in the maxilla. **(b)** Center of resistance of first molar. **(c)** Center of resistance of second molar. (L) Lingual; (B) buccal; (PM) premolar; (M) molar.

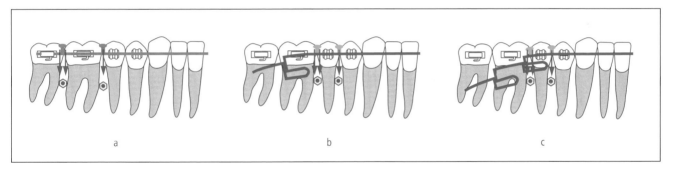

Fig 9-38 Second-order control. Clinically, control of the inclination of the occlusal plane is one of the most difficult problems in posterior intrusion. *(a)* Implants placed between the molars are very useful for controlling the second molars. Mechanics that intrude in a one-by-one sequence can increase the efficiency of the intrusion of mandibular molars. For example, *(b)* an L-loop or *(c)* a double L-loop results in effective and efficient second molar intrusion.

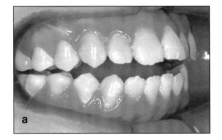
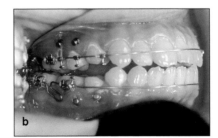
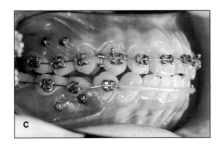
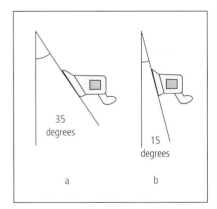

Figs 9-39a to 9-39c Strategy for intrusion in the mandible. **(a)** Prior to treatment. In general, the most posterior molars should be intruded more. **(b)** An L-loop made of 0.017 × 0.025-inch TMA wire with a tip-back bend, toe-in bend, and lingual crown torque is effective for controlling the second molar. **(c)** After intrusion.

Fig 9-40 Mechanics for third-order control. Bracket prescriptions with *(a)* sufficient lingual crown torque may be more useful than a *(b)* second molar tube with reduced lingual crown torque.

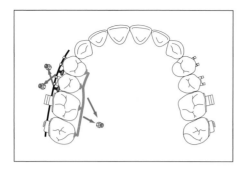

Fig 9-41 A limitation of unilateral intrusion is that crossarch splinting is less efficient than it is in bilateral intrusion. Therefore, the mechanics should have components with which to apply buccal and palatal intrusive forces.

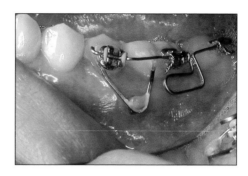

Fig 9-42 Because of patient discomfort, it is difficult to insert an implant on the lingual side in the mandible. Therefore, mandibular intrusion is more difficult to achieve than maxillary intrusion. The use of indirect anchorage is a good strategy for unilateral intrusion in the mandible.

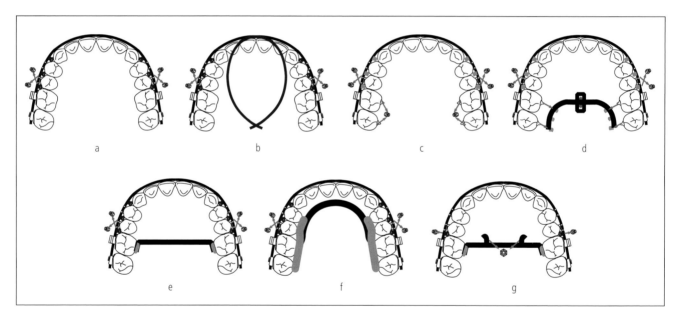

Fig 9-43 Control of the arch form and torque in intrusive mechanics. The use of crossarch splinting is stable. *(a)* Without crossarch splinting, using buccal intrusive force and full-size stiff wire of a passive form. During posterior intrusion, stiff wire of a passive form is not good at controlling arch form or torque. Even a full-size SS wire is not stiff enough for control, and arch expansion and bowing may occur. *(b)* Without crossarch splinting, using buccal intrusive force and a TMA wire with a bend. Posterior intrusion can be performed through buccal intrusive force applied from buccal implants with a constrictive bend and a compensating curve on a TMA wire without crossarch splinting. It looks simple and does not cause additional discomfort to the patient but is not efficient for intruding the second molar and does not simplify control of the arch form and torque. Careful monitoring and adjustment are also needed. The addition of a step bend may be helpful. *(c)* Without crossarch splinting, using buccal and palatal intrusive forces (I). The use of buccal and palatal intrusive forces is the most efficient means for intrusion and control of arch form and posterior torque. Palatal interdental implants are more comfortable for patients but limited in their ability to control the force application point. *(d)* Without crossarch splinting, using buccal and palatal intrusive forces (II). For application of palatal intrusive forces, midpalatal implants and a TPA can be used. This method is advantageous for controlling the line of action by changing the point of force application using multiple hooks on a TPA; however, the TPA may cause the patient discomfort. *(e)* With crossarch splinting. Crossarch splinting is a simple, easy way to control arch form. Either an active or a passive TPA can be used. Crossarch splinting causes additional discomfort to patients and may reduce the efficiency of tooth movement. To compensate for the reduced biomechanical efficiency of this technique, intrusive force should be applied posteriorly, near the second molars. *(f)* With crossarch splinting. Crossarch splinting of only the first molar is not sufficient for torque control. For proper torque control, at least the first and second molars must be included in the crossarch splinting. On the other hand, more splinting leads to less efficient movement. That is, when all posterior teeth are splinted, the inclination of the occlusal plane becomes more difficult to control. To compensate, an intrusive force should be applied posteriorly to control the second molar area. *(g)* With crossarch splinting and palatal intrusive force. To increase biomechanical efficiency, palatal intrusive force for palatal implants can be applied to the TPA. In this method, the palatal intrusive force should be applied posteriorly, near the second molars.

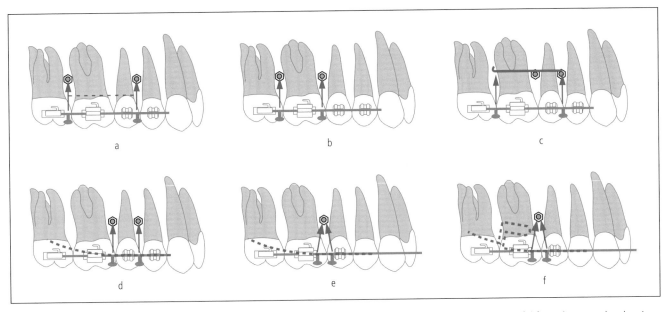

Fig 9-44 Control of the inclination of the occlusal plane in intrusive mechanics. For posterior intrusion to be successful from the second-order view-point, the inclination of the occlusal plane and the axes of individual teeth as well as vertical position have to be controlled. *(a)* The best way to control the anteroposterior inclination of an occlusal plane is to use two forces from two implants that are set apart; the production of moments is related to the amount of applied forces and the distances *(dashed red line)* between the forces. *(b)* To control the second molar, intrusive force should be applied posteriorly, near the second molar area. If the placement of implants between molars is not feasible, *(c)* a bonded extension arm or *(d)* a second-order bend can be used. *(e)* Two forces are essential to produce moments, even with a single implant. A step bend or *(f)* an L-loop can also be used to increase biomechanical efficiency.

Unilateral intrusion

Unilateral intrusion is more difficult than bilateral intrusion. For unilateral intrusion, mechanics should have components to apply intrusive forces from the buccal and lingual sides, because crossarch splinting is less effective in unilateral intrusion than in bilateral intrusion (Fig 9-41). Crossarch splinting in unilateral intrusion is only effective for controlling the arch form. In the case of mandibular unilateral intrusion, the second molar should be controlled three-dimensionally from the beginning of treatment. Close monitoring is necessary, and the use of indirect anchorage, which is more stable, may be recommended, although this may lower the treatment efficiency and take longer (Fig 9-42).

Bilateral intrusion

Posterior segments can be intruded bilaterally by various mechanics (Figs 9-43 to 9-55):

1. Intrusion using buccal and lingual intrusive forces with crossarch splinting
2. Intrusion using buccal and lingual intrusive forces without crossarch splinting
3. Intrusion using buccal intrusive force with crossarch splinting
4. Intrusion using buccal intrusive force without crossarch splinting

Crossarch splinting causes additional discomfort to patients but makes controlled tooth movement easier. Using a combination of buccal and lingual intrusive forces increases treatment efficiency.

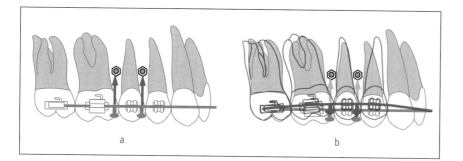

Fig 9-45 *(a)* Even with two forces applied, the use of stiff wire is not effective in controlling the second molar area or the inclination of the occlusal plane if intrusive force is applied away from the second molar. *(b)* Instead of creating a steeper occlusal plane, the force easily causes bowing because of the high resistance of the second molar.

Figs 9-46a to 9-46k Molar intrusion through single forces used without the application of moments (a statically determinate force system). Use of a single force for intrusion produces fast movement but may be ineffective for precise, three-dimensional control of individual teeth.

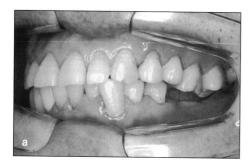

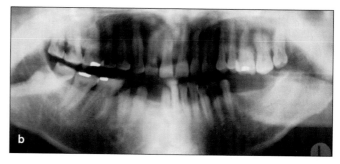

Figs 9-46a and 9-46b The available vertical space is insufficient for restoration of mandibular missing teeth with prosthodontic implants because of the extrusion of the opposing maxillary molars. Therefore, intrusion of the maxillary first and second molars is planned.

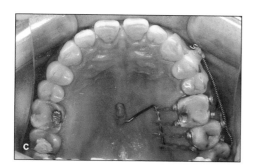

Fig 9-46c The mechanics are devised for molar intrusion. Two implants have been placed in the midpalatal suture area, and an extension arm is bonded to them. Three implants have also been placed in the buccal alveolus.

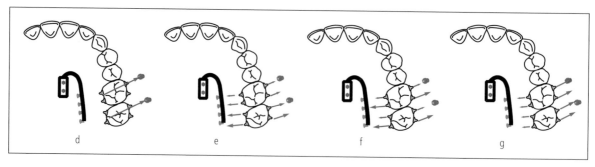

Figs 9-46d to 9-46g This mechanics system possesses all of the components for molar intrusion to control the vertical position, the arch form (buccolingual positions of individual teeth), the axis of individual teeth, the inclination of the occlusal plane, and the torque of individual teeth.

Fig 9-46h Through the use of single forces, the molars have been intruded.

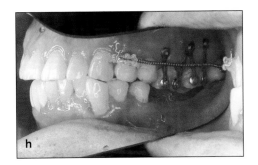

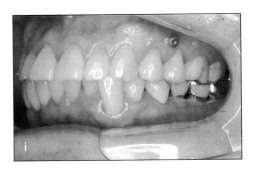

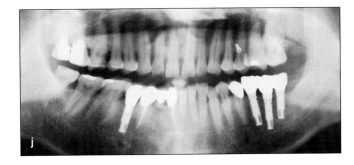

Figs 9-46i and 9-46j Vertical space for restorations has been secured.

Fig 9-46k At the 6-month follow-up after the end of active treatment, the results are well maintained.

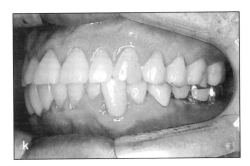

Figs 9-47a to 9-47d Molar intrusion with combined mechanics (ie, a combination of force-driven mechanics and shape-driven mechanics).

Fig 9-47a Maxillary second molar intrusion is planned to reestablish vertical space for restoration of mandibular missing teeth with prosthodontic implants.

Fig 9-47b An anchorage unit splinted with an implant is used for anchorage reinforcement. Buccal brackets and TMA wire with a step bend and tip-back bend are used to control vertical position, axis, and arch form.

Fig 9-47c Lingual intrusive force from a lingual extension arm is applied to control torque and increase efficiency.

Fig 9-47d The molars have been intruded and prosthodontic treatment has been completed.

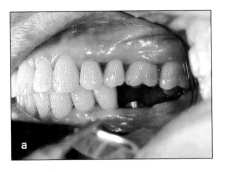

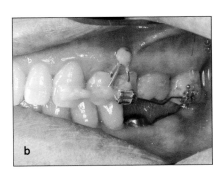

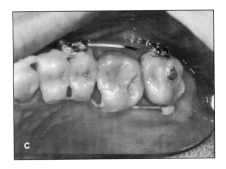

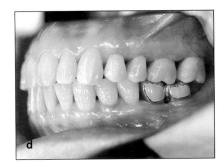

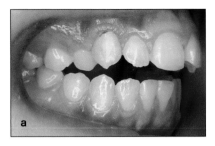
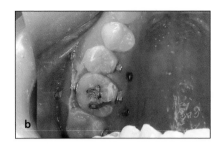
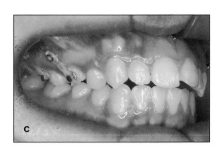

Figs 9-48a to 9-48c Intrusion using single buccal and palatal forces. Use of buccal and palatal intrusive forces is one of the most efficient ways to intrude molars. Furthermore, palatal interdental implants are more comfortable for patients but limited in their ability to control the point of force application. Therefore, a greater number of mini-implants may be needed to control the line of action, and implant position is very important for this type of mechanics. The line of action should be near the second molar. Control of the arch form and the angulation of each tooth is difficult. This method is also technique sensitive, so close monitoring and proper adjustment are needed. It is not fail-safe. The rate of intrusion for this type of mechanics is approximately 0.5 mm per month. **(a)** Clinical situation prior to treatment. **(b)** Treatment mechanics. **(c)** Clinical situation 4 months after treatment. The molars have been intruded in a relatively short period of time through the use of force-driven mechanics.

Figs 9-49a to 9-49d Molar intrusion with combined mechanics.

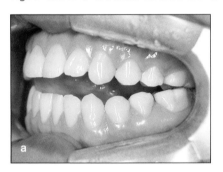
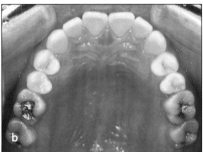

Figs 9-49a and 9-49b Clinical situation before treatment.

Fig 9-49c Buccal brackets and TMA wire with a second-order bend and toe-in bend are used to control vertical position, axis, and arch form.

Fig 9-49d Lingual intrusive force from a palatal interdental implant is applied to control torque and increase efficiency.

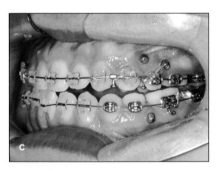
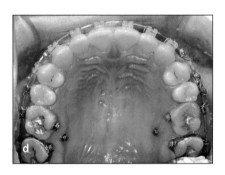

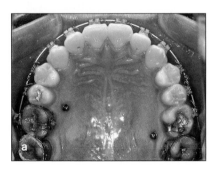
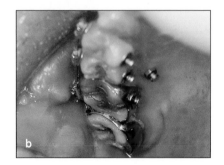
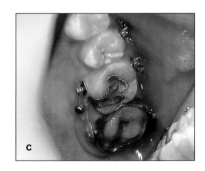

Fig 9-50a Control of the second molar is the core of posterior intrusion. It is better to apply force as posteriorly as possible to control the second molar. The palatal interdental implant has been placed between molars on the left side and between the second premolar and first molar on the right side because the palatal mucosa is thick.
Figs 9-50b and 9-50c Use of an implant between the second premolar and first molar on the right side provided less efficient torque control of the second molar.

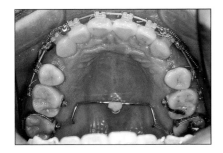

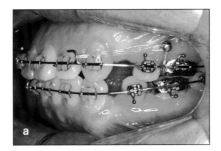

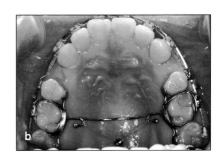

Fig 9-51 Midpalatal implants and an attached TPA can be used to apply palatal intrusive forces. This method is advantageous in controlling the line of action by changing the point of application using multiple hooks on the TPA, but the TPA may cause additional discomfort to the patient.

Figs 9-52a and 9-52b Intrusion with buccal and palatal single forces and crossarch splinting. Palatal intrusive force can be applied to hooks on the TPA from midpalatal implants. The TPA controls arch form effectively, and application of a palatal single force increases efficiency. The posterior teeth are splinted to one unit to control torque. The TPA should be located away from the palate so as not to impinge on the palate as intrusion proceeds. Palatal intrusive force should also be applied posteriorly, near the second molars. (Courtesy of Dr JK Lim, Seoul, Korea.)

Figs 9-53a to 9-53d Intrusion with a single force and crossarch splinting. Rigid splinting is not effective for controlling inclination of the occlusal plane. Therefore, implants between molars are necessary to apply force posteriorly.

Fig 9-53a To correct transverse discrepancies, rapid palatal expansion appliance will be used for expansion and for crossarch splinting. A rapid palatal expansion appliance will also be fabricated away from the palate in consideration of the amount of intrusion planned.

Figs 9-53b and 9-53c Fourth month after the start of treatment.

Fig 9-53d Six months after the start of treatment.

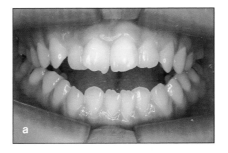

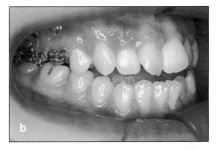

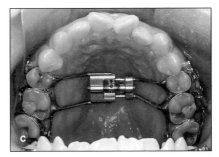

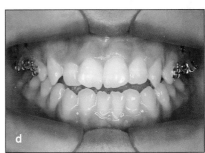

Figs 9-54a and 9-54b Intrusion with active crossarch splinting by precision lingual arch. An active-type Burstone precision lingual arch made of 0.032 × 0.032-inch TMA wire has been used to apply bilateral lingual crown torques on the first molar. The appliance is effective in controlling arch form and torque of the first molar but only weakly controls the torque of the remaining posterior teeth.

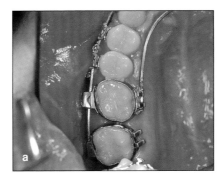

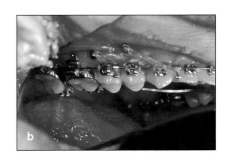

Figs 9-55a and 9-55b Intrusion using buccal intrusive force and a continuous arch.

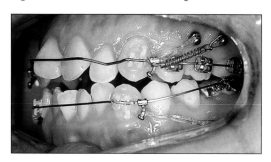

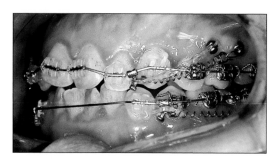

Fig 9-55a A second-order bend on TMA wire and buccal intrusive force to hooks on the main archwire of the premolar area have been placed to achieve molar intrusion. Hooks are positioned toward the occlusal surface to increase the vertical force vector.

Fig 9-55b Clinical situation after molar intrusion.

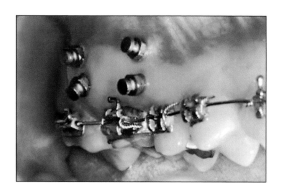

Fig 9-56 Molar intrusion with mini-implants has been applied, but the implants are inserted too far occlusally to match the desired level. New implants are inserted more apically, and the treatment is resumed.

Special considerations and monitoring

Proper diagnosis, treatment planning, and positioning of mini-implants are the first steps in posterior intrusion. Placement of mini-implants in the appropriate locations is the most critical procedure (Fig 9-56); appliances should be fabricated according to a precise treatment plan (Fig 9-57).

With any type of mechanics, three-dimensional monitoring and adjustment of tooth movement according to treatment progress are more important than selection of mechanics (Figs 9-58 to 9-65).

Periodontal control

Supragingival plaque creates an environment conducive to subgingival plaque as the teeth intrude. Proper oral hygiene, along with professional plaque control, is neces-sary for successful treatment. During intrusion of the posterior segment, close attention should be given to the most distal tooth, because angular bony change and pseudo-pocketing may occur.

Attachments

If possible, to preserve healthy periodontal tissues, bonded attachments are preferred to the use of bands on molars. Moreover, smaller attachments are easier to keep clean.

Alveolar trough

As with any type of tooth movement, intrusion should be performed within the envelope of the alveolar process or alveolar trough.[29] During intrusion, if excessive buccal tipping occurs, the risk of labial recession or dehiscence increases.

Figs 9-57a to 9-57d As the molars intruded, the TPA penetrated the palate. **(a and b)** Prior to intrusion. **(c and d)** During intrusion.

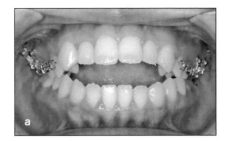
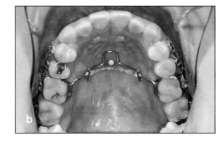
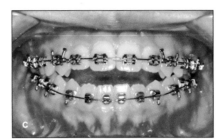
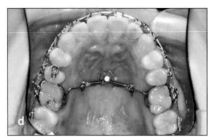

Figs 9-58a and 9-58b When only a single force is used, intrusion can occur differently on the left and right sides even though identical orthodontic force is applied. If the vertical positions on the **(a)** right and **(b)** left sides are different from each other, careful adjustment is needed because this results in frontal canting, which is difficult to correct.

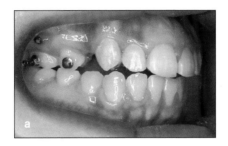
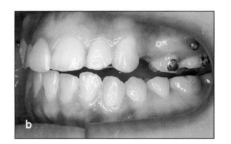

Figs 9-59a and 9-59b Canting of the occlusal plane can expand to the frontal plane as one side is more intruded than the other. **(a)** Frontal intraoral view. **(b)** Frontal facial view.

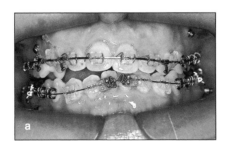
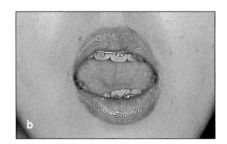

Figs 9-60a and 9-60b **(a)** Occlusal diagram. The change in arch form should be closely monitored from the first-order viewpoint. **(b)** Buccal intrusive force expands the arch, which is manifested as increased buccal overjet. In particular, the area where intrusive force is concentrated expands, and this force is easy to produce with the light wire. This tendency can be offset by a constriction bend or palatal intrusive force.

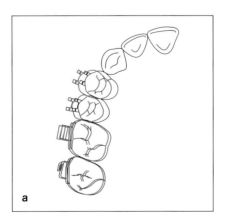
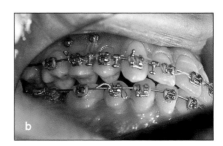

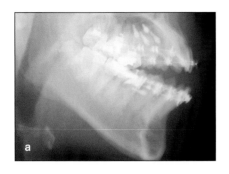

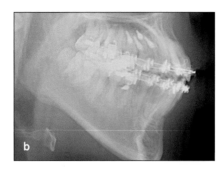

Fig 9-61a Because the patient did not cooperate in the use of maxillomandibular elastics, the anterior teeth were excessively intruded. As a result, the anterior vertical relationship and the smile line worsened.

Fig 9-61b The anterior vertical relationship was improved by intrusion of the posterior and anterior teeth.

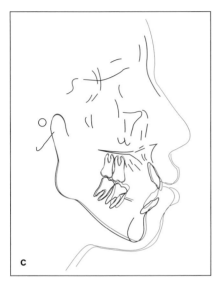

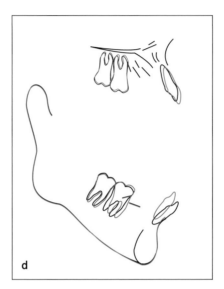

Figs 9-61c and 9-61d Cephalometric superimpositions of tracings of *(black)* Fig 9-61a and *(red)* Fig 9-61b.

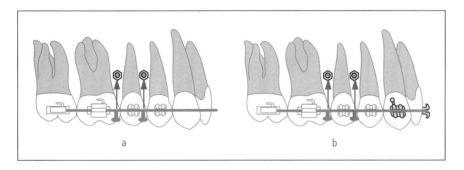

Fig 9-62 *(a)* The best way to prevent anterior teeth from being excessively intruded is to refrain from bonding brackets to anterior teeth until the molars are intruded up to the position of the treatment objective. *(b)* Bond brackets to anterior teeth only when the entire dentition must be intruded.

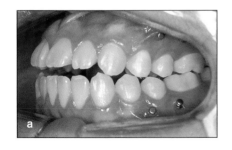

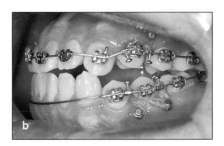

Figs 9-63a and 9-63b Intrusion occurs more easily in premolar areas than in molar areas because of the difference in the size of the root and the line of action, which is related to the position of the implant. Creation of a second-order bend or step bend may be useful for these situations.

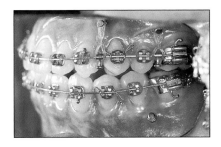

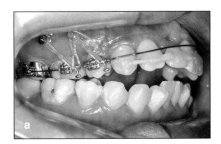

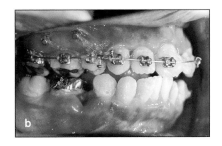

Fig 9-64 When the entire dentition must be intruded, it is most effective to use two implants that are set apart to produce moments that control the inclination of the occlusal plane. However, application of a single force is not enough to control the inclination of the occlusal plane.

Figs 9-65a and 9-65b From the viewpoint of the third-order control, buccal flaring of the teeth should be monitored carefully. Buccal intrusive force tends to intrude the buccal cusp first, so the palatal cusp appears to have fallen. The use of palatal intrusive force is the most effective for intrusive correction. **(a)** Prior to intrusion. **(b)** After intrusion.

Fig 9-66 For disocclusion of posterior teeth, coverage of just one or two teeth may not be sufficient. A vertical stop was formed on the second molar, but it has intruded instead of showing an increased vertical dimension. An anterior bite block should be used to disocclude the posterior teeth.

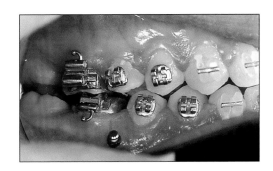

POSTERIOR EXTRUSION

Posterior extrusion can be classified into two types: posterior extrusion accompanied by an increase in facial vertical dimension, and posterior extrusion with unchanged facial vertical dimension. Extrusion that accompanies stretching of the overall soft tissue may result in relapse, as noted previously.[13]

Treatment planning

For posterior extrusion in conjunction with an increase in facial vertical dimension, disocclusion of the posterior teeth should be performed first. The problem of increasing the vertical dimension in a nongrowing patient is generally not a biomechanical issue but a physiologic one (Fig 9-66). That is, the evaluation of physiologic vertical dimension or freeway space must precede treatment.

There is no established protocol for diagnosis and treatment planning to increase the facial vertical dimension,[29,30] and the stability of increased facial vertical dimension is still controversial. Maintenance of an increased facial vertical dimension may be more difficult than the process of increasing the alveolar vertical dimension.

Biomechanics and mechanics

With implants, in contrast to conventional mechanics, extrusion is more difficult than intrusion because of the characteristics of implant mechanics. As in intrusion, in extrusion the molar must be controlled three-dimensionally.

Implants exhibit weak push mechanics (Fig 9-67). In addition, three-dimensional control should be maintained. That is, buccal extrusive force is not enough to accomplish extrusion, and buccal and lingual extrusive forces together are necessary for better torque control (Fig 9-68).

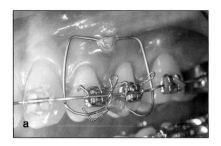 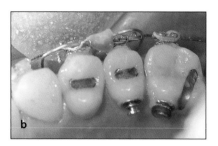

Fig 9-67a Implants are relatively poor at performing extrusive mechanics. Push springs extending from implants should be used for extrusive mechanics.

Fig 9-67b If push springs are used, a point contact should exist on the active parts.

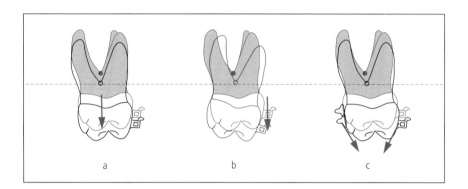

Fig 9-68 *(a)* To perform extrusion by bodily movement, an extrusive force should be applied through the center of resistance. *(b)* Only buccal extrusive force causes lingual tipping. *(c)* To obtain torque control, force should be applied from both the buccal and the lingual sides.

Correction of canting

Because of mini-implants, dental canting can be corrected nonsurgically. Dental or occlusal plane canting may be accompanied by skeletal canting or soft tissue canting. Therefore, diagnosis, treatment planning, and determination of the horizontal reference line are the critical factors in the correction of canting. Canting, including eye-level canting, is the most difficult situation to treat because the horizontal reference line is difficult to determine; eye-level canting is nearly impossible to correct.

To evaluate canting, it is necessary to examine not only the hard tissue but also the soft tissue three-dimensionally while the patient is at rest and smiling.[31,32] Centric relation on mounted casts is also useful for visualizing problems, as long as a thorough clinical examination of the face has been performed beforehand. However, centric relation mounting of casts can only allow visualization of the dental problem on the basis of the position of the facebow.

Dental canting is generally accompanied by discrepancies in the vertical and anteroposterior positions of the molars. If there are discrepancies in the molars, there are also discrepancies in the canines. For correction of canting, the anteroposterior position and axes of the canines and molars should be corrected altogether.

One-by-one correction

1. A database is established, and the treatment plan is developed accordingly. Additionally, the horizontal reference line is set.
2. The vertical position of molars is controlled.
3. The anteroposterior position of molars is controlled.
4. The axis, anteroposterior position, and vertical position of the canine are controlled.
5. The midline and frontal occlusal plane of the anterior teeth are controlled. To correct frontal canting, second-order and third-order angulation of individual teeth should also be corrected (Figs 9-69 and 9-70).

En masse correction

Complete-arch correction is performed with stiff rectangular archwire; in en masse correction, individual tooth movements may be slow, but total improvement is easier.

Fig 9-69 Canting is not a vertical problem only. To correct frontal canting, the vertical positions of the molars and the cusp tips (second-order angulation) of individual teeth should be corrected.

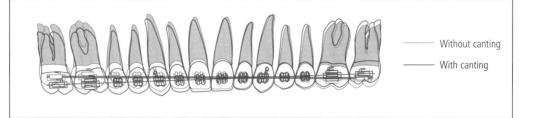

— Without canting
— With canting

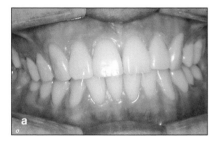
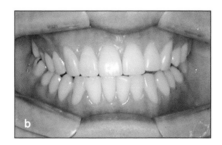
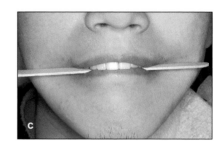

Figs 9-70a to 9-70c Movement of the whole dentition can resolve the problem shown in Fig 9-70a. The maxillary right posterior teeth are comparatively extruded.

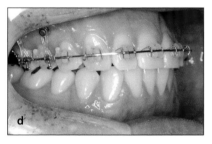
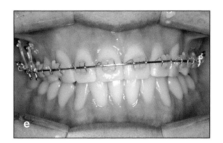
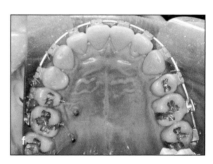

Figs 9-70d to 9-70f Intrusion of the maxillary right posterior segment through the use of buccal implants and palatal implants is used to correct the canting problem.

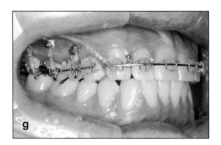
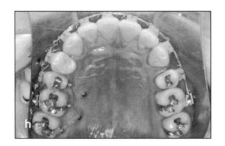
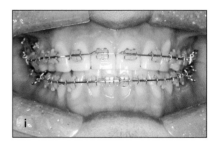

Figs 9-70g to 9-70i Sectional mechanics are used to increase the rate of tooth movement.

Figs 9-70j and 9-70k Clinical situation after canting correction by unilatral intrusion.

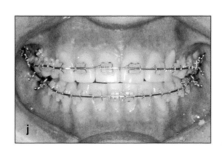
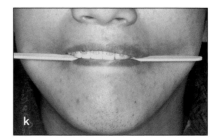

SUMMARY

During orthodontic treatment, control of the facial vertical dimension must be ensured in conjunction with control of the arch form (control of the buccolingual position of individual teeth); the torque of the individual teeth; the axis of the individual teeth; the inclination of the occlusal plane; and the anteroposterior position of the incisal edges. Orthodontic mini-implants can be used alone or with traditional mechanotherapy to accelerate and simplify treatment. These mechanics can be used to achieve intrusion or extrusion of the anterior and posterior teeth as well as correction of occlusal canting.

REFERENCES

1. Burstone CR. Deep overbite correction by intrusion. Am J Orthod 1977;72:1–22.
2. Weiland FJ, Bantleon HP, Droschl H. Evaluation of continuous arch and segmented arch leveling techniques in adult patients—A clinical study. Am J Orthod Dentofacial Orthop 1996;110:647–652.
3. Nanda R. Correction of deep overbite in adults. Dent Clin North Am 1997;41:67–87.
4. Shroff B, Yoon WM, Lindauer SJ, Burstone CJ. Simultaneous intrusion and retraction using a three-piece base arch. Angle Orthod 1997;67:455–461.
5. Park YC, Lee JS. Atlas of Contemporary Orthodontics, vol I. Seoul: Shinhung, 2001:250–261.
6. Graber TM, Vanarsdall RL, Vig KWL (eds). Orthodontics: Current Principles and Techniques. St Louis: Mosby, 2005:911–914.
7. Lindhe J, Karring T, Lang, NP. Clinical Periodontology and Implant Dentistry, ed 3. Copenhagen: Munksgaard, 1997:760–765.
8. Costopoulos G, Nanda R. An evaluation of root resorption incident to orthodontic intrusion. Am J Orthod Dentofacial Orthop 1996; 109:543–548.
9. Melsen B, Agerbaek N, Markenstam G. Intrusion of incisors in adult patients with marginal bone loss. Am J Orthod Dentofacial Orthop 1989;96:232–241.
10. McFadden WM, Engstrom C, Engstrom H, Anholm JM. A study of the relationship between incisor intrusion and root shortening. Am J Orthod Dentofacial Orthop 1989;96:390–396.
11. Baumrind S, Korn EL, Boyd RL. Apical root resorption in orthodontically treated adults. Am J Orthod Dentofacial Orthop 1996; 110:311–320.
12. Faltin RM, Faltin K, Sander FG, Arana-Chavez VE. Ultrastructure of cementum and periodontal ligament after continuous intrusion in humans: A transmission electron microscopy study. Eur J Orthod 2001;23:35–49.
13. Proffit WR, White RP, Sarver DM. Contemporary Treatment of Dentofacial Deformity. St Louis: Mosby, 2003:656–669.
14. Park YC, Lee JS. Atlas of Contemporary Orthodontics, vol I. Seoul: Shinhung, 2001:263–268.
15. Noroozi H, Moeinzad H. Extrusion-based leveling with segmented arch mechanics. Int J Adult Orthodon Orthognath Surg 2002;17: 47–49.
16. Denison TF, Kokich VG, Shapiro PA. Stability of maxillary surgery in openbite versus nonopenbite malocclusions. Angle Orthod 1989; 59:5–10.
17. Kim YH, Han UK, Lim DD, Serraon ML. Stability of anterior openbite correction with multiloop edgewise archwire therapy: A cephalometric follow-up study. Am J Orthod Dentofacial Orthop 2000;118:43–54.
18. Lo FM, Shapiro PA. Effect of presurgical incisor extrusion on stability of anterior open bite malocclusion treated with orthognathic surgery. Int J Adult Orthodon Orthognath Surg 1998;13:23–34.
19. Vermette ME, Kokich VG, Kennedy DB. Uncovering labially impacted teeth: Apically positioned flap and closed-eruption techniques. Angle Orthod 1995;65:23–32.
20. Proffit WR, Fields HW. Contemporary Orthodontics, ed 3. St Louis: Mosby, 1999:597–598.
21. Sherwood KH, Burch JG, Thompson WJ. Closing anterior open bites by intruding molars with titanium miniplate anchorage. Am J Orthod Dentofacial Orthop 2002;122:593–600.
22. Sugawara J, Baik UB, Umemori M, et al. Treatment and posttreatment dentoalveolar changes following intrusion of mandibular molars with application of a skeletal anchorage system (SAS) for open bite correction. Int J Adult Orthodon Orthognath Surg 2002; 17:243–253.
23. Park YC, Lee SY, Kim DH, Jee SH. Intrusion of posterior teeth using mini-screw implants. Am J Orthod Dentofacial Orthop 2003; 123:690–694.
24. Yao CC, Wu CB, Wu HY, Kok SH, Chang HF, Chen YJ. Intrusion of the overerupted upper left first and second molars by mini-implants with partial-fixed orthodontic appliances: A case report. Angle Orthod 2004;74:550–557.
25. Kuroda S, Katayama A, Takano-Yamamoto T. Severe anterior openbite case treated using titanium screw anchorage. Angle Orthod 2004;74:558–567.
26. Lee JS, Kim DH, Park YC, Kyung SH, Kim TK. The efficient use of midpalatal miniscrew implants. Angle Orthod 2004;74:711–714.
27. Yao CC, Lee JJ, Chen HY, Chang ZC, Chang HF, Chen YJ. Maxillary molar intrusion with fixed appliances and mini-implant anchorage studied in three dimensions. Angle Orthod 2005;75:754–760.
28. Engelking G, Zachrisson BU. Effects of incisor repositioning on monkey periodontium after expansion through the cortical plate. Am J Orthod 1982;82:23–32.
29. Turley PK. Orthodontic management of the short face patient. Semin Orthod 1996;2:138–153 [erratum 1997;3:73].
30. Watted N, Witt E, Bill JS. A therapeutic concept for the combined orthodontic surgical correction of angle Class II deformities with short-face syndrome: Surgical lengthening of the lower face. Clin Orthod Res 2000;3:78–93.
31. Bishara SE, Burkey PS, Kharouf JG. Dental and facial asymmetries: A review. Angle Orthod 1994;64:89–98.
32. Burstone CJ. Diagnosis and treatment planning of patients with asymmetries. Semin Orthod 1998;4:153–164.

TRANSVERSE CONTROL 10

MAXILLARY ORTHOPEDIC EXPANSION

There are three classic problems with regard to maxillary expansion: the first is unwanted tooth movement (buccal tipping)[1-6] during expansion, the second is how to achieve midpalatal suture separation in adult patients,[6-11] and the third is stability.[9,12,13] The skeletal achorage may be useful in solving these problems (Fig 10-1).[14-21] However, more research is needed to establish the treatment protocol for maxillary orthopedic expansion with mini-implants.

ASYMMETRIC TRANSVERSE CONTROL

Treatment planning, biomechanics, and mechanics

Asymmetric transverse problems may accompany skeletal problems; thus, precise diagnosis and treatment planning are extremely important. Specifically in patients with skeletal problems, satisfactory results or camouflage cannot be obtained through tooth movement alone.

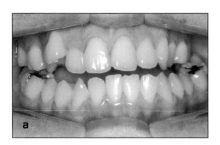

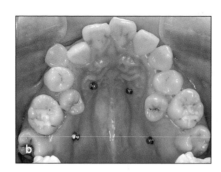

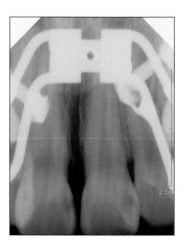

Figs 10-1a and 10-1b The patient is a 20-year-old woman whose chief complaint was an anterior crossbite and a prominent chin. She had a Class III profile with facial asymmetry and a severely constricted maxilla. The treatment objectives included establishment of a normal transverse skeletal relationship and improvement of facial esthetics. Treatment involved expansion of the maxilla and surgical correction of the skeletal discrepancy. A rapid maxillary expansion appliance with mini-implants was used. After implantation, the mini-implants and extension arms were bonded together with resin composite. The patient was instructed to turn the screws once a day immediately after placement of the rapid maxillary expansion appliance.

Fig 10-1c After 1 month of treatment, a suture opening is visible in a periapical radiograph.

Figs 10-1d and 10-1e After 2 months of treatment, the maxillary arch has expanded successfully.

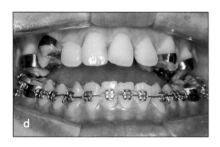

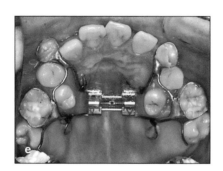

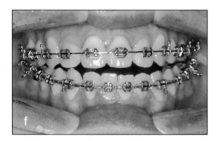

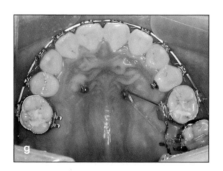

Figs 10-1f and 10-1g After 11 months of treatment, leveling and alignment are completed and the patient is ready for orthognathic surgery. Through the use of mini-implants, even without surgical assistance, skeletal dentoalveolar expansion of the maxilla has been achieved.

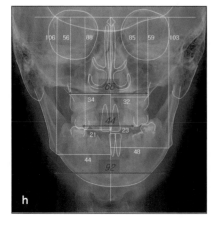

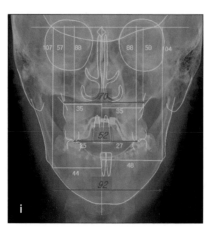

Fig 10-1h Anteroposterior cephalometric radiograph and analysis prior to expansion. The maxillary width is 26 mm less than the mandibular width.

Fig 10-1i Anteroposterior cephalometric radiograph and analysis after expansion. About 4 mm of skeletal expansion and an additional 4 mm of dental expansion have been obtained.

Figs 10-2a and 10-2b Bilateral expansion and rotation of the second molar are achieved with a precision lingual arch made of 0.032 × 0.032-inch titanium-molybdenum alloy (TMA) wire. **(a)** Before correction. **(b)** After correction.

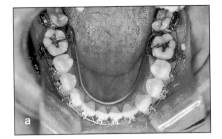

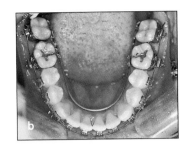

Figs 10-3a and 10-3b The scissor bite generally causes both horizontal and vertical problems. The second molars are out of position buccolingually and are extruded. Therefore, an intrusive force vector and a horizontal force vector are necessary for correction of the scissor bite. With mini-implants, unilateral and three-dimensional control is easy to achieve. **(a)** Pretreatment cast, lingual view. **(b)** Pretreatment cast, posterior view. (Courtesy of Dr JK Lim, Seoul, Korea.)

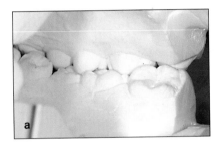

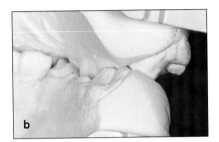

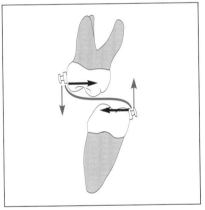

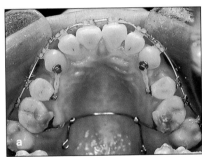

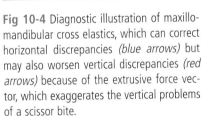

Fig 10-4 Diagnostic illustration of maxillomandibular cross elastics, which can correct horizontal discrepancies *(blue arrows)* but may also worsen vertical discrepancies *(red arrows)* because of the extrusive force vector, which exaggerates the vertical problems of a scissor bite.

Figs 10-5a and 10-5b A transpalatal arch (TPA) and an extension arm are useful for correcting a scissor bite, because these mechanics can improve both horizontal and vertical discrepancies. The extension arm is located apically; therefore, a single force from the extension arm has a horizontal, intrusive force vector, while a TPA maintains the molar width. However, excessive force can cause distortion of the arch form or mesial tipping of molars. **(a)** Before correction. **(b)** After correction.

The guidelines for selection of mechanics are similar as in other situations treated with implants. The Burstone lingual bracket and the active precision lingual arch are very effective for bilateral anchorage control (Fig 10-2). Although an active precision lingual arch is also effective for unilateral control, its treatment efficiency may be low, because it has a statically indeterminate force system.

The scissor bite is not only a transverse problem but also a vertical problem (Figs 10-3 to 10-5). A simple passive transpalatal arch (TPA) with extension arms is also effective for improving the asymmetric position of a molar (Fig 10-6).

The use of mini-implants makes the correction of asymmetric transverse dental problems possible. Mini-implants

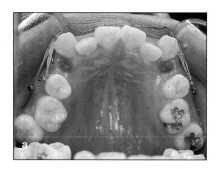

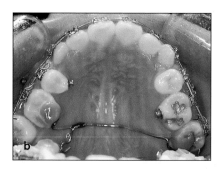

Fig 10-6a A TPA and an extension arm are useful for correcting problems of asymmetry. The maxillary right second molar shows a scissor bite while the maxillary left first molar shows a crossbite. Occlusal view after first premolar removal.

Fig 10-6b A TPA has been bonded to the molars because this properly maintains the arch form while a single force from an extension arm is applied to align the molars. After 5 months of treatment, most of the space is closed, the scissor bite has been corrected, and the arch form has been maintained.

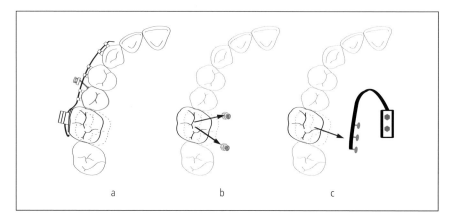

Fig 10-7 There are three ways to correct a single malaligned maxillary molar with implants. (a) A single buccal interdental mini-implant and indirect anchorage can be used. (b) Two interdental palatal mini-implants can be used to control the line of action. (c) Two midpalatal mini-implants and an attachment can be used.

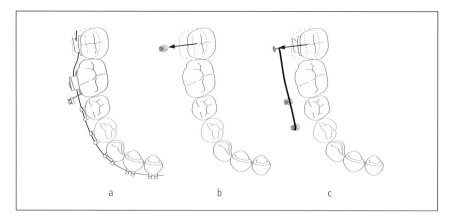

Fig 10-8 There are three ways to correct a single malaligned mandibular molar with implants. (a) A single buccal interdental mini-implant and indirect anchorage can be used. (b) A single buccal interdental mini-implant that is placed in the buccal shelf area can be used. (c) Two buccal mini-implants and an attachment can be used to control the line of action. Because there is more irritation with buccal extension arms in the mandibular arch than with lingual extension arms in the maxillary arch, buccal extension arms may be less stable in the mandibular arch.

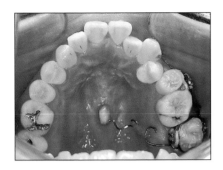

Fig 10-9 TPA extension on two midpalatal implants. For correction of scissor bite, two midpalatal implants have been inserted and an extension arm has been bonded to them to control the line of action. Constrictive and intrusive forces are applied to the second molar.

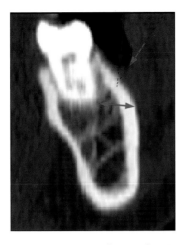

Fig 10-10a CT scan showing there is space available for implant placement *(green arrows)* on the buccal side of the mandibular second molar area. *(purple arrow)* Recommended placement angle; *(red arrow)* avoidable placement angle.

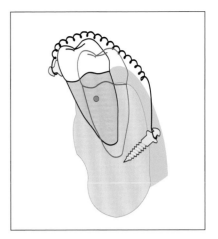

Fig 10-10b For treatment of the type of situation shown in Fig 10-10a, a single buccal mini-implant can be placed in the buccal shelf area. Using a closed technique with an extension wire, an expansion force and intrusive force are applied to the second molar for correction of scissor bite.

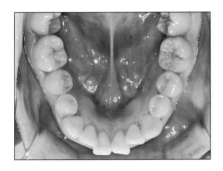

Fig 10-11a The scissor bite of the mandibular left second molar requires correction.

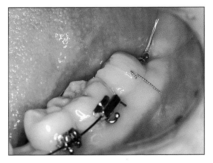

Fig 10-11b To correct the scissor bite, a single buccal mini-implant is placed. A lingual button is bonded, and a single force is applied by an extension wire from the implant. A single force is biomechanically effective and efficient and can therefore improve a scissor bite quite rapidly.

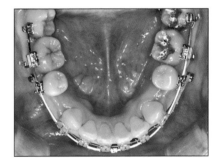

Fig 10-11c After 3 months of treatment, the scissor bite is corrected. Brackets are then bonded so that treatment can be continued according to the plan. (Figs 10-11a to 10-11c courtesy of Dr JK Lim, Seoul, Korea.)

can be used for direct anchorage or indirect anchorage (Figs 10-7 to 10-9). If an intrusive force vector is required for correction, orthodontic force applied directly from implants is recommended (Figs 10-10 to 10-13).

If an intrusive force vector is not required for vertical correction, the use of indirect anchorage is suggested, but this may not provide absolute anchorage. Moreover, the fact that molars are more difficult to move because they have large roots and are loaded by occlusal forces should be considered. Therefore, for treatment efficiency, the use of single forces is better than the use of brackets and wires, particularly for molars with large roots (see Figs 10-11 to 10-13). The use of a provisional bite-opening appliance may be necessary to correct a scissor bite or a crossbite.

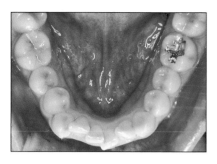

Fig 10-12a The mandibular right second molar is in scissor bite.

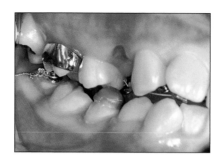

Fig 10-12b Before correction of the scissor bite, the posterior occlusion is disoccluded by bonding of glass-ionomer cement on a mandibular premolar that will be extracted for treatment. With the closed technique, a single buccal mini-implant is used to correct the scissor bite.

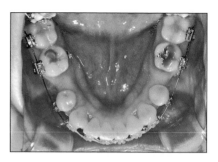

Fig 10-12c After correction of the scissor bite, brackets are bonded and treatment is continued according to general procedures. (Figs 10-12a to 10-12c courtesy of Dr JK Lim, Seoul, Korea.)

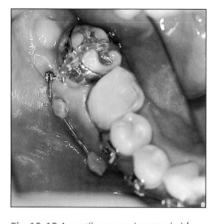

Fig 10-13 A cantilever arm is extended from two orthodontic implants, so that the line of action can be maneuvered to pass through the center of resistance of the second molar to correct the scissor bite.

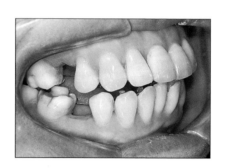

Fig 10-14a A fixed bite block should be used on the occlusal surface of the mandibular molar with care. (From Park et al.[22] Reprinted with permission.)

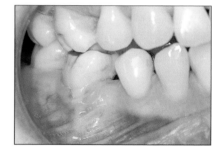

Fig 10-14b Premature contact causes traumatic occlusion and increases the risk of recession and loss of attachment. (From Park et al.[22] Reprinted with permission.)

Periodontal considerations

Tooth movement outside the alveolar trough or envelope of the alveolar process increases the risk of dehiscence or recession, and traumatic occlusion on the molars exacerbates the situation.

Occlusal force

Traumatic occlusion increases tooth mobility, the risk of recession, and loss of attachment. For correction of a scissor bite or a crossbite, posterior disocclusion may be necessary (see Fig 10-12); it can also reduce the dis-

comfort experienced by some patients. A removable bite block or fixed bite-raising appliance made with core resin or resin-reinforced glass-ionomer cement can be used to raise the bite temporarily. As treatment progresses, occlusal adjustment should be performed (Fig 10-14).

Intrusive force

Orthodontic force applied from implants should have a direct, generally intrusive force vector. This is favorable for correction of scissor bite but is unfavorable in some other situations. Therefore, the intrusive force component should be controlled.

REFERENCES

1. Proffit WR. Contemporary Orthodontics, ed 3. St Louis: Mosby, 2000.

2. Chung CH, Goldman AM. Dental tipping and rotation immediately after surgically assisted rapid palatal expansion. Eur J Orthod 2003; 25:353–358.

3. Bassarelli T, Dalstra M, Melsen B. Changes in clinical crown height as a result of transverse expansion of the maxilla in adults. Eur J Orthod 2005;27:121–128.

4. Lagravere MO, Major PW, Flores-Mir C. Long-term dental arch changes after rapid maxillary expansion treatment: A systematic review. Angle Orthod 2005;75:155–161.

5. Koudstaal MJ, van der Wal KG, Wolvius EB, Schulten AJ. The Rotterdam palatal distractor: Introduction of the new bone-borne device and report of the pilot study. Int J Oral Maxillofac Surg 2006;35:31–35.

6. Byloff FK, Mossaz CF. Skeletal and dental changes following surgically assisted rapid palatal expansion. Eur J Orthod 2004;26: 403–409.

7. Betts NJ, Vanarsdall RL, Barber HD, Higgins-Barber K, Fonseca RJ. Diagnosis and treatment of transverse maxillary deficiency. Int J Adult Orthodon Orthognath Surg 1995;10:75–96.

8. Kanekawa M, Shimizu N. Age-related changes on bone regeneration in midpalatal suture during maxillary expansion in the rat. Am J Orthod Dentofacial Orthop 1998;114:646–653.

9. Handelman CS, Wang L, BeGole EA, Haas AJ. Nonsurgical rapid maxillary expansion in adults: Report on 47 cases using the Haas expander. Angle Orthod 2000;70:129–44.

10. Anttila A, Finne K, Keski-Nisula K, Somppi M, Panula K, Peltomaki T. Feasibility and long-term stability of surgically assisted rapid maxillary expansion with lateral osteotomy. Eur J Orthod 2004;26: 391–395.

11. Knaup B, Yildizhan F, Wehrbein H. Age-related changes in the mid-palatal suture. A histomorphometric study. J Orofac Orthop 2004; 65:467–474.

12. Koudstaal MJ, Poort LJ, van der Wal KG, Wolvius EB, Prahl-Andersen B, Schulten AJ. Surgically assisted rapid maxillary expansion (SARME): A review of the literature. Int J Oral Maxillofac Surg 2005;34:709–714.

13. Vanarsdall RL. Transverse dimension of long-term stability. Semin Orthod 1999;5:171–180.

14. Parr JA, Garetto LP, Wohlford ME, Arbuckle GR, Roberts WE. Sutural expansion using rigidly integrated endosseous implants: An experimental study in rabbits. Angle Orthod 1997;67: 283–290.

15. Pinto PX, Mommaerts MY, Wreakes G, Jacobs WV. Immediate postexpansion changes following the use of the transpalatal distractor. J Oral Maxillofac Surg 2001;59:994–1000.

16. Gerlach KL, Zahl C. Transversal palatal expansion using a palatal distractor. J Orofac Orthop 2003;64:443–449.

17. Harzer W, Schneider M, Gedrange T. Rapid maxillary expansion with palatal anchorage of the hyrax expansion screw—Pilot study with case presentation. J Orofac Orthop 2004;65:419–424.

18. Ramieri GA, Spada MC, Austa M, Bianchi SD, Berrone S. Transverse maxillary distraction with a bone-anchored appliance: Dento-periodontal effects and clinical and radiological results. Int J Oral Maxillofac Surg 2005;34:357–363.

19. Gerlach KL, Zahl C. Surgically assisted rapid palatal expansion using a new distraction device: Report of a case with an epimucosal fixation. J Oral Maxillofac Surg 2005;63:711–713.

20. Kircelli BH, Pektas ZO, Uckan S. Orthopedic protraction with skeletal anchorage in a patient with maxillary hypoplasia and hypodontia. Angle Orthod 2006;76:156–163.

21. Harzer W, Schneider M, Gedrange T, Tausche E. Direct bone placement of the hyrax fixation screw for surgically assisted rapid palatal expansion (SARPE). J Oral Maxillofac Surg 2006;64:1313–1317.

22. Park YC, Hwang HS, Lee JS. Atlas of Contemporary Orthodontics, vol II. Seoul: Shinhung, 2003.

PREPROSTHODONTIC ORTHODONTIC TREATMENT OR ADJUNCTIVE TOOTH MOVEMENT

PREPROSTHODONTIC ORTHODONTIC TREATMENT

Among patients requiring preprosthodontic orthodontic treatment, some present several missing teeth, while others exhibit entire dentitions that have been damaged. It is difficult to obtain anchorage from remaining teeth in such cases, so conventional orthodontic treatment may be limited. The mini-implant can provide orthodontic anchorage regardless of the condition of the dentition, and it is very useful for preprosthodontic orthodontic treatment (Fig 11-1). Furthermore, the range of tooth movement is greater if mechanics can be accomplished utilizing rigid anchorage, and, in addition, greater esthetic and functional improvement in periodontal conditions can be achieved. Therefore, proper treatment planning becomes more involved to maximize the benefit from the increased potential of orthodontic treatment with regard to esthetics, function, and prosthodontic strategy.

As a preliminary stage of prosthodontic rehabilitation for missing teeth or as an adjunctive treatment, orthodontics can largely fulfill the following roles:

1. The repositioning of teeth, including abutment teeth for tooth replacement (Fig 11-2)
2. The creation of horizontal and vertical space for prosthodontic restorations
3. The esthetic and functional improvement of periodontal conditions through tooth movement
4. The formation of alveolar bone[1–6] (Figs 11-3 to 11-6)

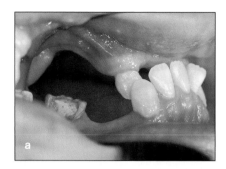

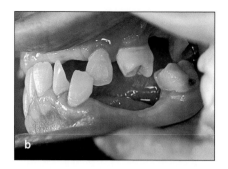

Figs 11-1a and 11-1b Forced eruption of the canine and strategic rearrangement of the abutment teeth are required for prosthodontic treatment of a patient with cleidocranial dysostosis. Many teeth are missing, and thus anchorage is difficult to obtain.

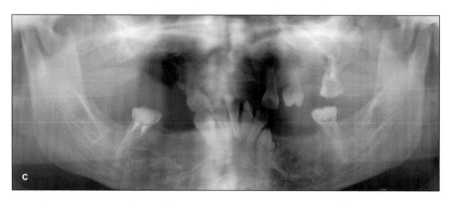

Fig 11-1c Pretreatment panoramic radiograph.

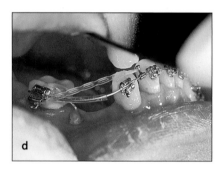

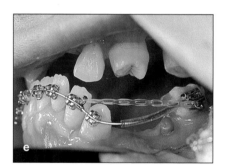

Figs 11-1d and 11-1e Results after 6 months of treatment. A mini-implant has been placed in the mandible and connected to the first molar to force eruption of the canine and to serve as anchorage for anterior alignment.

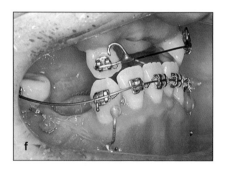

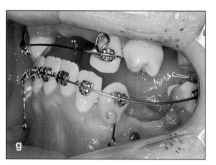

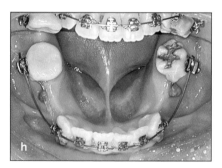

Figs 11-1f to 11-1h Results after 14 months of treatment. **(f)** Right lateral view. **(g)** Left lateral view. **(h)** Occlusal view.

Figs 11-2a to 11-2d A woman with a history of loss of the maxillary central incisors and right canine in an automobile accident 4 years previously was referred for the correction of improper relationships in the premolar area prior to prosthodontic treatment.

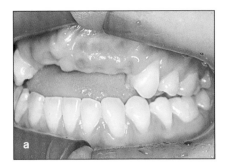
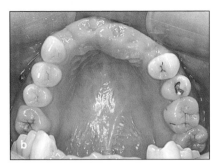
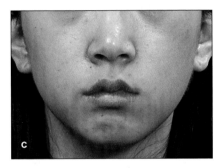
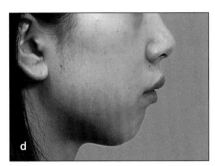

Figs 11-2e to 11-2h The posterior teeth have been intruded and the right premolar has been protracted to improve the long face. The right premolar has replaced the canine, so there is no need for restoration of the canine. The occlusion and facial esthetics are improved.

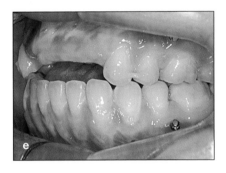
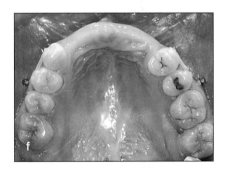
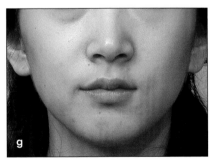
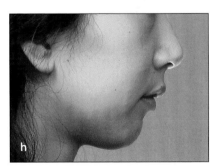

Fig 11-2i A provisional removable appliance has been placed after the completion of orthodontic treatment.

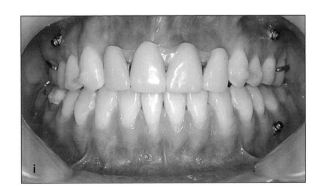

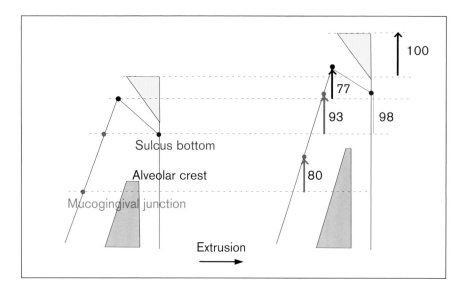

Fig 11-3 Vertical alveolar bone formation. Orthodontic tooth movement can indirectly create or remodel alveolar bone and gingiva.[1] *(gray)* Alveolar crest of bone; *(yellow)* enamel at the cementoenamel junction.

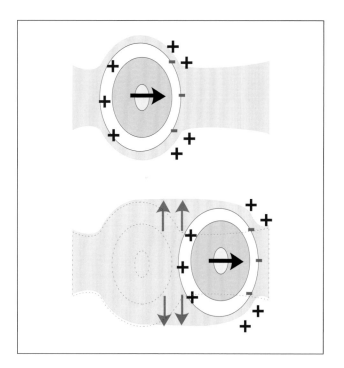

Fig 11-4 Lateral alveolar bone remodeling can occur.[2,3] Moving teeth in a narrowed ridge with direct bone resorption may achieve lateral expansion of the ridge through compensatory bone formation. In this way, orthodontic tooth movement can indirectly reshape alveolar bone. This principle could be useful in cases requiring implant placement in pretreatment in a narrowed ridge. If a tooth is moved into the narrowed area, an implant could be placed in the site where a previous tooth had existed, and the need for bone grafting might be eliminated or minimized. However, this kind of lateral expansion may have adverse effects on the vertical level of periodontal attachment, particularly in the mandible. *(blue plus sign)* Compensating bone formation; *(red minus sign)* direct bone resorption.

In treatment planning, periodontal conditions should be considered first. Compromised periodontal support may not be appropriate for long-term maintenance.

The treatment plan must also be realistic. Rigid anchorage is needed to protract molars to any position, and this process requires considerable time. According to Roberts' study,[7] the maximal rate of translation of the midroot area through dense cortical bone is about 0.5 mm per month for the first few months; the rate then declines to less than 0.3 mm per month until the first molar extraction site is closed. Additionally, there is a wide range in the rates of mesial movement of mandibular molars among individual patients. That is, rigid anchorage is not the determining factor in successful treatment, particularly in mandibular molar protraction (Figs 11-7 and 11-8).

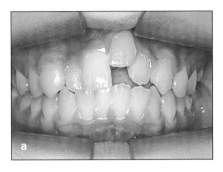
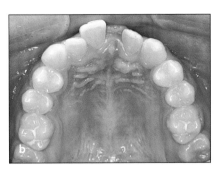
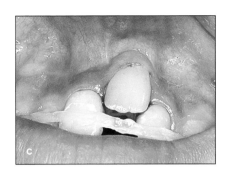

Figs 11-5a to 11-5c An 11-year-old boy experienced complete avulsion and transplantation of the maxillary left central incisor when he was 9 years old. He has an extensive periodontal defect, and esthetics are poor. The left central incisor is now ankylosed and its prognosis is poor. The treatment plan is to recover the lost vertical height of periodontal tissue through surgical luxation of the ankylosed tooth and orthodontic extrusion to level the alveolar bone and teeth.

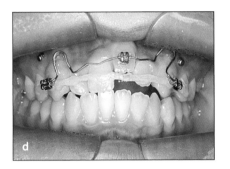
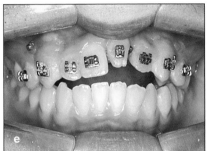
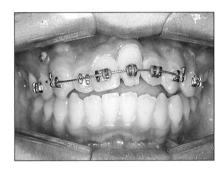

Figs 11-5d and 11-5e The first attempt has failed and adjacent teeth have been intruded.

Fig 11-5f On the second attempt with luxation and vertical movement, the extrusive force is applied after surgical repositioning.

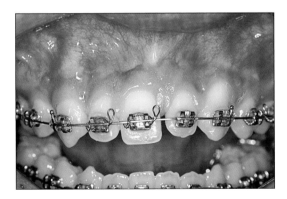
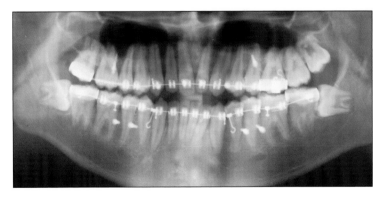

Fig 11-5g After the tooth has been extruded to the maximum level and extracted, the extraction space is closed with the adjacent teeth and the periodontal defect has been eliminated.

Fig 11-5h Panoramic radiograph at the completion of extrusion and space closure.

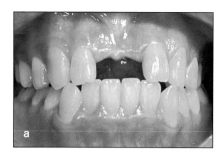
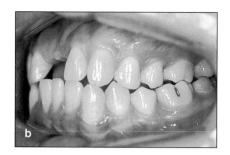

Figs 11-6a and 11-6b Prosthodontic implants will be used to restore both central incisors in a patient who lost the teeth at the age of 9 years in an automobile accident. Because 11 years have passed since the loss of the teeth, the ridge resorption is severe. There are two treatment options: implant placement in the central incisor areas with bone grafting, or orthodontic movement of the lateral incisors to the central incisor positions and implant placement in the lateral incisor areas. After discussion with the patient and consultation with the prosthodontist, the second option has been chosen.

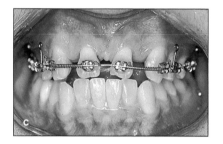
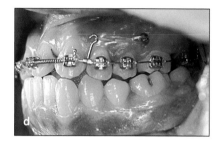
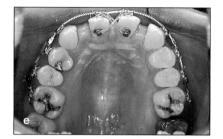

Figs 11-6c to 11-6e As the lateral incisors move, the ridge is expanded laterally.

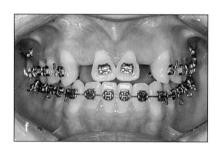
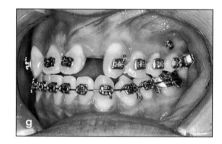

Figs 11-6f and 11-6g Lateral incisors are moved into the central incisor positions.

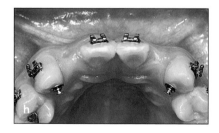
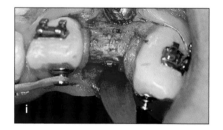
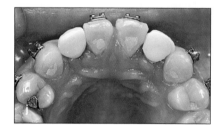

Figs 11-6h to 11-6j The bone width needed for implant placement has been achieved via lateral expansion by orthodontic movement. Prosthodontic implants are placed without bone grafting.

Fig 11-7 Mandibular molar protraction should be planned carefully, especially in patients with insufficient soft and hard tissues. Note high frenum and lack of attached gingiva.

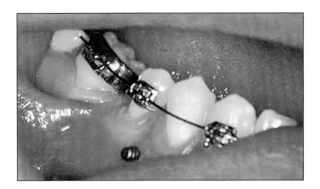

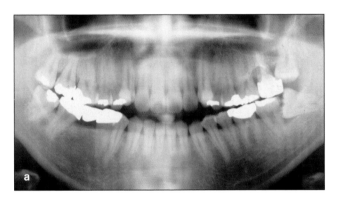

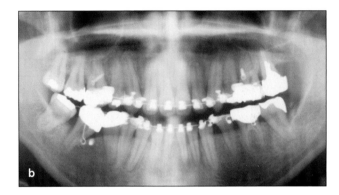

Figs 11-8a and 11-8b Because of the poor periodontal health conditions, the prosthodontic pontic is removed, and an attempt is made to close the pontic space through orthodontic treatment.

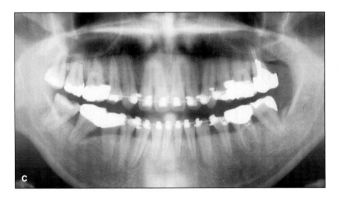

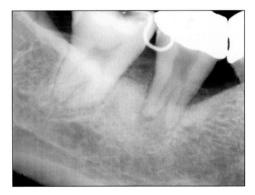

Figs 11-8c and 11-8d The space has nearly been closed by orthodontic treatment, but the periodontal health of the second molar does not appear to be adequate. Molar protraction to the edentulous area is especially difficult in the mandible. In contrast to the maxilla, the mandible is composed of high-density bone; furthermore, the turnover rate of the mandible is significantly lower than that of the maxilla. Therefore, the "with the bone" technique shown in Fig 11-5 must be planned with extreme care in the mandible.

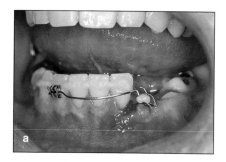

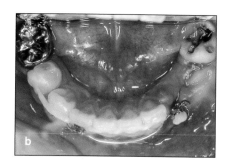

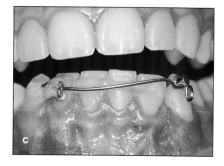

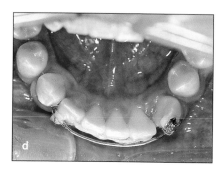

Figs 11-9a and 11-9b The classic strategy in anchorage control, which includes many teeth as anchor parts and uses minimal force, may be effective. However, with a prolonged treatment period, even a small force may develop unwanted effects. To control anchorage, the anterior teeth are splinted with fiber-reinforced resin composite, and a minimal extrusive force of 50 g is exerted by a cantilever spring to force the eruption of the canine.

Figs 11-9c and 11-9d As the treatment period has prolonged, the anterior anchorage unit has rotated.

ADJUNCTIVE TREATMENT

Adjunctive orthodontic treatment is tooth movement carried out to facilitate other dental procedures necessary to control disease and restore function.[8] It can be part of multidisciplinary restorative treatment or used for the improvement of local periodontal discrepancies.

Treatment planning

The classic treatment principle in adjunctive orthodontic treatment is to improve a particular aspect of the occlusion rather than to comprehensively alter it. The concept of "passive bracketing" or "passive wiring" was important in conventional adjunctive orthodontic treatment from the aspect of anchorage control.[8,9] "Minimal" treatment has been recommended to control anchorage and to minimize patient discomfort[8,9] (Fig 11-9).

However, because anchorage problems have been solved through the use of mini-implants, anchorage-centered strategies should be reevaluated. As long as the patient accepts the treatment and the result is likely to be stable, all other problems can be addressed during the necessary treatment period required to solve the chief complaint.

Molar uprighting

After consideration of the periodontal conditions of the molar in question and its relationship to opposing teeth, the type of tooth movement required should be planned accordingly.[10,11]

Molar protraction

The mandibular molars are supported by high-density bone, which requires considerable treatment time for protraction, as Roberts[7,12] indicated. Moreover, mandibular molar protraction becomes less predictable when the molar is being moved to an edentulous area with an atrophic and narrower alveolar bone, and when the protracted molar is fully developed and root formation is complete. Alveolar bone loss, gingival recession, and dehiscence may result from protraction, and there is greater likelihood for side effects to occur with longer treatment periods (see Fig 11-8).

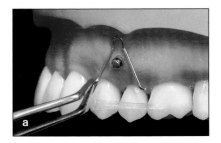
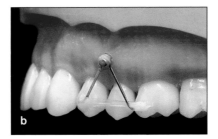
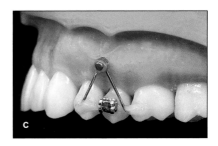

Figs 11-10a to 11-10c Procedure for preparation of the anchorage unit splinted with the implant. This procedure may look somewhat complicated, but if done properly, it can be widely applied and easily used. **(a)** The implant is placed. The implant head should be exposed adequately to allow the addition of resin. Sandblasting of the implant head is optional; it is generally unnecessary but can increase bonding strength at the interface. A 0.016 × 0.022-inch SS wire is bent so that it is able to hook mechanically to the neck of the implant. The wire should be located for connection of the implant and the teeth. Both ends are attached with flowable resin. **(b)** Flowable resin is also placed on the teeth to be used for anchorage, and then the fiber-reinforced resin composite is placed and polymerized. The wire prepared for splinting is placed, and flowable resin is used to fix both ends of the wire to the teeth. The wire should be passively positioned to prevent unnecessary application of stress to the implant. The implant and the wire are united with flowable resin. This area is reinforced by the addition of hard resin, such as the resins used for core buildup or resins that contain fillers. Occlusal force is loaded on the teeth and then delivered to the joint between the implant and the wire, which may cause bonding failure. **(c)** The fiber-reinforced resin composite is reinforced with hard resins, and a bracket is then attached. A twin bracket is recommended, because it is advantageous for producing moments.

Figs 11-11a and 11-11b The connection wire must have a shape that provides mechanical forms that can resist the principal orthodontic load even without resin. The connection wire should also be positioned passively. **(a)** For intrusion cases, the connection wire should be made to resist extrusion of the anchor part. **(b)** For extrusion cases, the connection wire should be made to resist intrusion of the anchor part.

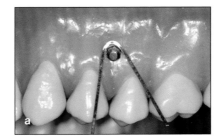
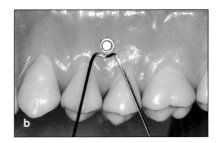

Molar intrusion

Treatment plans that include either an occlusal reduction procedure or molar intrusion should be determined after examination of the alveolar bone condition, pulpal conditions (whether teeth are endodontically treated or not), and the location of the furcation.

Mechanics: Anchorage unit splinted with the implant

An anchorage unit splinted with the implant (Fig 11-10) is very useful for movement of several teeth. Although additional chair time is required to bend a wire and bond an attachment (Figs 11-10 and 11-11), this unit can provide stable anchorage for three-dimensional control of the teeth. This type of mechanics requires some effort

but leads to smoother progression of treatment, because it is mostly rigid three-dimensionally, as opposed to two-dimensionally. Three-dimensional anchorage is particularly useful during the movement of one or two teeth in a situation that requires a long treatment period (Figs 11-12 and 11-13).

Therefore, these mechanics are indicated in the following cases:

1. When only one or two teeth should be moved over a long period of time
2. When only one or two teeth should be moved without the movement of any other teeth

For example, molar intrusion before prosthodontic treatment is one good indication. These mechanics may be detrimental to oral hygiene, so they are not suitable for patients with high caries indices.

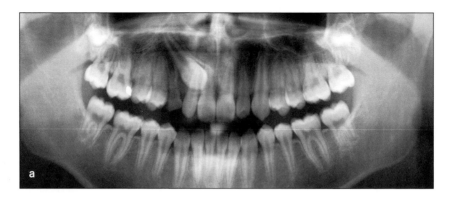

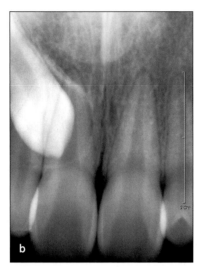

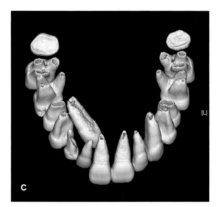

Figs 11-12a to 11-12c The maxillary right canine is impacted. **(a)** Panoramic radiograph. **(b)** Periapical film. **(c)** Computed tomography scan reconstruction.

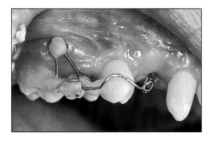

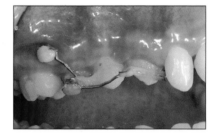

Fig 11-12d For extrusion of the impacted canine, an implant, fiber-reinforced resin composite, a bracket, and one cantilever spring made of 0.017 × 0.025-inch TMA are used.

Fig 11-12e Slight movement of the anchor part has developed due to bonding failures between the connecting SS wire and implant. For this reason, the first molar is excluded from the anchorage unit. When possible, bending of the wire is preferable to create a form that provides mechanical resistance when an orthodontic force is applied.

Fig 11-13a An anchorage unit splinted with the implant is also useful in molar protraction. Both first molars in an 18-year-old woman have been diagnosed as hopeless.

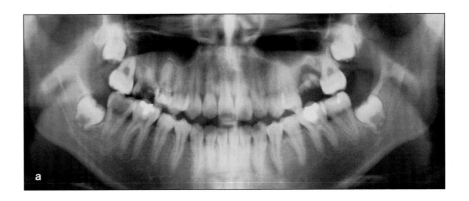

Figs 11-13b and 11-13c The second molars are to be protracted with an anchorage unit splinted to an implant. Crossarch splinting with a 0.0175-inch twist-flex wire is also used for anchorage reinforcement.

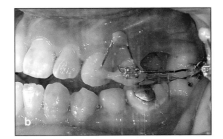
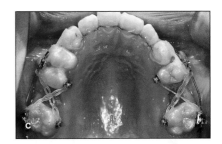

Figs 11-13d and 11-13e Appearance after 5 months of treatment.

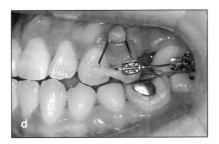
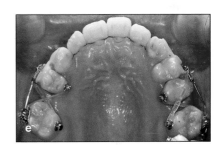

Treatment considerations

The active and reactive units of teeth must be clarified in absolute terms. If even a slight movement of the reactive unit (anchor part) is not permitted by the treatment plan, anchorage should be reinforced by the inclusion of more teeth, because indirect anchorage of implants cannot provide absolute anchorage.

In general, patients who need prosthodontic treatment also need periodontal treatment, because the periodontal condition of the other teeth tends to be inadequate. Much attention must be given to the maintenance of oral hygiene and periodontal control. For successful treatment, periodontal control is the most important issue, particularly in adults in whom orthodontic adjunctive treatment is required.

Treatment protocol

First, the implant is placed. The implant head should be exposed adequately to allow the addition of resin. Sandblasting of the implant head is optional; it is generally unnecessary but can increase bonding strength at the interface. A 0.016 × 0.022-inch stainless steel (SS) wire is bent so that it is able to hook mechanically to the neck area of the implant according to the type of tooth movement required.

After placement of flowable resin on the teeth to be included in the anchorage, the fiber-reinforced resin composite is placed and polymerized to connect the teeth. The wire is positioned to connect the implant to the teeth (see Fig 11-10a), and both ends of the wire are fixed to the teeth with flowable resin (see Fig 11-10b). The wire should be passively positioned to avoid application of unnecessary stress on the implant.

The implant and the wire are united with flowable resin (see Fig 11-10b). This area is then reinforced by the addition of hard resins, such as the resins used for core buildup or resins that contain fillers. Occlusal force is loaded on the teeth and then delivered to the joint between the implant and the wire, which may cause bonding failure.

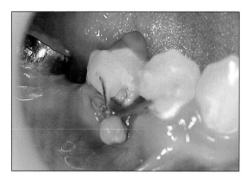

Fig 11-14 Dental caries has developed because of poor oral hygiene.

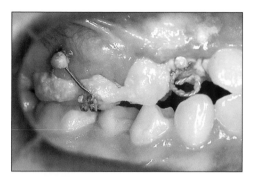

Fig 11-15 As with other types of mechanics, this type of splint is contraindicated in patients with high caries indices or poor oral hygiene. The appliances will be removed because of inadequate maintenance of oral hygiene.

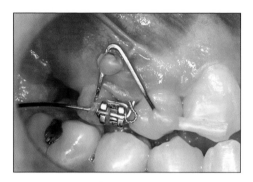

Fig 11-16a Bonding failure may occur.

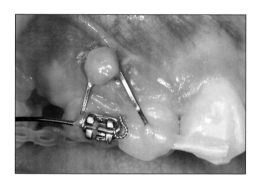

Fig 11-16b The repair process encompasses sandblasting of the interface and the implant head, application of metal conditioner or porcelain conditioner, and application of resin for repair.

The fiber-reinforced resin composite also should be reinforced with hard resins, and a bracket is then attached (see Fig 11-10c). A twin bracket is recommended because it is advantageous for producing moments.

The splinting wire should have two-point contacts with the tooth unit of the anchorage to resist rotation effectively. The wire should create a form that provides mechanical resistance to the principal orthodontic force (see Figs 11-11a and 11-11b).

Treatment monitoring

The anchorage unit is not perfectly rigid in these mechanics because of the characteristics of indirect anchorage. Although implants are used, indirect anchorage has the potential to allow loss of anchorage. The tooth may move approximately 1 mm if excessive force or moments are applied. Therefore, a conventional strategy of anchorage control should be considered. For example, the minimal amount of force should be used, and treatment should progress as steadily as possible.

As mentioned previously, maintenance of oral hygiene is difficult because of the complexity of the mechanics. Patients should be instructed to maintain rigorous oral hygiene; oral hygiene around the mechanics should be closely monitored (Figs 11-14 and 11-15). If needed, an oral irrigator should be prescribed for patients whose home care is not satisfactory.

At recall appointments, the clinician should assess oral hygiene, determine the presence or absence of bonding failure (Fig 11-16), and look for potential movement of the anchorage unit.

SUMMARY

The mini-implant can provide orthodontic anchorage regardless of the condition of the dentition; for this reason, it is very useful for preprosthodontic orthodontic treatment. The mini-implant can also be incorporated in multidisciplinary restorative treatment or used for the improvement of local discrepancies. Among its adjunctive uses are molar uprighting, molar protraction, and molar intrusion.

An anchorage unit splinted with the implant can provide stable anchorage for three-dimensional control of the teeth. Three-dimensional anchorage is particularly useful during movement of one or two teeth in a situation that requires a long treatment period.

REFERENCES

1. Kajiyama K, Murakami T, Yokota S. Gingival reactions after experimentally induced extrusion of the upper incisors in monkeys. Am J Orthod Dentofacial Orthop 1993;104:36–47.
2. Melsen B. Current Controversies in Orthodontics. Chicago: Quintessence, 1991:149–152.
3. Melsen B. Current Controversies in Orthodontics. Chicago: Quintessence, 1991:224–226.
4. Salama H, Salama M. The role of orthodontic extrusive remodeling in the enhancement of soft and hard tissue profiles prior to implant placement: A systematic approach to the management of extraction site defects. Int J Periodontics Restorative Dent 1993;13:312–333.
5. Mantzikos T, Shamus I. Forced eruption and implant site development: Soft tissue response. Am J Orthod Dentofacial Orthop 1997;112:596–606.
6. Mantzikos T, Shamus I. Case report: Forced eruption and implant site development. Angle Orthod 1998;68:179–186.
7. Roberts WE, Arbuckle GR, Analoui M. Rate of mesial translation of mandibular molars using implant-anchored mechanics. Angle Orthod 1996;66:331–338.
8. Proffit WR. Contemporary Orthodontics, 2nd ed. St Louis: Mosby-Yearbook, 1993:307.
9. Park YC, Hwang HS, Lee JS. Atlas of Contemporary Orthodontics vol II. Seoul: Shinhung, 2003:210–215.
10. Roberts WW III, Chacker FM, Burstone CJ. A segmental approach to mandibular molar uprighting. Am J Orthod 1982;81:177–184.
11. Park YC, Lee JS. Atlas of Contemporary Orthodontics, vol I. Seoul: Shinhung, 2001:237–243.
12. Roberts WE, Marshall KJ, Mozsary PG. Rigid endosseus implant utilized as anchorage to protract molars and close an atrophic extraction site. Angle Orthod 1990;60:135–152.

INDEX